W9-CCK-575

Atherosclerosis and Oxidant Stress

Atherosclerosis and Oxidant Stress:
A New Perspective

Edited by

Jordan L. Holtzman, M.D., Ph.D.

Professor, Departments of Pharmacology and Medicine
and Division of Environmental Health Sciences
University of Minnesota
Minneapolis, Minnesota

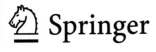 Springer

Jordan L. Holtzman, M.D., Ph.D.
Professor, Departments of Pharmacology and Medicine
  And Division of Environmental Health Sciences
University of Minnesota
Minneapolis, Minnesota

ISBN-13: 978-0-387-72345-7   e-ISBN-13: 978-0-387-72347-1

Library of Congress Control Number: 2007925438

Printed on acid-free paper.

9 8 7 6 5 4 3 2 1

springer.com

Preface

During the twentieth century we saw a veritable revolution in medicine. Some of the most notable advances have been in the elucidation of the risk factors for and treatment of cardio- and cerebral vascular disease. Identifying these factors through epidemiological studies has led to the development of guidelines for a healthy life style and therapies to control this major killer of the elderly. As a result of these efforts at the present time cardiovascular disease, rather than being the leading cause of death in the United States, has dropped to second behind cancer. Beginning with such seminal studies as the Seven Countries study and the Framingham program, these major advances have resulted from a collaboration among several disciplines, including epidemiology, clinical trials, cell biology, and basic biochemistry. The combined findings from these disparate disciplines have served as the foundation for the institution of public health measures, such as smoking cessation campaigns and new dietary recommendations, as well as the development of medications to prevent disease through the control of such major risk factors as hypertension and hyperlipidemia. One of the major insights into the underlying cause of vascular injury is that it is initiated by oxidant injury to the vessel wall. The current volume is organized around the role of oxidant damage in this disease process. We have sought to present the most recent studies from various disciplines which can serve as the basis for further improvements in our understanding and control of cardio- and cerebral vascular disease.

Contents

Contributors

Shari S. Bassuk, ScD, Epidemiologist, Division of Preventive Medicine, Brigham and Women's Hospital, 900 Commonwealth Avenue, Boston, MA 02215, Tel: (617) 278-0814, sbassuk@rics.bwh.harvard.edu

Thomas S. Bowman, MD MPH, VA Boston Healthcare System, Division of Aging, Brigham and Women's Hospital, 1620 Tremont Street, Boston, MA 02120, tsbowman@partners.org

Thomas P. Erlinger, MD, MPH, Adjunct Associate Professor of Medicine, University of Texas Medical Branch at Galveston, 1601 Rio Grance, Suite 340, Austin, TX 78701, Tel: (512) 324-8930, Terlinger@seton.org

James S. Forrester, MD, Division of Cardiology, Cedars-Sinai Medical Center, 8700 Beverly Boulevard, Los Angeles, CA 90048, Tel: (310) 855-3893, forrester@cshs.org

J. Michael Gaziano, MD, MPH, VA Boston Healthcare System, Division of Aging, Brigham and Women's Hospital, 900 Commonwealth Avenue, Boston, MA 02215, jmgaziano@partners.org

Myron D. Gross, PhD, Associate Professor, Department of Laboratory Medicine and Pathology and Epidemiology, MMC 609, University of Minnesota, 420 Delaware Street S.E., Minneapolis, MN 55455, Tel: (612) 624-5417, Fax: (612) 625-8950, Gross001@umn.edu

Michael A. Hill, Ph.D., Dalton Cardiovascular Research Center, Department of Medical Pharmacology and Physiology, University of Missouri, 134 Research Park Drive, Columbia, MO 65211, hillmi@missouri.edu

Jordan L. Holtzman, MD, PhD, Professor, Department of Pharmacology and Medicine, and Division of Environmental Health Sciences, University of Minnesota, Minneapolis, MN, Tel: (612) 624-9883, Fax: (612) 824-8304, Holtz003@umn.edu

Alicia J. Jenkins, MBBS, MD, FRACP, FRCP, The University of Melbourne, Department of Medicine, St. Vincent's Hospital, 41 Victoria Parade, Fitzroy, Victoria 3065, Australia, jenkinsa@medstv.unimelb.edu.au

Chih-Hao Lee, PhD, Department of Genetics and Complex Diseases, Harvard University School of Public Health, 665 Huntington Avenue, Boston, MA 02115, Tel: (617) 432-5778, clee@hsph.harvard.edu

Edgar R. Miller, III, PhD, MD, Associate Professor of Medicine and Epidemiology, Johns Hopkins Medical University, 2024 East Monument Street, Suite 1-500M, Baltimore, MD 21205, Tel: (410) 502-6444, Fax: (410) 5026446, ermiller@jhmi.edu

Kimberly P. Miller, Ph.D., Food and Drug Administration, Center for Drug Evaluation and Research, Division of Reproductive and Urologic Products, 10903 New Hampshire Avenue, Bldg. 22, Rm. 5347, Silver Spring, MD 20993

Kenneth S. Ramos, PhD, Distinguished Professor and Chairma, Department of Biochemistry and Molecular Biology, and Director, Center for Genetics and Molecular Medicine, University of Louisville Health Sciences Center, Louisville, KY 40292, Tel: (502) 852-5217, Fax: (502) 852-6222, Kenneth. ramos@louisville.edu

Shannon M. Reilly, Department of Genetics and Complex Diseases, Harvard University School of Public Health, 665 Huntington Avenue, Boston, MA 02115, smreilly@fas.harvard.edu

Kevin G. Rowley, PhD, Senior Research Fellow, Onemda VicHealth Koori Health Unit, Centre for Health and Society, School of Population Health, The University of Melbourne VIC 3010, Victoria 3010, Australia, rowleyk@medstv.unimelb.edu.au

Ernesto L. Schiffrin, MD, PhD, FRSC, FRCPC, FACP, Physician-in-Chief, Department of Medicine, Sir Mortimer B. Davis-Jewish General Hospital. Canada Research Chair and Director, Hypertension and Vascular Research Unit, Lady Davis Institute for Medical Research. Professor and Vice-Chair (Research), Department of Medicine, McGill University, Ernesto.schiffrin@mcgill.ca

Rhian M. Touyz, MD, PhD, Kidney Research Centre, University of Ottawa, Ottawa Health Research Institute, Ottawa, Ontario, Canada, Tel: (613) 562-5800 ext. 824, Fax: (613) 562-5487, rtouyz@uottawa.ca

Chapter 1
The Pathogenesis of Atherosclerosis and Plaque Instability

James S. Forrester

Despite the dramatic reduction in cardiac events reported in the lipid lowering trial, a substantial body of evidence from sources as diverse as epidemiology, clinical trials and cell biology suggests that the atherogenesis involves processes far more complex than elevation in serum lipids (Table 1.1). Until the 1980s the central focus of pathologists was the debate over whether coronary thrombosis is a premortem or postmortem event. In the late 1980s, however, coronary angioscopy in symptomatic patients focused attention on plaque rupture. Angioscopy in patients at the time they were experiencing clinical syndromes definitively demonstrated that the culprit lesion in patients with stable angina was an atheroma with a smooth surface, whereas those with unstable angina had a disrupted endothelial surface, with or without thrombus formation.[1,2] Although these data established the causal importance of intimal disruption in acute coronary syndromes, there was no understanding of its pathologic basis.

In the early 1990s, vascular pathologists identified three characteristic histologic features of unstable plaque: a large lipid core, an abundance of inflammatory cells, and a thin fibrous cap.[3] The differences in both size of the lipid core and macrophage volume between stable and disrupted plaques are striking. For instance, Felton et al. studied 334 human aortic plaques. In the aortae with disrupted plaque, the unstable lesions had fourfold greater cross-sectional area occupied by lipid, an eightfold greater area occupied by macrophages, and a fibrous less than a third as thick as that found in stable atheroma.[4] Nonetheless, there was very limited insight into what biologic processes were responsible for the development of these three characteristics. At the turn of the century, therefore, there emerged a clear need to identify the cellular biologic processes which lead to the three unique histologic features of the unstable plaque.

In this chapter, we describe our current understanding of the cellular processes responsible for creation of the atheroma and its evolution to instability and rupture. These processes can be described didactically as a series of discrete steps (Fig. 1.1). This schema simplifies a complex process because a diverse group of mediators drive each step and each of the cell mediators affect more than one step in the plaque destabilization.

J.L. Holtzman (ed.), *Atherosclerosis and Oxidant Stress: A New Perspective.*
© Springer 2008

Table 1.1 Inferential evidence from diverse sources, which suggest that the lipid hypothesis is insufficient as a theory of atherogenesis

Inferential evidence	Source
Major variation in death rates at same serum cholesterol level	Fourfold difference in cardiac mortality among countries in the same quartile of serum cholesterol[53]
Predicted vs observed trial outcomes	35% greater reduction in events with statin therapy than predicted from an epidemiologic model[54]
Substantial reduction in cardiac events with a diet that does not lower LDL	30–70% short-term reduction in events post infarction with diets that have little or no effect on LDL [55]
Reduced cardiac events with triglyceride lowering, with no change in LDL	22% reduction in events in the VA HIT trial using gemfibrozil[56]

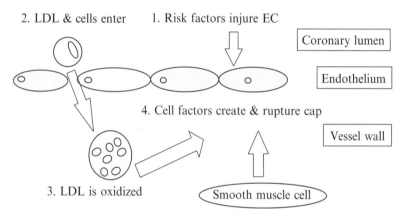

Fig. 1.1 The steps in atheroma destabilization. Activated endothelial cells express adhesion molecules that attract leukocytes that enter the blood vessel wall. LDL in the vessel wall is oxidized, and taken up by macrophages. The activated cells in the vessel wall express cytokines that maintain the inflammatory process. Proteases digest the fibrous cap, and smooth muscle cells undergo apoptosis, leading to rupture of the fibrous cap (see text)

Creation of the Lipid Core

The starting point for atheroma formation and plaque destabilization is endothelial activation. (In this chapter we use the term "activation" rather than "dysfunction," since cells frequently are responding normally to a noxious stimulus.) The activators of endothelial cells are the traditional risk factors for coronary heart disease (CHD) including hypercholesterolemia, smoking, and hypertension. But many other less well-recognized factors such as homocystinemia, immune complexes, and a wide spectrum of infectious agents also are capable of activating the endothelium.[5,6] The response of the endothelium to these stresses is quite rapid. For instance, forearm vascular reactivity increases substantially in the 4-h period following ingestion of a fatty meal.[7] Conversely, chronic low density lipoprotein (LDL) lowering improves vascular reactivity,[8] and acute LDL apheresis can increase stress-induced coronary blood flow by 30% within 24 h of the procedure.

Endothelial cell activation is characterized by upregulation of leukocyte adhesion molecules and selectin adhesion receptors. This response may be particularly prominent at branching points of blood vessels, where the loss of normal laminar flow reduces the local expression of endothelium-derived nitric oxide, which suppresses adhesion molecule expression.[8–10] In response, circulating white cells adhere and roll along the endothelial surface. After attachment, the cells express pseudopods and enter the blood vessel wall through the endothelial gap junctions. This movement is facilitated by monocyte chemoattractant protein-1 and other chemoattractants.[11]

The importance of this initial step at the blood cell-blood vessel interface in the initiation of atheroma formation is illustrated by studies in atherosclerosis-prone transgenic mice: animals deficient in platelet and endothelial selectins have 40% smaller lesions.[12] In man adhesion molecule and selectin expression on plaques is twofold greater than on the normal arterial endothelium,[13] and serum adhesion molecule concentration correlates directly with carotid intimal thickness as measured by ultrasound.[14]

Cholesterol moves in and out of the blood vessel wall attached to transport proteins. It enters as low density lipoprotein, with apolipoprotein B as its carrier. In the presence of local inflammation, the LDL that enters the blood vessel wall undergoes oxidation by oxygen-free radicals. Although the data from cell culture studies and animal models suggest that oxidation plays a central role in atherogenesis and plaque instability, the data in man is more inferential. Antibodies against LDL are found in atherosclerotic lesions, and human plasma contains antibodies that react with oxidized LDL.[15] Further, Hasegawa et al. found that the level of plasma oxidized LDL increases with increasing age and is significantly higher in patients with atherosclerosis than controls.[16] The process begins with peroxidation of polyunsaturated fatty acids in the LDL lipid.[17,18] These modified lipids are no longer recognized by the LDL receptor, but are recognized by the scavenger receptor of the monocytes that have entered the blood vessel wall. This receptor is not under sterol-mediated feedback control. Consequently, the monocytes avidly ingest cholesterol, and in the process become tissue macrophages. The differentiation from monocyte to macrophage is augmented by macrophage colony stimulating factor. Filled with lipid, these cells, appropriately named foam cells, become trapped as tissue macrophages in the sub-endothelial proteoglycan substrate of the extracellular matrix. Over time, the predominant lipids in the evolving atheroma become free cholesterol and cholesterol esters.

Lipid accumulation in the vessel wall is neither unidirectional nor relentless. It is balanced by reverse cholesterol transport, i.e., movement of cholesterol out of the blood vessel wall. This process also involves transport proteins and lipoprotein carriers. Reverse cholesterol transport begins with efflux of cholesterol from cell membranes to phospholipid acceptor particles in the interstitial fluid, the most important of which are nascent HDL particles, which are composed of phospholipid

apo A-I. Cholesterol in the nascent HDL is esterified by lecithin cholesterol acyl-
transferase (LCAT) to cholesterol esters. Cholesteryl ester transfer protein (CETP)
exchanges the cholesteryl ester for the triglyceride, decreasing HDL-C. Cholesterol
is then transported to the liver where it is excreted into the bile.

As a generality, as serum LDL increases, there is a compensatory increase in
reverse cholesterol transport. For instance, de la Llera Moya found that patients in
the highest decile of plasma LDL had a 30% greater rate of reverse cholesterol
transport than those in the lowest decile.[19] On the other hand, plasma HDL concentration correlates only roughly with the level of reverse cholesterol transport. Thus,
because HDL also inhibits adhesion molecule expression, is an antioxidant and
blocks matrix metalloproteinase expression, it has a number of potentially antiatherogenic actions.[20,21]

When lipid accumulation exceeds reverse cholesterol transport, the lipid core
enlarges, creating the first histologic characteristic of the unstable plaque, the large
lipid core. In compensation the external diameter of the vessel wall increases. This
phenomenon has major clinical importance: serial angiographic studies before and
after plaque rupture in man have that about half of the vulnerable plaques with large
lipid cores are not flow limiting prior to plaque rupture. Thus unstable lesions are
not necessarily severely stenotic, and conversely angiographically severe stenoses
are not necessarily unstable.[22]

Local Inflammation in the Vessel Wall

Tissue macrophages, activated by oxidized LDL and/or other pro-oxidant stimuli,
initiate and maintain a local inflammatory reaction by expression of cytokines.[23,24]
In the wall of the vessel with an unstable plaque, every cell type is activated (Table
1.2). The endothelial cell expresses adhesion molecules. Degranulating mast cells
increase 15-fold and become TNF-alpha positive, serving as a potent stimulus to
continuing endothelial cell activation.[25,26] The smooth muscle cell changes from the
contractile to the secretory phenotype, expressing extracellular matrix proteins,
particularly collagen that forms the fibrous cap.[27] This stabilizing effect, however,
is countered by activated T-lymphocytes that express gamma interferon inhibiting
extracellular matrix expression.[28] In summary, the complete spectrum of inflammatory
cytokines has now been identified in unstable human plaque.[29-32] These cytokines

Table 1.2 Cell activation in the unstable plaque

Cell type	Unstable vs. Stable atheroma
Smooth Muscle	Two-fold increase in volume of synthetic organelles (42% vs. 21%)[27]
Macrophage	Eightfold greater volume of cells[4]
Mast	17:1 ratio of degranulated to granulated cells[25]
T-Lymphocyte	Along with macrophage, the predominant cell at rupture site[29]

There are major histologic and functional differences between stable and unstable human
atheroma, even within the same vessel.

have multiple overlapping actions. For instance TNF-alpha also promotes oxidative stress, TGF-beta stimulates the production of lipoprotein-trapping proteoglycans, colony stimulating factors cause macrophage replication, and interferon gamma suppresses smooth muscle replication.[33] Cytokines that promote cap formation and stabilization, like platelet-derived growth factor and insulin-like growth factor, are also expressed,[34] but in the unstable plaque the balance between these competing factors favors collagen breakdown rather than synthesis.

Reflecting the abundance and diversity of inflammatory cytokines, the temperature of unstable lesions is increased. For instance, in unstable angina patients the culprit lesion is on average 0.6°C higher than in patients with stable angina, and in patients with myocardial infarction it is 1.0°C higher.[35] There is a direct correlation between plaque temperature and macrophage volume. In summary, the unstable plaque is the body's inflammatory process as it is expressed in the unique tissue of the blood vascular wall.

The process of plaque destabilization, however, is more complex than local inflammation alone. Systemic inflammation also plays an important, albeit less clearly defined role. Remarkably, local plaque temperature also correlates with the systemic level of circulating cell adhesion molecules, cytokines, and plasma c-reactive protein (CRP).[36] Further, the presence of chromic infection and elevated CRP increases the risk of new atheroma formation fivefold.[37] Chronic infection increases the risk of mortality in patients with established CHD by about 40%. A meta-analysis of seven studies involving 1,053 cases of non-fatal myocardial infarction or CHD death, with a mean follow-up of 6 years. The risk ratio of CHD for people in the upper tertile of plasma CRP compared to the bottom tertile was 1.7.[38] Thus a reasonable speculation is that systemic inflammation aggravates local inflammation.

Thinning of the Fibrous Cap

The balance between connective tissue synthesis and breakdown determines the integrity of the fibrous cap that isolates the lipid core. The strength of the cap reflects extracellular matrix proteins expressed by smooth muscle cells. Opposing this action are the activated inflammatory cells, particularly macrophages, T-lymphocytes, and mast cells.[39] Collagen digestion is accomplished by proteases, particularly the family of metalloproteinases (MMPs), expressed predominantly by macrophages.[40] Indeed, in human unstable plaques macrophage density correlates with decreased mechanical strength.[41] MMP expression is intimately related to LDL oxidation. In macrophages oxidized LDL doubles MMP expression whereas native LDL has no effect.[42] Expression of MMP is also upregulated by tumor necrosis factoralpha and interleukin-1.[43,44] The redundancy of the mechanisms responsible for plaque instability is illustrated by the spectrum of other compounds that induce MMP expression, including plasmin, oxygen radicals, and Chlamydial heat shock protein.[45,46]

Table 1.3 Destabilizing effects of cell products identified in unstable atheroma

	Important action in unstable plaque	Other actions
TNF-α[36]	Upregulates adhesion molecules	Increases thrombogenicity
IL-1β[39]	Activates endothelial cells	Causes SMC apoptosis
MMP[27]	Digests collagen	Digests elastin
Tenascin[45]	Stimulates MMP expression	SMC apoptosis
TGF-β[29]	Stimulates collagen synthesis	Stimulates lipid trapping proteoglycans
TF[48]	Promotes thrombin generation	Promotes MMP expression
IGF-δ[44]	Suppresses collagen expression	Causes SMC apoptosis

The cell products in unstable plaque each have multiple actions that contribute to stabilization. In addition, there is substantial overlap among the effects of cytokines. This redundancy makes it unlikely that targeting a single cytokine will be an effective approach. (Reproduced with permission from Forrester J. Ann Int Med 2002;137:823–833).

Concomitant with destruction of collagen in the unstable plaque, there is suppression of its synthesis. Smooth muscle cell function is suppressed by interferon-gamma from T-lymphocytes.[47,48] The smooth muscle cells in advanced lesions also made susceptible to apoptosis by TNF-alpha and interferon-gamma. In our laboratory Wallner et al. have also shown that the extracellular protein tenascin-C, which is not present in the normal vessel wall, is strongly expressed by macrophages in unstable plaque.[49,50] Tenascin stimulates MMP expression and causes smooth muscle cell apoptosis (Table 1.3).

Erosion of the fibrous cap culminates in plaque rupture, with release of tissue factor, followed by platelet adhesion and thrombus formation. As we observed by angioscopy a decade or more ago, if the thrombus is partially occlusive, it causes the syndrome of unstable angina, whereas complete occlusion causes myocardial infarction. Plaque rupture most commonly occurs at the plaque shoulder, where T-lymphocytes and macrophages predominate and smooth muscle cells are less common.[51] Interestingly, tissue factor content in unstable plaque is twice that in stable plaques, and correlates directly with both macrophage volume,[52] providing the final link the inflammatory process, plaque rupture and coronary thrombosis.

The pathogenesis of the three histologic characteristics of unstable plaque, so poorly understood just a decade ago, can now be defined. The formation of a large lipid core begins with LDL entry into the vessel wall. In the presence of chronic systemic or local vascular inflammation, created or amplified by a spectrum of risk factors, the endothelium is activated. Activated endothelial cells attract monocytes to enter the vessel wall. Within the vessel wall, the monocytes encounter oxidized LDL, the product of oxidative stress, also a manifestation of inflammatory activation. The monocytes avidly ingest oxidized LDL, becoming trapped in the subendothelium as tissue macrophages. As macrophages ingest LDL and later die, a large necrotic lipid core is created. The abundance of inflammatory cells in the unstable plaque is maintained and amplified by cytokine-induced cell activation. The third histologic characteristic of the unstable plaque is the thin fibrous cap. This results from extracellular matrix breakdown by proteases. At the same time collagen synthesis is diminished by cytokine-induced suppression of SMC function and promotion of SMC apoptosis. When the fibrous cap ruptures, most commonly at the shoulders, it exposes both tissue factor and collagen to the flowing blood stream. Both are prothrombotic.

In science, the tools we have for measuring it often determine the way we perceive reality. For CHD these perceptions have also determined management. In the 1980s, revascularization therapy had its origin in angiography. In the 1990s thrust of LDL lowering statin therapy had as its basis the correlation of elevated blood lipids and cardiac events. Today the ability to measure endothelial reactivity, oxidative stress, cholesterol transport, and serum and tissue cytokines provide the basis for an expanded view of management of CHD. Based on cell biology of plaque rupture, we can now identify at least five therapeutic targets for plaque stabilization: endothelial passivation, very aggressive LDL lowering, inhibition of LDL oxidation, acceleration of reverse cholesterol transport, and inhibition of inflammation. If these approaches are additive, substantial further reduction in coronary events should be possible in the coming decade.

References

1. Forrester JS, Litvack F, Grundfest W, Hickey A. A perspective of coronary disease seen through the arteries of living man. Circulation 1987;75:505–513.
2. Sherman CT, Litvack F, Grundfest W, Lee M, Hickey A, Chaux A, Kass R, Blanche C, Matloff J, Morgenstern L, Forrester JS. Coronary Angioscopy in patients with unstable angina pectoris. N Engl J Med 1986;315(15):913–919.
3. Davies MJ. The composition of coronary-artery plaques. N Engl J Med 1997;336(18): 1312–1314.
4. Felton CV, Crook D, Davies MJ, Oliver MF. Relation of plaque lipid composition and morphology to the stability of human aortic plaques. Arterioscler Thromb Vasc Biol 1997;17(7):1337–1345.
5. Shechter M, Sharir M, Forrester J, Bairey-Merz CN. Is There a benefit to lowering low-density lipo protein below 100 Mg/Dl in patients with coronary artery disease. JACC 1999;33:271A.
6. Mellwig KP, Baller D, Gleichmann U, Moll D, Betker S, Weise R, Notohamiprodjo G. Improvement of coronary vasodilatation capacity through single LDL apheresis. Atherosclerosis 1998;139(1):173–178.
7. Vogel RA. Cholesterol Lowering and Endothelial Function. Am J Med 1999;107(5):479–487.
8. Topper JN, Cai J, Falb D, et al. Identification of vascular endothelial genes differentially responsive to fluid mechanical stimuli: cyclooxygenase-2, manganese superoxide dismutase, and endothelial cell nitric oxide synthase are selectively up-regulated by steady laminar shear stress. Proc Natl Acad Sci USA 1996;93:10417–10422.
9. De Caterina R, Libby P, Peng HB, et al. Nitric oxide decreases cytokine-induced endothelial activation: nitric oxide selectively reduces endothelial expression of adhesion molecules and proinflammatory cytokines. J Clin Invest 1995;96:60–68.
10. Nagel T, Resnick N, Atkinson WJ, et al. Shear stress selectively upregulates intercellular adhesion molecule-1 expression in cultured human vascular endothelial cells. J Clin Invest 1994;94:885–891.
11. Qiao JH, Tripathi J, Mishra NK, et al. Role of macrophage colony-stimulating factor in atherosclerosis: studies of osteopetrotic mice. Am J Pathol 1997;150:1687–1699.

12. Dong ZM, Chapman SM, Brown AA, Frenette PS, Hynes RO, Wagner DD. The combined role of P and E-selectins in atherosclerosis. J Clin Invest 1998;102(1):145–152.

13. Van der Wal AC, Das PK, Tigges AJ. Adhesion molecules on the endothelium and mononuclear cells in human atherosclerotic lesions. Am J Pathol 1992;141:1427–1433.

14. Rohde L, Lee RT, Rivero J, Jamacochian M, Arroyo L, Briggs W, Rifai N, Libby P, Creager M, Ridker P. Circulating cell adhesion molecules are correlated with ultrasound-based assessment of carotid atherosclerosis. Arterioscler Thromb Vasc Biol 1998;18(11):1765–1770.

15. Avogaro P, Bigitolo BG, Cassolato G. Presence of a modified low density lipoprotein in humans. Arteriosclerosis 1998;8:79–87.

16. Hasegawa A, Toshima S, Nakano A, Nagai R. Oxidized LDL in patients with coronary heart disease and normal subjects. Nippon Rinsho 1999;57(12):2754–2758.

17. Steinberg D. Low density lipoprotein oxidation and its pathobiological significance. J Biol Chem 1997;272:20963–20966.

18. de la Llera Moya M, Atger V, Paul JL, Fournier N, Moatti N, Giral P, Friday KE, Rothblat G. A cell culture system of screening human serum for ability to promote cellular cholesterol efflux. Arterioscler Thromb 1994;14:1056–1065.

19. Woollett LA, Kearney DM, Spady DK. Diet modification alters plasma HDL cholesterol concentrations but not the transport of HDL esters to the liver in the hamster. J Lipid Res 1997;38:2289–2302.

20. Barter PJ. Inhibition of endothelial cell adhesion molecular expression by high density lipoproteins. Clin Exp Pharmacol Physiol 1997;24(3/4):286–287.

21. Bonnefont-Rousselot D, Therond P, Beaudeux JL, Peynet J, Legrand A, Delattre J. High density lipoproteins (HDL) and the oxidative hypothesis of atherosclerosis. Clin Chem Lab Med 1999;37(10):939–948.

22. Forrester JS, Shah PK. Lipid lowering vs. revascularization: an idea whose time (for testing) has come. Circulation 1997;96(4):1360–1362.

23. Galis Z, Sukhova G, Kranzhofer R, Clark S, Libby P. Macrophage foam cells from experimental atheroma constitutively produce matrix-degrading proteinases. Proc Natl Acad Sci USA 1995;92:402–406.

24. Barath P, Jakubowski A, Fishbein M, Grundfest W, Litvack F, Forrester J. Are mast cells the culprit in coronary plaque destabilization? J Am Coll Cardiol 1988;9:II-52.

25. Kaartinen M, Penttila A, Kovanen P. Mast cells in rupture-prone areas of human coronary atheromas produce and store TNF-α. Circulation 1996;94:2787–2792.

26. Chen Y-H, Chen Y-L, Lin S-J, Chou C-Y, Mar G-Y, Chang M-S, Wang S-P. Electron microscopic studies of phenotypic modulation of smooth muscle cells in coronary arteries of patients with unstable angina pectoris and post-angioplasty restenosis. Circulation 1997;95:1169–1175.

27. Libby P. Molecular bases of the acute coronary syndromes. Circulation 1995;91(11): 2844–2850.

28. van der Wal AC, Becker AE, van der Loos CM, Das PK. Unstable plaques, endothelial function, and coronary artery thrombosis: site of intimal rupture or erosion of thrombosed coronary atherosclerotic plaques is characterized by an inflammatory process irrespective of the dominant plaque morphology. Circulation 1994;89:36–44.

29. Barath P, Fishbein MC, Cao J, Berenson J, Helfant RH, Forrester JS. Detection and localization of tumor necrosis factor gene expression in human atheroma. Am J Cardiol 1990;65:297–302.

30. Sukhova G, Schonbeck U, Rabkin E, Schoen F, Poole A, Billinghurst R, Libby P. Evidence for increased collagenolysis by interstitial collagenases-1 and −3 in vulnerable human atheromatous plaques. Circulation 1999;99(19):2503–2509.

31. Anguera I, Miranda-Guardiola F, Bosch X, Filella X, Sitges M, Marin JL, Betriu A, Sanz G. Elevation of serum levels of the anti-inflammatory cytokine. interleukin-10 and decreased risk of coronary events in patients with unstable angina. Am Heart J 2002;144:811–817.

32. Bobik A, Agrotis A, Kanellakis P, Dilley R, Krushinsky A, Smirnov V, Tararak E, Condron M, Kostolias G. Distinct patterns of transforming growth factor-β isoform and receptor expression in human atherosclerotic lesions. Circulation 1999;99:2883–2891.

33. Ross R. Atherosclerosis is an inflammatory disease. Am Heart J 1999;138:S419–S420.
34. Casscells W, Hathorn B, David M, Krabach T, Vaughn WK, McAllister HA, Bearman G, Willerson JT. Thermal detection of cellular infiltrates in living atherosclerotic plaques: possible implications for plaque rupture and thrombosis. Lancet 1996;347:1447–1449.
35. Malik IS, Haskard DO. Soluble adhesion molecules in ischaemic heart disease. Eur Heart J 1999;20:990–991.
36. Kiechl S, Egger G, Mayr M, Wiedermann CJ, Bonora E, Oberhollenzer F, Muggeo M, Xu Q, Wick G, Poewe W, Willeit J. Chronic infections and the risk of carotid atherosclerosis: prospective results from a large population study. Circulation 2001;103(8):1064–1070.
37. Danesh J. Smoldering arteries: low-grade inflammation and coronary heart disease. JAMA 1999;282(22):2169–2171.
38. Shah PK, Falk E, Badimon JJ, Fernandez-Ortiz A, Mailhac A, Villareal-Levy G, Fallon JT, Regnstrom J, Fuster V. Human monocyte-derived macrophages induce collagen breakdown in fibrous caps of atherosclerotic plaques: potential role of matrix-degrading metalloproteinases and implication for plaque rupture. Circulation 1995;95:1565–1569.
39. Brown DL, Hibbs MS, Kearney M, Loushin C, Isner JM. Identification of 92-kd gelatinase in human coronary atherosclerotic lesions: association of active enzyme synthesis with unstable angina. Circulation 1995;95:2125–2131.
40. Lendon CL, Davies MJ, Born GVR, Richardson PD. Atherosclerotic plaque caps are locally weakened when macrophage density is increased. Atherosclerosis 1991;87:87–90.
41. Xu XP, Meisel SR, Ong HM, Kaul S, Cercek B, Rajavashisth TB, Sharifi B, Shah PK. Oxidized low-density lipoprotein regulates matrix metalloproteinase-9 and is tissue inhibitor in human monocyte-derived macrophages. Circulation 1999;99:993–998.
42. Saren P, Welgus HG, Kovanen PT. TNF-alpha and IL-beta selectively induce expression of 92-kDa gelatinase by human macrophages. J Immunol 1996;157:4159–4165.
43. Rajavashisth TB, Xu X-P, Jovinge S, Meisel S, Xu X-O, Chai N-N, Fishbein MC, Kaul S, Cercek B, Sharifi B, Shah PK. Membrane type 1 matrix metalloproteinase expression in human atherosclerotic plaques: evidence for activation by proinflammatory mediators. Circulation 1999;99(24):3103–3109.
44. Rajagopalan S, Meng XP, Ramasamy S, Harrison DG, Galis ZS: Reactive oxygen species produced by macrophage-derived foam cells regulate the activity of vascular matrix metalloproteinases in vitro: implications for atherosclerotic plaque stability. J Clin Invest 1996;98:2572–2579.
45. Kol A, Sukhova GK, Lichtman AH, Libby P. Chlamydial heat shock protein 60 localizes in human atheroma and regulates macrophage tumor necrosis factor-α and matrix metalloproteinase expression. Circulation 1998;98:300–307.
46. Bennett MR, Evan GI, Schwartz SM. Apoptosis of human vascular smooth muscle cells derived from normal vessels and coronary atherosclerotic plaque. J Clin Invest 1995;95:2266–2274.
47. Henderson EL, Geng Y-J, Sukhova GK, Whittemore AD, Knox J, Libby P. Death of smooth muscle cells and expression of mediators of apoptosis by T lymphocytes in human abdominal aneurysms. Circulation 1999;99:96–104.
48. Wallner K, Li C, Shah PK, Fishbein MC, Forrester JS, Kaul S, Sharifi B. Tenascin-C is expressed in macrophage-rich human coronary atherosclerotic plaque. Circulation 1999;99(10):1284–1289.
49. LaFleur DW, Chiang J, Fagin JA, Forrester JS, Shah PK, Sharifi BG. Smooth muscle cells interact with tenascin through its fibrinogen-like domain. FASEB 1998;12(4):A479.
50. Falk E, Shah P, Fuster V. Coronary plaque disruption. Circulation 1995;92:657–671.
51. Toschi V, Gallo R, Lettino M, Fallon JT, Gertz SD, Fernandez-Ortiz A, Chesebro JH, Badimon L, Nemerson Y, Fuster V, Badimon JJ. Tissue factor modulates the thrombogenicity of human atherosclerotic plaques. Circulation 1997;95:594–599.
52. Forrester JS, Kaul S, Bairey-Merz N. The aggressive lipid lowering controversy. J Am Coll Cardiol 2000;36:1419–1425.

53. Packard CJ. Relationship Between LDL-C Changes and CHD Event Reduction with Pravastatin In the West of Scotland Coronary Prevention Study (WOSCOPS). Circulation 1997;96(suppl I):I–107.
54. deLorgeril M, Salen P, Martin J-L, Monjaud I, Delaye J, Mamelle N. Mediterranean Diet, Traditional Risk Factors, and the Rate of Cardiovascular Complications After Myocardial Infarction. Circulation 1999;99:779–785.
55. Rubins HB, Robins SJ, Collins D, Fye CL, Anderson JW, Elam MB, Faas FH, Linares E, Schaefer EJ, Schectman G, Wilt T, Wittes J. Gemfibrozil for the Secondary Prevention of Coronary Heart Disease in Men with Low Levels of High-Density Lipoprotein Cholesterol. New Engl J Med 1999;341(6):410–418.
56. Relation of gemfibrozil treatment and lipid levels with major coronary exacts; VA-HIT; a randomized controlled trial 2001;285:1585–1591.

Chapter 2
Epidemiological Studies on Atherosclerosis: The Role of the Mediterranean Diet in the Prevention of Cardiovascular Disease

Edgar R. Miller III and Thomas P. Erlinger

Introduction

The Seven Countries Study, reported by Ancel Keys in 1970,[12] was the first substantive epidemiological evidence to support the hypothesis that multiple dietary factors determine coronary heart disease (CHD) risk. This seminal longitudinal study of populations in Europe, Asia, and the United States was conducted with rigorous, standardized dietary data collection and meticulously tracked clinical outcomes. A striking finding was the apparent large CHD risk reduction associated with consumption of a "Crete," a.k.a. "Mediterranean" diet. Since this report, further research has attempted to confirm these findings and characterize features of the diet which may account for the substantial reduction in CHD risk.

The purpose of this chapter is to characterize the "Mediterranean diet" as it was originally described, review observational studies that confirm CHD risk reduction with adherence to the diet, and report the results of clinical trials conducted to determine the effectiveness of the Mediterranean-style diet at reducing cardiovascular disease risk. In the process, we describe the food composition and nutrient profile of the Mediterranean diets. Finally, we report results of feeding studies that provide insight into probable mechanisms that mediate risk reduction: including effects on oxidative stress markers and traditional cardiovascular disease (CVD) risk factors including lipids and blood pressure.

Several limitations to our characterization of the Mediterranean diet exist. First, dietary patterns are exceedingly difficult to describe, in part, because of substantial heterogeneity of the diets that fall under a common rubric (e.g. Mediterranean diets) and because of secular trends. The classically described "Crete" diet associated with reduced CVD risk is being supplanted by contemporary versions of these diets that often reflect Western culture. This chapter focuses, to the extent possible, on modifications of the original dietary pattern. Second, health outcomes, such as CHD mortality, are often unavailable and, when available, are not directly comparable across studies. Hence, recent observational studies that examine the association of the Mediterranean dietary patterns and CVD risk may have different endpoints. Despite these caveats, the health benefits of Mediterranean-style diets

J.L. Holtzman (ed.), *Atherosclerosis and Oxidant Stress: A New Perspective.*
© Springer 2008

appear robust and research has advanced our understanding of the mechanisms that may account for the CVD risk reduction.

The Mediterranean Diet and Risk of CVD

In view of the numerous cultures and agricultural patterns of the Mediterranean region, the 'Mediterranean' diet cannot be characterized by a specific nutrient profile; rather, this term is applied to a dietary pattern. In this context, the dietary pattern, extensively described in the Seven Countries Study remains a historical reference point (Table 2.1).

This study, which began in the mid-1950s, was the first to systematically examine the relationship between diet and risk of CVD across geographically and culturally distinct populations. The countries were the United States, Finland, The Netherlands, Italy, Yugoslavia, Greece, and Japan. Over the course of 5years of follow-up, CHD mortality varied widely among these countries with the highest average annual age-adjusted incidence occurring in Finland (47/10,000) and the US (47/10,000), and the lowest in Greece (8/10,000), Japan (9/10,000), and Italy (7/10,000).[12] Results suggest that consumption of a Mediterranean diet, similar to that of Crete in the 1960s, was associated with one of the lowest risks of CHD in the world. This reduced risk can be attributed, in part, to differences in dietary patterns. Compared to the diet of the US cohort in the Seven Countries Study, the Cretan diet in 1960 was higher in bread, legumes, fruit, olive oil (monounsaturated fat), wine, and fish. Smaller differences were observed for vegetables, cereals, and potatoes. One common finding was the low consumption of non-fish meats in the Crete compared to the US diet. Key features of the traditional Mediterranean diet are summarized in Table 2.2.

Over time, the diet of Crete has changed remarkably and is now characterized by higher intake of saturated fat and cholesterol, and reduced intake of monounsaturated fats.[5] At the same time, total fat consumption has fallen. These trends have been accompanied by a steady rise in CHD risk during 25 years of follow-up of the Cretan cohort.[16] Today, the Cretan diet increasingly resembles a western diet; there has been a concurrent rise in CHD risk. Hence, the reference Mediterranean diet should be anchored to its original description and characterization.

Observational Study Results

Since the publication of the Seven Countries study, others have examined the association between the consumption of Mediterranean dietary pattern and risk of CHD. Notably, the characterization of the diet has required development of a Mediterranean-diet score that incorporates salient characteristics of this diet.[29] A scale of 0–9 was created and indicates the degree of adherence to the traditional Mediterranean diet.

Table 2.1 Characteristics of the 1960 Crete, a.k.a "Mediterranean diet," compared with the average diet consumed by the United States men (age 40–59 years) and diets tested within the setting of randomized clinical trails

Dietary pattern	Typical US diet men age 40–59 (1997–1999) (Zhou[31])	Crete 1960[12]	Mediterranean-like diets		DASH/Prudent American[2]	OMNI/Carbohydrate diet[3]	OMNI/Protein diet[3]	OMNI/Unsaturated fat diet[3]
			Lyon Diet Heart Study clinical trial (de Lorgeril[8])	Indo-Mediterranean Diet Heart Study[25]				
Source of diet information	24h dietary recall	Food record	Unspecified diet survey	7-day detailed food diary	Analyses of composited meals and from menus	Analyses of composited meals and from menus	Analyses of composited meals and from menus	Analyses of composited meals and from menus
Fat (%kcal)	33.3	41.9	30.4	26.3	25.6	27	27	37
Saturated (%kcal)	10.8	8.9	8	8.2	7	6	6	6
Polyunsaturated (% kcal)	7.0	4.4	4.6	8.1	6.8	8	8	10
Monounsaturated (% kcal)	12.4	26.8	17.	10	9.9	13	13	21
Protein (% kcal)	15.6	12.5	16.2	14.2	17.9	15	25	15
% protein from plant	32					36	48	36
Carbohydrates (% kcal)	48.4	43	53.4	59.5	56.5	58	48	48
Fiber (g/1,000 kcal)	8.2	15.2	9.6	23.9	14.8	14.3	14.3	14.3
Cholesterol (mg/1,000 kcal)	133	74.5	104	62	72	71	71	71
Alcohol (% kcal)	2.7	2.7	5.8			<2	<2	<2

(continued)

Table 2.1 (continued)

| Dietary pattern | Typical US diet men age 40–59 (1997–1999) (Zhou 2000) | Mediterranean-like diets | | | DASH/ Prudent American[2] | OMNI/ Carbohydrate diet[3] | OMNI/Protein diet[3] | OMNI/ Unsaturated fat diet[3] |
		Crete 1960[12]	Lyon Diet Heart Study clinical trial (de Lorgeril 1994)	Indo-Mediterranean Diet Heart Study[25]				
Description		High in fruits, vegetables, bread, cereals, potatoes, beans, nuts, and seeds; includes olive oil, dairy products, fish, poultry, wine, and eggs; and is reduced in red meat	Emphasizes bread, root vegetables, green vegetables, fish, poultry, and is reduced in red meat. Butter and cream replaced with margarine rich in Alpha-linolenic acid	Emphasizes low total fat (<30%), saturated fat (<10%) and cholesterol (<300 mg/ day.) In addition, emphasizes fruits, vegetables, nuts, whole grains, and oils rich in linolenic acid	Emphasizes fruits, vegetables, and low-fat dairy products; includes whole grains, poultry, fish, and nuts; and is reduced in red meat and sweets	Similar to DASH except for slightly reduced protein	Approximately 50% of protein from plants (legumes, grains, nuts, and seeds)	Emphasized Monounsaturated fat-included olive oil, canola, safflower oils, and a variety of nuts and seeds to meet targeted fatty acid distribution

Table 2.2 Dietary features characteristic of the traditional Mediterranean diet[29]

High intake of vegetables, legumes, fruits, nuts, and whole-grain non-refined cereals
High intake of olive oil
Low intake of saturated fats
Moderately high intake of fish
Low to moderate intake of dairy products (mostly yogurt and cheese)
Low intake of meat and poultry
Regular but moderate intake of alcohol (primarily wine with meals)

A value of 0 or 1 was assigned to each of nine components with the use of sex-specific median as a cut-off. For beneficial components (vegetables, legumes, fruits and nuts, cereal, high monounsaturated fat intake, and fish), persons whose consumption was below the median were assigned a value of 0, and persons whose consumption was above the median were assigned a value of 1. For components presumed to be detrimental (meat, poultry, and dairy products), persons whose consumption was below the median were assigned a value of 1, and persons whose consumption was at or above the median were assigned a value of 0. For alcohol, a value of 1 was assigned for those who consumed between 5 and 25 g/day and 0 to those with more or less consumption.

In a prospective study of 22,043 adults in Greece followed for 44 months, there was a reduction in total mortality (adjusted hazards ratio (HR) = 0.75, 95% confidence interval (CI), 0.64–0.87) and in death due to CHD (HR = 0.67, 95% CI, 0.59–0.98) associated with a two point increment in the Mediterranean diet score.[29] A subgroup analysis of those with prevalent CVD at baseline, showed that adherence to the diet by two units was associated with a 27% lower total mortality (HR = 0.73, 95% CI, 0.58–0.93) and 31% lower risk of cardiac deaths (HR = 0.69, 95% CI, 0.52–0.93).[28] Hence, the diet was associated with a reduced risk of CVD in both those with and without prevalent disease. This Greek population was part of the European Prospective Investigation into Cancer and Nutrition (EPIC) cohort study that reported results for the entire cohort of 74,607 men and women from 10 European countries. In the entire cohort, using a similar scoring technique, each 2 point increment in the diet score was associated with a reduction of 8% in total mortality (95% CI, 3–12%).[30]

The Healthy Ageing Longitudinal study in Europe (HALE), examined singly the effects of consumption of the Mediterranean diet, and in combination with being physically active, moderate alcohol use, and nonsmoking on 10 year all-cause and CHD mortality in 2,339 men and women ages 70–90 from 11 European countries.[13] Adherence to the Mediterranean diet was associated with a significant reduction in all-cause mortality (HR = 0.77, 95% CI, 0.68–0.88). Adherence to the Mediterranean diet combined with additional diet and lifestyle factors lowered the all-cause mortality rate (HR = 0.35, 95% CI, 0.28–0.44). In total, lack of adherence to this low risk pattern was associated with a population attributable risk of 60% for all deaths, 64% for deaths from coronary heart disease, and 61% from cardiovascular diseases.

Clinical Trial Results – Variations to the Mediterranean Diet

The interpretations of the findings from these and other observational studies suggest that partial adoption of the Mediterranean diet is associated with reductions in CVD across many populations, in the young and old, and those with and without prevalent disease ages. Since observational studies do not establish a cause and effect relationship, a stronger test of the hypothesis for a relationship between the effects of the Mediterranean diet on CVD risk is in the setting of a clinical trial. Two trials designed to test the effects of variations of the Mediterranean diet on clinical CVD outcomes were the Lyon Diet Heart Study[8] and the Indo-Mediterranean Diet Heart Study.[25] Both randomized trials were conducted in participants with established CVD.

The Lyon Diet Heart Study

The Lyon Diet Heart Study was designed to evaluate the impact of a Mediterranean diet on the risk of cardiovascular mortality in persons at high risk for CHD.[8] The diet was based on the 1960 Cretan diet as defined by the Seven Countries Study, but the intervention also included supplementation with margarine rich in alpha-linolenic acid (ALA). Participants were advised to eat more bread, root vegetables, green vegetables, fish, and fruit. In addition, participants were asked to reduce their intake of red meat and pork. Finally, participants were asked to replace butter and cream with the supplemental margarine rich in ALA that was provided by the study. Estimated energy intake (% kcal) from fats was 30.5% from total fat, 8.3% from saturated fats, 0.8% from n-3 fatty acids, and 3.6% from n-6 fatty acids. Mean cholesterol intake was 217 mg/day. After a mean follow-up of 27 months, there was a 70% reduction in total mortality (20 deaths in control group vs. 8 deaths in experimental group) and a 73% reduction in the combined endpoint of cardiovascular deaths and non-fatal myocardial infarctions among persons assigned to the Mediterranean diet intervention compared to the control group (33 events in control group vs. 8 events in experimental group).

While the results of this trial were impressive, several issues deserve comment. First, a beneficial effect of the intervention was observed very early in the trial, well before significant regression of atherosclerotic plaque might occur. This would suggest that mechanisms other than prevention of atherosclerosis, per se, might be responsible for the beneficial effects of the study diet. Experimental evidence suggests that ALA could have anti-thrombotic and anti-arrythmogenic effects.[10,22] Hence, the impact of the intervention in preventing atherosclerosis is uncertain. A second and related issue is whether the Lyon Diet Heart Study diet can prevent CHD to the same extent as a traditional Mediterranean diet and other diets associated with a very low incidence of CHD. Despite the impressive relative risk reductions associated with the Lyon

Diet Heart Study diet, it is quite possible that the absolute risk of CHD might still exceed that associated with other dietary patterns. Third, it is difficult to separate the effects of the diet from the effects of the ALA supplements that were provided to participants. Dietary advice was given infrequently in the trial, whereas the ALA rich oils were supplied free of charge to participants. Behavioral intervention studies suggest that the frequency of dietary advice provided in the Lyon Diet Heart Study was insufficient to substantially change diet. In contrast, provision of the free ALA supplements might have been sufficient to accomplish this aspect of the intervention.

Indo-Mediterranean Diet Heart Study

A recently completed trial conducted in India, the Indo-Mediterranean Diet Heart Study,[25] complements findings from the Lyon Diet Heart Study. The study population consisted primarily of men (~90%) who were at high-risk for either a first myocardial infarction or a recurrence; approximately 60% had a history of myocardial infarction at baseline, and 35% had a recent (<4 weeks) myocardial infarction. In contrast to the Lyon Diet Heart Study, two-thirds of participants were vegetarian at baseline. All participants were given advice to reduce their intake of fat, saturated fat, and cholesterol (<30% kcal from fat, <10% kcal from saturated fat, and <300 mg cholesterol/day). Those participants in the intervention arm were also advised to increase their consumption of fruits, vegetables, and nuts and to use mustard seed and soybean oil (3–4 servings/day), both of which are rich in ALA.

It is noteworthy that approximately 60% of calories came from carbohydrates, of which a substantial proportion was presumably from fruit, vegetable, and grain consumption. In contrast to the Lyon Diet Heart Study, consumption of the Indo-Mediterranean diet resulted in significant reductions in total and LDL cholesterol, and an increase in HDL-cholesterol. In addition, blood pressure and body mass index were reduced with the Indo-Mediterranean diet compared to controls. A common feature of both the Lyon Diet Heart study and Indo-Mediterranean Diet Heart study was the emphasis on ALA consumption. In the latter study, increased consumption was achieved by emphasizing foods and oils rich in ALA (nuts, soybean oil, and mustard seed oil).

After 2 years of follow-up, there was a 50% reduction in total cardiovascular endpoints (fatal myocardial infarction, non-fatal myocardial infarction, and sudden cardiac death) in the intervention group (39 events) compared to the control group (76 events). Both non-fatal myocardial infarction and sudden death were reduced in the intervention group; however, there was no significant difference in fatal myocardial infarction. These results are consistent with results from the Lyon Diet Heart Study, where there were significant reductions in sudden death and non-fatal myocardial infarctions. Still, these impressive results are somewhat surprising, because, at baseline, two-thirds of participants were vegetarians.

Clinical Feeding Study Results

The Lyon Diet Heart study and the Indo-Mediterranean diet trial relied on behavior modification strategies to promote adoption of the Mediterranean diet plans to participants. Compliance with dietary recommendations was hard to assess and effects of on-traditional CVD risk factors hard to ascertain. In fact, in the Lyon Diet Heart study, end-of study assessment of the traditional CVD risk factors including blood pressure and lipids, were not different between groups.[8] This finding was unexpected as emphasis on unsaturated fatty acids rather than saturated or trans-fatty acids would be expected to beneficially affect serum lipid levels.[23] Likewise, dietary patterns emphasizing fruits and vegetables have been shown to substantially lower blood pressure and are discussed next.[2] Hence determining the effects of the Mediterranean diet on traditional CVD risk factors, including blood pressure and lipids, and on markers of oxidative stress, may be best determined in a different setting: clinical feeding studies. Feeding trials are conducted under ideal conditions of monitoring and compliance where all components of diet are controlled. Three seminal feeding trials described below were designed to examine effects of dietary patterns on blood pressure and lipids and allows for true estimates of the effects of changes of dietary patterns on traditional CVD risk factors.

The Dash Trials

The Dietary Approaches to Stop Hypertension (DASH) and DASH-sodium trials[2,24] tested the effects of a carbohydrate-rich diet that emphasizes fruits, vegetables, and low-fat dairy products and that is reduced in saturated fat, total fat, and cholesterol on blood pressure, total cholesterol, and LDL cholesterol. This diet is rich in potassium, magnesium, calcium, and fiber, and is reduced in total fat, saturated fat, and cholesterol; it is also slightly increased in protein. Effects of this diet were compared against a group randomized to a "control" diet which had a nutrient composition that is typical of that consumed by many Americans (Table 2.2). Its potassium, magnesium, and calcium levels were comparatively low, while its macronutrient profile and fiber content corresponded to average US consumption. A "fruits and vegetables" diet tested in the original DASH trial was rich in potassium, magnesium, and fiber but otherwise similar to the control diet. All three diets contain similar amounts of sodium (approximately 3,000 mg/day) and both studies used isocaloric feeding to avoid the influence on weight loss and calorie restriction on these CVD risk factors.

In the original DASH study, among all participants, the DASH diet significantly lowered mean systolic BP by 5.5 mmHg and mean diastolic BP by 3.0 mmHg.[2] The fruits and vegetables diet also significantly reduced BP but to a lesser extent, about 50% of the effect of the DASH diet. The reductions in hypertensive individuals (11.6/5.3 mmHg) (Fig. 2.1) were striking and were significantly greater than the corresponding effects in non-hypertensive individuals (3.5/2/2 mmHg). The effects occurred rapidly and were apparent after only 2 weeks. The DASH-sodium trial

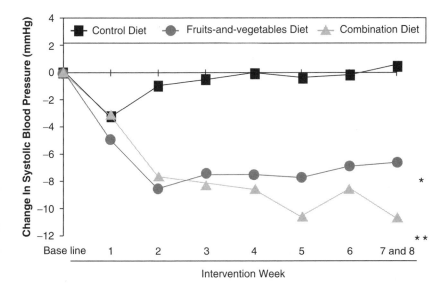

Fig. 2.1 DASH diet results: change in systolic blood pressure (mmHg) in hypertensive participants randomized to diets[6]

confirmed these results and further documented the effect of sodium intake on blood pressure in those who consumed the control and DASH diets. In addition to BP reduction, the DASH diet also reduced serum homocysteine levels[1] and had favorable effects on blood lipids.[21]

The DASH trials results give important insight into the effects of dietary patterns on CVD risk factors. Similarities between the Mediterranean dietary pattern and DASH diets include the high daily servings of fruits and vegetables (8–10 servings/day), the emphasis on whole-gain foods, fish, and nuts. Both diets are low in saturated fat and high in fiber. These factors and the concomitant increases in potassium, magnesium, and calcium may in part account for a substantial proportion of the observed CVD risk reduction with consumption of the Mediterranean diet and may be mediated through effects on traditional CVD risk factors and reductions in oxidative stress. However, unlike the Mediterranean dietary pattern which has a high fat content (41% – primarily monounsaturated fat) the DASH diet is reduced in total fat (27%).

OMNI Heart Trial

Results of DASH trials were important in providing an estimate of the magnitude of effects of diet on blood pressure, total cholesterol, and LDL cholesterol. However, the diet also lowered HDL-cholesterol and had no effect on triglycerides, traditional risk factors that are associated with CVD risk. These carefully conducted trials can provide insight into components of the Mediterranean dietary pattern which

Table 2.3 The change from baseline on serum LDL-cholesterol, HDL-cholesterol, triglycerides, and blood pressure in participants after consuming each of the OMNI-Heart diets for 6 weeks

OMNI Heart – Lipid results (mg/dL)

		Mean change from baseline in each diet		
LDL-C	Baseline	CARB	PROT	UNSAT
All	129.2	−11.6	−14.2	−13.1
LDL-C ≥ 130	156.7	−19.8	−23.6	−21.9
LDL-C < 130	105.2	−4.4	−6.1	−5.4
HDL-C	50.0	−1.4	−2.6	−0.3
Triglycerides	101.5	0.1	−16.4	−9.3

Omni-Heart blood pressure results (mmHg)

		Mean change from baseline in each diet		
Systolic BP	Baseline	CARB	PROT	UNSAT
All	131.2	−8.2	−9.5	−9.3
HTN Only	146.5	−12.9	−16.1	−15.8
PreHTN Only	127.5	−7.0	−8.0	−7.7
Diastolic BP	77.0	−4.1	−5.2	−4.8

might reduce CVD risk either through traditional CVD risk factors or through effects which lower oxidative stress.

The OMNI-Heart trial, the third in the series of clinical feeding studies, tested whether partial replacement of carbohydrate with either unsaturated fat or protein can improve blood pressure and lipid risk factors.[3] The OMNI-Heart trial was a randomized, 3 periods, crossover, feeding trial designed to determine the effects on blood pressure and serum lipids of three healthful diets. Each feeding period lasted 6 weeks and body weight was held constant. Each diet was reduced in saturated fat. The three diets (characterized in Table 2.2) include: a carbohydrate-rich diet, similar to the DASH diet (CARB diet); a diet rich in proteins (PROT), approximately half from plant sources; and a diet rich in unsaturated fat (UNSAT), predominantly monounsaturated fat. The UNSAT diet not only had all the DASH diet similarities previously described, but also was higher in fat (37%), predominantly monounsaturated fat (21%) primarily from olive and canola oils, approaching levels characteristic of the Mediterranean diet. Participants were 164 healthy adults with prehypertension of Stage 1 hypertension. Results of the OMNI trial are presented in Table 2.3. Reductions in blood pressure and lipids from baseline were substantial. The magnitude of blood pressure reduction across all diets is similar to that which can be achieved with medication treatment.

Mediterranean Diet Effects on Oxidative Stress

The direct relationship between traditional CVD risk factors and risk of atherosclerosis is well established. Dietary modifications which lower blood pressure and lipids provide a likely explanation for much of the risk reduction. However, oxidative stress, including oxidation of LDL-c (oxLDL) appears to be an important, if not obligatory step in the pathogenesis of atherosclerosis and may accelerate this process.[26] Hence, measurement of oxidative stress using biomarkers may offer insight into mechanisms of CVD risk reduction beyond that which is predicted by lipids or other CVD risk factors alone.

Oxidative stress markers commonly used, including nonspecific in vitro assays to determine the susceptibility of lipids to oxidation (i.e. lag time, thiobarbituric acid substances, malondialdehyde, oxygen radical absorbing capacity (ORAC) or assays that measure, in vivo, end-product of oxidative damage to lipids (e.g., breath ethane or urinary isoprostanes). Formation of these oxidation products is dependant on free radical activity (i.e. metabolic rate), substrate concentration (i.e. lipids), and antioxidant activity (both endogenous and dietary). Hence, alterations in dietary patterns can give important insight into the benefit or harm of nutrients when linked to subsequent changes in markers of oxidative stress.

In the DASH trial, consumption of the DASH diet reduced breath ethane exhalation (an in vivo marker of oxidized n-3 polyunsaturated acids)[17] and reduced urinary isoprostanes (an in vivo degradation product of arachidonic acid). These findings provide indirect evidence for reduced oxLDL in vivo. In addition, consumption of the DASH diet was previously shown to prevent an expected rise in urinary isoprostanes induced by acute hyperlipidemia.[15] Consumption of the DASH diet resulted in increasing serum antioxidants and the ORAC of serum (Fig. 2.2).

A limitation of the ORAC assay is the inability to determine which component(s) of the diet provides the greatest activity in protecting against oxidative stress. However, consumption of the DASH diet resulted in increased serum levels of several carotenoids including lutein, cryptoxanthin, zeaxanthin and β-carotene,

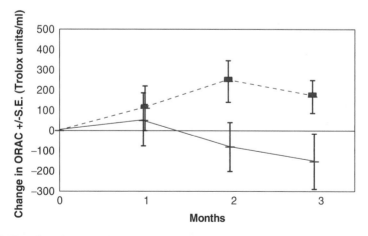

Fig. 2.2 The effect of consumption of the DASH diet (squares) compared with the typical American Diet (hatch-mark) on the oxygen radical absorbing capacity (ORAC) of serum over 3 months[18,20,31]

important lipid soluble antioxidants. A proportionate increase in lipid peroxidation products derived from a higher polyunsaturated fat intake, can be diminished by supplementation of diet with plant-based sources of antioxidants such as flavenoids.[11] In addition, supplementation of diet with carotenoid-rich vegetable products has been shown to enhance lipoprotein carotenoid concentrations and reduce lipid peroxidation in healthy men consuming a diet controlled for fat intake.[4] Consumption of a diet high in fruit and vegetable has also been shown to increase endogenous enzymatic antioxidant activity (erythrocyte glutathionione peroxidase activity) and resistance of plasma lipoproteins to oxidation.[9] Finally, reduced oxidative stress observed in the DASH trial may, in part, be explained by the higher serum content of these dietary antioxidants and enhanced antioxidant enzymatic activity.

Additional benefits of consumption of the Mediterranean diet may be related to a predominance of monounsaturated fat in the diet. Monounsaturated fats are more resistant to oxidation than polyunsaturated fats.[19,14] A higher proportional polyunsaturated fatty acid intake results in an increased number of double bonds (targets of oxidation) which has previously been linked to greater oxidation in vitro.[7] The Mediterranean diet, compared with the typical US diet, is greatly reduced in polyunsaturated fatty acids. Hence, enrichment of diet with monounsaturated fatty acids will reduce the rate of oxidized lipids.[27] Finally, olive oil is enriched with several compounds that constitute the unsaponified fraction of the oil, (hydrocarbons, sterols, and polyphenols), that prevent the oil from oxidation and underlie its exceptional stability.[19]

Collectively, these studies suggest that the consumption of the Mediterranean style diet may lower risk of CVD, independent of traditional CVD risk factors, via the increased antioxidants and reduced oxidative stress.

Summary and Conclusion

The Mediterranean dietary patterns are associated with lower CHD rates and with improved CHD risk factors. In the interpretation of observational data, it is often difficult to separate the effects of diet from other factors, e.g., smoking and physical inactivity, that likely account, in part, for observed differences in CHD risk. Nonetheless, the totality of evidence documenting a beneficial impact of Mediterranean dietary patterns on CHD risk is remarkable and consistent in both the original Seven Countries Study and in recent studies of populations with Western variants of the original diet. Cardiovascular disease risk reduction by consumption of the Mediterranean diet may be mediated through demonstrated effects on traditional CVD risk factors of through effects of factors which reduce oxidative stress.

Overall, such findings have tremendously important public health implications. Despite broad variation in geography, lifestyle, and locally available foods, it is evident that for most populations, a Mediterranean style diet that reduces CHD risk is readily available. The public health challenge is achieving population-wide adoption of beneficial dietary patterns in the setting of powerful influences that promote unhealthy lifestyles.

References

1. Appel LJ, Miller ER III, Jee SH, Stolzenberg-Solomon R, Lin PH, Erlinger T. Effect of dietary patterns on serum homocysteine: results of a randomized, controlled feeding study. Circulation 2000;102:852–857.
2. Appel LJ, Moore TJ, Obarzanek E, Vollmer W, Svetkey LP, Sacks F, Bray G, Vogt TM, Cutler JA, Simons-Morton D, Lin H-P, Karanja N, Windhauser MM, McCullough M, Swain J, Steele P, Evans MA, Miller ER III, Harsha DW, for the DASH Collaborative Research Group. A clinical trial of the effects of dietary patterns on blood pressure. N Eng J Med 1997;336:1117–1124.
3. Appel LJ, Sacks FM, Carey V, Obarzanek E, Swain J, Miller ER III, Conlin PR, Erlinger TP, Rosner BA, Laranjo N, Charleston J, McCarron P, Proschan MA, Bishop L. The effect of protein, monounsaturated fat, and carbohydrate intake on blood pressure and serum lipids: results of the OmniHeart randomized trial. JAMA 2005;294:2455–2464.
4. Bub A, Watzl B, Abrahamse L, Delincee H, Adam S, Wever J, Muller H, Rechkemmer G. Moderate intervention with carotenoid-rich vegetable products reduces lipid peroxidation in men. J Nutr 2000;130:2200–2206.
5. Costacou T, Bamia C, Ferrari P, Riboli E, Trichopoulou A. Tracing the Mediterranean diet through principal components analyses in the Greek population. Eur J Clin Nutr 2003;75:1378–1385.
6. Conlin PR, Chow DC, Miller ER III, Svetky LP, Lin P-H, Harsha DW, Moore TJ, Sacks FM, Appel LJ. The effect of dietary patterns on blood pressure control in hypertensive patients: results from the dietary approaches to stop hypertension (DASH) trial. Am J Hypertens 2000;13:949–955.
7. DeLany JP, Windhauser MM, Champagne CM, Bray GA. Differential oxidation of individual dietary fatty acids in humans. Am J Clin Nutr 2000;72:905–911.
8. de Lorgeril M, Salen P, Martin JL, Monjaud I, Boucher P, Mamelle N. Mediterranean dietary pattern in a randomized trial: prolonged survival and possible reduced cancer rate. Arch Intern Med 1998;158:1181–1187.
9. Dragsted LO, Pedersen A, Hermetter A, Basu S, Hansen M, Haren GR, Kall M, Brienholt V, Castenmiller JM, Stagsted J, Jakobsen J, Skibsted L, Ramsumussen SE, Loft S, Sandrstrom B. The 6-day study: effects of fruit and vegetables on markers of oxidative stress and antioxidant defense in healthy nonsmokers. Am J Clin Nutr 2004;79:1060–1072.
10. Freese R, Mutanen M, Valsta LM, Salminen I. Comparison of the effects of two diets rich in monounsaturated fatty acids differing in their linoleic/alpha-linolenic acid ratio on platelet aggregation. Thromb Haemost 1994;71:73–77.
11. Fremont L, Gozzelino MT, Franchi MP, Linard A. Dietary flavenoids reduce lipid peroxidation in rats fed polyunsaturated or monounsaturated fat diets. J Nutr 1998;128:1495–1502.
12. Ancel K. Coronary Heart Disease in Seven Countries. New York: American Heart Association Monograph Number 29, 1970.
13. Knoops KTB, de Groot LCPGM, Kromhout D, Perrin A-E, Moreisas-Varela, Menotti A, van Staveren WA. Mediterennanean diet, lifestyle factors, and 10 year mortality in elderly European men and women. JAMA 2004;292:1433–1439.
14. Kratz M, Cullen P, Kassner F, Fobker M, Abuja PM, Assmann G, Wahrburg U. Effects of dietary fatty acids on the composition and oxidizability of low-density lipoprotein. Eur J Clin Nutr 2002;56:72–81.
15. Lopes HF, Martin KL, Nashar K, Morrow JD, Goodfriend TL, Egan BM. DASH diet lowers blood pressure and lipid-induced oxidative stress in obesity. Hypertension 2003;41:422–430.
16. Menotti A, Kromhout D, Blackburn H, Fidanza F, Buzina R, Nissinen A. Food intake patterns and 25-year mortality from coronary heart disease: cross-cultural correlations in the seven countries study. The Seven Countries Study Research Group. Eur J Epidemiol 1999;15:507–515.
17. Miller ER III, Appel LJ, Risby TH. The effects of dietary patterns on measures of lipid peroxidation: results from a randomized clinical trial. Circulation 1998;98:2390–2395.

18. Miller ER III, Erlinger TP, Sacks FM, Svetkey LP, Charleston J, Lin P-H, Appel LJ. A dietary pattern that lowers oxidative stress increases antibodies to oxidized LDL: results from a randomized controlled feeding study. Atherosclerosis 2005;183:175–182.

19. Moreno JJ. Effect of olive oil minor components on axidative stress and arachidonic acid mobalization and metabolism by Macrophages raw 264.7. Free Rad Biol Med 2003;35:1073–1081.

20. Moreno JJ, Mitjavila MT. The degree of unsaturation of dietary fatty acids and the development of atherosclerosis (review). J Nutr Biochem 2003;14:182–195.

21. Obarzanek E, Sacks FM, Vollmer WM, Bray GA, Miller ER III, Lin PH, et al. Effects on blood lipids of a blood pressure-lowering diet: the dietary approaches to stop hypertension (DASH) trial. Am J Clin Nutr 2001;74(1):80–89.

22. Renaud S, Lanzmann-Petithory D. Dietary fats and coronary heart disease pathogenesis. Curr Atheroscler Rep 2002;4(6):419–424.

23. Sacks F. Dietary factors. Clinical trials in cardiovascular disease: A Companion to Bruanwald's heart disease. Philadelphia: W.B. Saunders Company, 1999, pp.423–431.

24. Sacks FM, Svetkey LP, Volmer WM, Appel LJ, Bray GA, Harsha D, Obarzanek E, Conlin PR, Miller ER III, Simons-Mortons D, Karanja N, Lin P-H, for the DASH-sodium collaborative research group. A clinical trial of the effects on blood pressure of reduced dietary sodium and the DASH dietary pattern (The DASH-sodium trial). New Eng J Med 2001;344:3–10.

25. Singh RB, Dubnov G, Niaz MA, Ghosh S, Singh R, Rastogi SS, et al. Effect of an Indo-Mediterranean diet on progression of coronary artery disease in high risk patients (Indo-Mediterranean Diet Heart Study): a randomized single-blind trial. Lancet 2002;360:1455–1461.

26. Steinberg D, Parthasarathy S, Carew TE, Khoo JC, Witztum JL. Beyond cholesterol: modifications of low-density lipoprotein that increase atherogenicity. N Eng J Med 1989;320:915–924.

27. Tsimikas S, Philis-Tsimikas A, Alexopoulos S, Sigari F, Lee C, Reaven PD. LDL isolated from Greek subjects on a typical diet or from American subjects on an oleate-supplemented diet induces less monocyte chemotaxis and adhesion when exposed to oxidative stress. Atheroscler Thromb Vasc Biol 1999;19:122–130.

28. Trichopoulou A, Bamia C, Trichopoulou D. Mediterranean diet and survival among patients with coronary heart disease in Greece. Arch Intern Med 2005;165:929–935.

29. Trichopoulou A, Costacou T, Bamia C, Trichopoulou D. Adherence to a Mediterranean diet and survival in a Greek population. N Engl J Med 2003;348:2599–2608.

30. Trichopoulou A, Orfanos P, Norat T, Bueno-de-Mesquita B, Ocke M, Peeters PH, van der Schouw YT, Boeing H, Hoffman K, Boffetta P, Nagel G, Masala G, Krogh V, Panico S, Tumino R, Vineis P, Bamia C, Naska A, Benetou V, Ferrari P, Slimani N, Peru G, Martinez-Garcia C, Navarro C, Rodriguez-Barranco M, Dorronsors M, Spencer E, Key T, Bingham S, Khaw K-T, Kesse E, Clavel-Chapelon F, Boutron-Ruault M-C, Berglund G, Wirfalt E, Hallmans G, Johansson I, Tjonneland A, Olsen K, Hundborg H, Riboli E, Trichopoulou D. Modified Mediterranean diet and survival: EPIC-elderly prospective cohort study. BMJ 2005(published 8 April 2005 online).

31. Zhou BF, Stamler J, Dennis B, Moag-Stahlberg A, Okuda N, Robertson C, Zhao L, Chan Q, Elliott P, for the INTERMAP Research Group. Nutrient intakes of middle-aged men and monen in China, Japan, United Kingdom, and United States in the late 1990's: the INTERMAP study. J Hum Hypertension 2003;17:623–630.

Chapter 3
Interventional Trials of Antioxidants

Thomas S. Bowman, Shari S. Bassuk, and J. Michael Gaziano

Introduction

Prospective observational studies have found consistent associations between higher intakes of fruit and vegetables and reduced rates of coronary heart disease (CHD)[1-4] and ischemic stroke.[1,5,6] The exact mechanisms for these apparent protective effects are not entirely clear. It is possible that higher fruit and vegetable intake replaces fat and cholesterol intake, but alternatively, the observed beneficial effects may be due to micronutrients contained in the fruits and vegetables. Micronutrients with antioxidant properties might be responsible for the lower rates of cardiovascular disease (CVD) associated with fruit and vegetable consumption.

Laboratory research has identified a possible mechanism – the inhibition of oxidative damage – by which antioxidants might reduce the risk of atherosclerosis and CVD. In addition, many cross-sectional, case-control, and cohort studies have found an association between antioxidant vitamin consumption and a reduced risk of CVD. These results suggest that antioxidants such as vitamin E, beta-carotene, and vitamin C may be involved in the prevention of CVD but do not provide a definitive answer. Several large-scale, randomized trials of antioxidant supplements have now been completed and are not entirely consistent. In this chapter, we discuss the rationale for conducting large-scale trials of antioxidant supplements and review completed and ongoing trials.

Basic Laboratory Research

Oxidative processes may play an important role in the pathogenesis of many chronic diseases, including atherosclerosis, cancer, arthritis, eye disease, and reperfusion injury during myocardial infarction (MI). Data from in vitro and in vivo studies suggest that oxidative damage to low-density lipoprotein (LDL) promotes several steps in atherogenesis,[7] including endothelial cell damage,[8,9] foam cell accumulation,[10-12] and growth[13,14] and synthesis of autoantibodies.[15] In addition, animal studies suggest that free radicals may directly damage arterial

J.L. Holtzman (ed.), *Atherosclerosis and Oxidant Stress: A New Perspective.*
© Springer 2008

Table 3.1 Natural defense mechanisms against oxidative damage

Compartmentalization of oxidative metabolism

Binding of molecular oxygen and reactive species to proteins to prevent random oxidative reactions

Binding of transition metals (e.g., iron and copper) to transport and storage proteins to prevent involvement in free radical reactions

Enzymatic antioxidants (e.g., superoxide dismutase, catalase, and glutathione peroxidase)

Nonenzymatic antioxidants (e.g., vitamin C, vitamin E, beta-carotene, urate, bilirubin, and ubiquinols)

Mechanisms to repair or dispose of damaged DNA, proteins, lipids, and carbohydrates

endothelium,[16] promote thrombosis,[17] and interfere with normal vasomotor regulation.[18] Oxidative damage may enhance atherogenesis by a cascade of reactions.

Several systems have evolved in aerobic organisms to minimize the damaging effects of uncontrolled oxidation (Table 3.1). Mechanisms exist to prevent the formation of unintended free radicals, and oxidative metabolism is carefully compartmentalized with oxygen and its highly reactive species tightly bound to enzymes. Metal ions such as copper and iron are bound to storage or transport proteins to prevent catalytic reactions with oxygen species that could lead to the formation of free radicals. In addition, enzymatic (e.g., superoxide dismutase, catalase, glutathione peroxidase) and nonenzymatic (e.g., vitamins E and C, urate) antioxidants scavenge free radicals, thereby minimizing the damage they can cause once they have been formed. Lastly, there are mechanisms for repairing the damage resulting from unintended oxidative reactions.

Antioxidant vitamins represent one of the many nonenzymatic antioxidant defense mechanisms. Vitamin E (of which alpha-tocopherol is the major component), beta-carotene (a provitamin A), and vitamin C (ascorbic acid) are among the most abundant and most widely studied natural antioxidants. However, there are many other dietary compounds that may function as antioxidants. In vitro data have demonstrated the possible role of these antioxidants in preventing or slowing various steps in atherogenesis by inhibiting the oxidation of LDL or other free radical reactions. These antioxidants have also been shown to prevent experimental atherogenesis in many but not all animal models of atherosclerosis.

Observational Epidemiology

While molecular mechanisms exist to explain potential benefits of antioxidants, clinical outcomes are needed to evaluate the benefit in humans. Observational studies can use information about diet and vitamin intake to identify potential protective effects of antioxidants. Results from cross-sectional, case-control, and cohort studies suggest that antioxidant consumption reduces the risk of developing heart disease and stroke[19] with the strongest data in favor of vitamin E.[20]

Several large cohort studies have evaluated the relationship between vitamin E intake and incidence of CHD. The largest of these is the Nurses' Health Study (NHS), a cohort study of more than 87,000 U.S. female nurses aged 34–59 years with no history of CVD.[21] Dietary antioxidant intake and use of antioxidant vitamin supplements were ascertained through a semiquantitative food frequency questionnaire administered at baseline in 1980 with information on antioxidant supplements updated biennially. After 8 years, women in the highest quintile of vitamin E intake had a 34% lower risk of CHD (nonfatal MI and fatal CHD) compared with those in the lowest quintile (P for trend < 0.001). It was vitamin E supplementation – not dietary intake – that was associated with lower risk. Participants who took at least 100 IU of vitamin E supplements per day for more than 2 years experienced reductions of 40% or more in the risk of CHD, after adjustment for age and cardiac risk factors.

These results were consistent with the Health Professionals Follow-up Study (HPFS), an observational study of nearly 40,000 US male health professionals aged 40–75 years who did not have CHD, diabetes, or hypercholesterolemia.[22] After adjustment for cardiac risk factors, the relative risk (RR) of CHD for those in the highest vs. lowest quintile of vitamin E intake was 0.60 (95% confidence interval (CI) 0.44–0.81; P for trend = 0.01). Further analysis revealed that the protective association was strongest for vitamin E consumed in supplements. Men who took at least 100 IU per day for at least 2 years had a multivariate RR of 0.63 (95% CI, 0.47–0.84) for CHD compared with men who did not take vitamin E supplements. A weak association was found for dietary vitamin E intake alone; among men who did not take vitamin supplements, the RR comparing the extreme quartiles was 0.79 (95% CI, 0.54–1.15, P for trend = 0.11).

The Iowa Women's Health Study evaluated the association between antioxidant vitamin intake and CHD mortality over 7 years among 34,486 postmenopausal women with no history of CVD.[23] In contrast to the NHS and HPFS findings, vitamin E intake from food but not from supplements was strongly associated with a lower risk of CHD mortality. Women in the highest quintile of dietary vitamin E intake, without any supplementation, had a RR of 0.38 compared with those in the lowest quintile (P for trend = 0.004). Controlling for other dietary factors associated with vitamin E intake, such as intake of linoleic acid, folate, and fiber did not affect the results. Similarly, a Finnish study also found a significant inverse association between dietary intake of vitamin E and CHD mortality among 2,385 women 30–69 years of age over a 14-year period.[23]

The relationship between vitamin E and CVD has also been examined in two elderly cohorts. The Established Populations for Epidemiologic Studies of the Elderly program, a 10-year study of 11,178 U.S. men and women aged 67–105 years, found a decreased risk of CHD mortality (RR = 0.53; 95% CI, 0.34–0.84) and overall mortality (RR = 0.66; 95% CI, 0.53–0.83) among those taking vitamin E supplements.[24] However, no association between dietary vitamin E intake (using the semiquantitative food frequency questionnaire) and MI was observed in the Rotterdam Study which followed 4,802 Dutch men and women aged 55–95 years with no history of MI over 4 years.[25]

In contrast to studies of vitamin E intake, studies of vitamin E blood levels, conducted as nested case–control studies within large cohorts, have generally yielded null results. For example, a study of 734 men in the Multiple Risk Factor Intervention Trial found no association between serum vitamin E levels and risk of nonfatal MI or CHD death over a 20-year follow-up period.[26]

Rationale for Randomized Trials

Observational results suggest that antioxidants may have protective effects, but these studies have important limitations. For example, uncontrolled confounding from unknown or unmeasured confounders can be similar in magnitude to the observed health effects, and antioxidant consumption may be merely a marker for a different cardioprotective factor (e.g., exercise, diet) that is responsible for the observed health benefits. In addition, intakes of individual dietary antioxidants tend to be highly correlated with each other, making it difficult to determine the specific benefit of a particular antioxidant. Because of these limitations, randomized trials of adequate power, length of follow-up, and therapeutic dose are necessary to sort out the effects of antioxidants. By assigning subjects randomly to treatment or placebo, potential confounders should be evenly distributed between the two groups.

Antioxidant vitamins are commonly used nutritional supplements, and their use is rapidly increasing. Evaluation of the benefits and risks of antioxidants is essential for determining the place of these supplements in clinical medicine. Large-scale randomized trials could provide positive results to justify the rational use of certain antioxidants, and null results could limit the unneeded use of supplements and allow for a focus on proven therapies.

In 1991, the U.S. National Heart, Lung, and Blood Institute's (NHLBI) conference, "Antioxidants in the Prevention of Human Atherosclerosis" concluded that large-scale randomized trials were required to test the hypothesis that dietary antioxidants reduce the risk of CVD and recommended the initiation of randomized trials to examine the role of vitamin C, vitamin E, and beta-carotene in the primary and secondary prevention of CVD.[27] Antioxidant use in the general population was increasing at that time, and researchers realized that randomized trials would have to start soon so that enough people would be willing to be assigned to a placebo group. In this chapter, we review the large-scale clinical trials of vitamin E alone, beta-carotene alone, vitamin C, and combination antioxidants in both the primary and secondary prevention of CVD.

Vitamin E Primary Prevention Trials

Clinical trials of vitamin E have focused on alpha-tocopherol, the major component of vitamin E and the predominant antioxidant in circulating lipoproteins.[28] Large randomized trials that examined vitamin E alone in the primary prevention of CVD are summarized in Table 3.2.

Table 3.2 Completed and ongoing randomized clinical trials of vitamin E supplementation in the primary prevention of cardiovascular disease (CVD)

Study	Population; Country	Agent(s)[a]	Duration (years)	Endpoint	Effect of vitamin E supplementation RR (95% CI)
Alpha-Tocopherol, Beta-Carotene Cancer Prevention Trial (ATBC)	29,133 male smokers aged 50–69 years; Finland	Beta-carotene (20 mg/d), vitamin E (50 mg/d), or both	6	CVD mortality Fatal ischemic heart disease Fatal ischemic stroke Fatal hemorrhagic stroke	0.98 (0.89–1.08) 0.95 (0.85–1.05) 0.84 (0.59–1.19) 1.50 (1.03–2.20)
Primary Prevention Project (PPP)	4,495 men and women aged ≥50 years, with ≥1 CVD risk factor; Italy	Vitamin E (300 mg/d); aspirin (100 mg/d); open-label design	3.6	CVD mortality + MI + stroke CVD mortality Nonfatal MI Nonfatal stroke	1.07 (0.74–1.56) 0.86 (0.49–1.52) 1.01 (0.56–2.03) 1.56 (0.77–3.13)
Women's Health Study (WHS)	39,876 female health professionals aged ≥45 years; United States	Beta-carotene (50 mg every other day), vitamin E (600 IU every other day), aspirin (100 mg every other day), or a combination (2 × 2 × 2 factorial design)	10.1	CVD mortality + MI + stroke CVD mortality MI Stroke	0.93 (0.82–1.05) 0.76 (0.59–0.98) 1.01 (0.82–1.23) 0.98 (0.82–1.17)
Physicians' Health Study II (PHS II)	15,000 male physicians aged ≥55 years; United States	Vitamin E (400 IU every other day), beta-carotene (50 mg every other day), vitamin C (500 mg/d), multivitamin (daily), or a combination (2 × 2 × 2 × 2 factorial design)	8	CVD mortality + MI + stroke	Ongoing

[a]All trials were placebo controlled, except for the Primary Prevention Project (PPP), which used an open-label design.

The Alpha-Tocopherol, Beta-Carotene (ATBC) Cancer Prevention Study was the first large-scale randomized trial of antioxidant vitamins in a well-nourished population. This 2 × 2 factorial trial tested the effect of synthetic vitamin E (50 mg/d) and beta-carotene (20 mg/d) in the prevention of lung cancer among 29,133 Finnish male smokers aged 50–69 years.[29] After a median of 6.1 years, vitamin E supplementation did not reduce the risk of lung cancer (the primary endpoint). There was also no clear reduction in risk of death due to ischemic heart disease (RR = 0.95; 95% CI, 0.85–1.05) or ischemic stroke (RR = 0.84; 95% CI, 0.59–1.19) although the risk of developing angina was lower among those assigned to vitamin E (RR = 0.91; 95% CI, 0.83–0.99).[30] It was initially thought that the lack of convincing beneficial effect may have been due to inadequate dosing of vitamin E or a short follow-up time, but post-trial results with 8 more years of follow-up found no effect of alpha-tocopherol on total mortality (RR = 1.01; 95% CI, 0.96–1.05).[31]

The Primary Prevention Project (PPP) was an open-label 2 × 2 factorial trial of vitamin E (300 mg/d) and low-dose aspirin in 4,495 Italian men and women with one or more of the following CVD risk factors: hypertension, hypercholesterolemia, diabetes, obesity, family history of premature MI, or age ≥65 years.[32] Since there was convincing evidence that aspirin was beneficial, the trial was stopped early after a mean follow-up of 3.6 years. At that time, vitamin E had no effect on any prespecified endpoint including the main combined endpoint of CVD death, nonfatal MI, and nonfatal stroke (RR = 1.07; 95% CI, 0.74–1.56). The negative result may have been due to insufficient statistical power or inadequate dosing of vitamin E.

In the Vitamin E Atherosclerosis Prevention Study (VEAPS), 353 men and women aged ≥40 years with an LDL ≥130 mg/dL and no evidence of CVD were randomized to vitamin E (400 IU) or placebo, and followed every 3 months for an average of 3 years.[33] Vitamin E supplementation increased plasma vitamin E levels, decreased circulating oxidized LDL and decreased LDL oxidative susceptibility, but there was no difference in the primary endpoint of progression of common carotid artery intima-media thickness. In this group of low-risk participants, vitamin E did not reduce the progression of subclinical atherosclerosis.

The Women's Health Study (WHS) was designed to test whether vitamin E supplementation decreases the risk of CVD and cancer among a cohort of initially healthy women.[34] Beginning in 1992, this clinical trial enrolled 39,876 U.S. female health professionals and evaluated the effect of vitamin E (600 IU every other day) on CVD events with a mean follow-up of 10.1 years.[35] For the primary combined CVD outcome (nonfatal MI, nonfatal stroke, or CVD death), vitamin E supplementation did not have a significant effect (RR = 0.93; 95% CI, 0.82–1.05). For individual endpoints, vitamin E did not have an effect on MI (RR = 1.01; 95% CI, 0.82–1.23), stroke (RR = 0.98; 95% CI, 0.82–1.17), or total mortality (RR = 1.04; 95% CI, 0.93–1.16); however, there was a reduction in CVD death (RR = 0.76; 95% CI, 0.59–0.98). The WHS was the largest trial to date to evaluate clinical outcomes over an extended time period, and the results of this important study did not support the use of vitamin E supplementation for the prevention of CVD among healthy women.

In summary, trials of vitamin E supplementation have provided inconsistent results in the primary prevention of CVD, with a recent large study (WHS) that failed to show convincing CVD benefit for long-term use of vitamin E. One ongoing clinical trial, the Physicians' Health Study II (PHS II), is a large study assessing several antioxidants, including vitamin E (400 IU every other day) and results are expected in 2007.[36] The PHS II will provide additional data to help identify the potential benefits and possible risks of vitamin E supplementation in the primary prevention of CVD.

Vitamin E Secondary Prevention Trials

Patients with established CVD may have high oxidative stress and be at a higher risk for a clinical event. As a result, antioxidant use may be most beneficial in the secondary prevention of CVD. Randomized trials of vitamin E alone in the secondary prevention of CVD are summarized in Table 3.3.

Early small trials used surrogate endpoints to test the effects of supplemental vitamin E in patients with established atherosclerotic disease. In a trial of 100 patients over 4 months, 1,200 IU/d of vitamin E supplementation following percutaneous transluminal coronary angioplasty led to a 30% reduction in the risk of restenosis, but this did not reach statistical significance ($P = 0.06$).[37] A study of 120 men and women with intermittent claudication randomized to antioxidants or placebo over 2 years found little improvement in lower limb function and similar rates of cardiovascular events and death,[38] and the ATBC trial found that 50 mg/d of vitamin E had no preventive effect on the development of claudication (RR = 1.05; 95% CI, 0.98–1.14).[39]

Studies of vitamin E for the prevention of angina pectoris have had mostly negative results. A placebo-controlled trial of 3,200 IU/d of vitamin E in stable angina patients led to a nonsignificant trend toward an improved angina pain score in a 9-week placebo-controlled trial[40] while a trial of large dose vitamin E (1,600 IU/d) in 48 patients with angina found no benefit on exercise capacity, left ventricular function or angina symptoms.[41] These small studies of short duration may not have been adequately powered to detect small-to-moderate benefits of antioxidant therapy, but even among 1,795 smokers with angina followed over 4 years in the ATBC trial there was no evidence of a beneficial effect with low-dose vitamin E supplementation (RR = 1.06; 95% CI, 0.85–1.33).[42]

In the Cambridge Heart Antioxidant Study (CHAOS), vitamin E in two doses (400 or 800 IU/d) was tested vs. placebo over a median of 510 days in 2,002 patients with CHD.[43] Those assigned to vitamin E had a lower risk of nonfatal MI (RR = 0.23; 95% CI, 0.11–0.47), but they also had a nonsignificant increase in CVD deaths (RR = 1.18; 95% CI, 0.62–2.27). The study's primary endpoint was combined nonfatal MI and CVD death, and vitamin E reduced this risk (RR = 0.53; 95% CI, 0.34–0.83). Because of the relatively small number of study participants, the randomization process left imbalances in the treatment groups, with the placebo

Table 3.3 Completed and ongoing randomized clinical trials of vitamin E supplementation in the secondary prevention of cardiovascular disease (CVD)

Study	Population; Country	Agent(s)[a]	Duration (years)	Endpoint	Effect of vitamin E supplementation RR (95% CI)
Cambridge Heart Antioxidant Study (CHAOS)	2,002 men and women with atherosclerosis, mean age = 62 years; United Kingdom	Vitamin E (400 or 800 IU/d)	1.4	CVD mortality + MI Nonfatal MI CVD mortality	0.53 (0.34–0.83) 0.23 (0.11–0.47) 1.18 (0.62–2.27)
Alpha-Tocopherol, Beta-Carotene Cancer Prevention Trial (ATBC) substudy	1,862 male smokers aged 50–69 with prior MI; Finland	Vitamin E (50 mg/d), beta-carotene (20 mg/d), or both	6	Major coronary event Nonfatal MI CHD mortality	0.90 (0.67–1.22) 0.62 (0.41–0.96) 1.33 (0.86–2.05)
Gruppo Italiano per lo Studio della Sopravvivenza nell'Infarto miocardico Prevenzione trial (GISSI)	11,324 men and women with prior MI; Italy	Vitamin E (300 mg/d), n-3 polyunsaturated fatty acids (1 g/d), or both; open-label design	3.5	CVD mortality + MI + stroke CVD mortality	0.98 (0.87–1.10) 0.80 (0.65–0.99)[b]
Heart Outcomes Prevention Evaluation trial (HOPE)	9,541 men and women age ≥55 years, at high risk of CVD; N. America, S. America, Europe	Vitamin E (400 IU/d), Ramipril 10 mg/d	4.5	CVD mortality + MI + stroke CVD mortality MI Stroke	1.05 (0.95–1.16) 1.05 (0.90–1.22) 1.02 (0.90–1.15) 1.17 (0.95–1.42)
HOPE – The Ongoing Outcomes (HOPE-TOO)	3,994 men and women originally in the HOPE trial	Vitamin E (400 IU/d)	7.0	CVD mortality + MI + stroke Heart failure Hospitalization for heart failure	1.04 (0.96–1.14) 1.13 (1.01–1.26) 1.21 (1.00–1.47)

Study	Population	Intervention	Years	Endpoints	RR (95% CI)
Secondary Prevention with Antioxidants of Cardiovascular disease in Endstage renal disease (SPACE)	196 hemodialysis patients with CVD, mean age = 65 years; Israel	Vitamin E (800 IU/d)	1.4	MI + ischemic stroke + peripheral vascular disease + unstable angina	0.46 (0.27–0.78)
				MI	0.30 (0.10–0.80)
Women's Antioxidant Cardiovascular Study (WACS)	8,171 female health professionals aged ≥45 years, with CVD or ≥3 coronary risk factors; United States	Vitamin E (600 IU every other day), other antioxidant[c], or a combination (2 × 2 × 2 factorial design)	9.4	MI + stroke + revascularization + CVD mortality	0.94 (0.85–1.04)

[a] All trials were placebo controlled, except for the GISSI trial which used an open-label design.
[b] Secondary 4-way analysis.
[c] Beta carotene (50 mg/d), vitamin C (500 mg/d); or combination of folic acid (2.5 mg/d), vitamin B6 (50 mg/d), and vitamin B12 (1 mg/d).

group having more men, lower total cholesterol levels, lower systolic blood pressures, and fewer diabetics. There is no clear explanation for the striking difference in results for nonfatal MI and CVD death. CHAOS was the first large prospective clinical trial to produce some results in favor of the oxidation theory in atherosclerosis.

In the Gruppo Italiano per lo Studio della Sopravvivenza nell'Infarto miocardico (GISSI) Prevention Trial, 11,324 patients with a history of acute MI within the last 3 months were randomized in an open-label design to vitamin E (300 mg daily), n-3 polyunsaturated fatty acids (1 g daily), both, or neither over 3.5 years.[44] The primary analysis included nonfatal MI, nonfatal stroke, and CVD death, and vitamin E did not have an effect on this combined endpoint (RR = 0.98; 95% CI, 0.87–1.10). However, vitamin E supplementation did have a statistically significant effect on the secondary endpoint of CVD death (RR = 0.80; 95% CI, 0.65–0.99), in contrast to the results of the CHAOS study.

The Heart Outcomes Prevention Evaluation (HOPE) study randomized 9,541 participants with CVD or diabetes and at least one other CVD risk factor (hypertension, hypercholesterolemia, smoking, low HDL, or microalbuminuria) into a study of vitamin E (400 IU daily), the angiotensin-converting enzyme inhibitor ramipril, both agents, or neither.[45] The study was stopped early after a mean follow-up of 4.5 years because of the beneficial effects of ramipril. Vitamin E had no effect on the primary combined endpoint of MI, stroke, and CVD death (RR = 1.05; 95% CI, 0.95–1.16), and secondary analysis of various CVD endpoints (e.g., unstable angina, revascularization) also failed to show any reduced risk with vitamin E supplementation. The HOPE study had high rates of compliance and used large doses of vitamin E, and an extension of the trial, HOPE-The Ongoing Outcomes (HOPE-TOO) continued to follow nearly 4,000 participants for a median duration of 7.0 years.[46] In HOPE-TOO, vitamin E supplementation did not reduce major CVD events (RR = 1.04; 95% CI, 0.96–1.14), and there was an increased risk of heart failure (RR = 1.13; 95% CI, 1.01–1.26) and hospitalization for heart failure (RR = 1.21; 95% CI, 1.00–1.47) associated with long-term vitamin E supplementation.

Because antioxidants may have an earlier and more pronounced effect in patients with high oxidative stress, the Secondary Prevention with Antioxidants of Cardiovascular Disease in Endstage Renal Disease (SPACE) trial randomized 196 hemodialysis patients with CVD to large doses of vitamin E (800 IU daily) or placebo.[47] After a median follow-up of 519 days, vitamin E was associated with significant reductions in the combined endpoint of MI (fatal and nonfatal), ischemic stroke, peripheral vascular disease, and unstable angina (RR = 0.46; 95% CI, 0.27–0.78). Those in the vitamin E group were less likely to have an MI (RR = 0.30; 95% CI, 0.10–0.80), but there was no significant difference in other secondary endpoints including total mortality (RR = 1.09; 95% CI, 0.70–1.70). The results of this small trial with relatively short follow-up were consistent with the CHAOS trial and suggest that high doses of vitamin E may have a role in selected patients with high oxidative stress. A subsequent 9.4-year trial among 8,171 female health professionals at increased risk of CVD either because of a prior history of CVD (i.e., prior MI, angina, stroke, TIA, coronary revascularization, carotid endarterectomy, peripheral arterial disease), the Women's Antioxidant Cardiovascular Study (WACS), found no overall effect of vitamin E (600 IU every other day) on the combined endpoint of MI, stroke, revascularization, or CVD death (RR = 0.94; 95% CI, 0.85–1.04) or on the individual components of this endpoint. However, in subgroup analyses by prior CVD (vs. 3 or more risk factors), there were significant reductions in the combined endpoint (RR = 0.88; 95% CI, 0.78–0.98) and in MI (RR = 0.75; 95% CI, 0.56–0.99) among those with prior CVD.[48]

A 2003 meta-analysis of large randomized vitamin E trials found no benefit in total mortality (RR = 1.02; 95% CI, 0.98–1.06) or CVD death (RR = 1.00; 95% CI, 0.95–1.06) from supplementation in a wide range of doses in various study groups,[49] and the authors concluded that vitamin E supplementation in primary or secondary prevention of CVD could not be routinely recommended. However, they were unable to assess particular groups with high oxidative stress and antioxidants may work best in individuals with high rates of lipid peroxidation.[50] The clinical trials of vitamin E do not disprove the oxidation hypothesis in atherosclerosis, and future studies may need to be conducted in younger subjects (i.e., prior to a lifetime of lipid oxidation) or high-risk subgroups (perhaps using a marker to identify high oxidative stress) most likely to benefit from antioxidant therapy.[51]

Beta-carotene Primary Prevention Trials

Results from large-scale randomized trials of beta-carotene in the primary prevention of CVD have been disappointing. These trials are summarized in Table 3.4. In the previously described ATBC trial among Finnish male smokers, participants assigned to 20 mg/d of beta-carotene had an increased risk of ischemic heart disease mortality (RR = 1.12; 95% CI, 1.00–1.25) and no reduction in the risk of angina (RR = 1.06; 95% CI, 0.97–1.16). For the primary endpoint of lung cancer, an increased risk was noted after 4 years (RR = 1.18; 95% CI 1.03–1.36), but this association disappeared after 6 years of post-trial follow-up (RR = 1.06; 95% CI 0.94–1.20).[31] There were no late preventive effects of beta-carotene.

The Skin Cancer Prevention Study randomized 1,805 men and women with a history of skin cancer to 50 mg of beta-carotene daily or placebo.[52] After a median treatment period of 4.3 years and median follow-up of 8.2 years, there was no significant reduction in CVD mortality (RR = 1.15; 95% CI, 0.81–1.63), cancer mortality (RR = 0.86; 95% CI, 0.56–1.32), or total mortality (RR = 1.05; 95% CI, 0.83–1.32) associated with beta-carotene supplementation.

The Physicians' Health Study (PHS I) was a randomized, double-blind, placebo-controlled trial of beta-carotene (50 mg every other day) and low-dose aspirin among 22,071 U.S. male physicians aged 40–84 years, of whom 11% were current smokers and 39% were former smokers.[53] After 12 years of follow-up, those assigned to beta-carotene experienced no benefit with respect to CVD mortality

Table 3.4 Completed and ongoing randomized clinical trials of beta-carotene alone in the primary prevention of cardiovascular disease (CVD)

Study	Population; Country	Agent(s)[a]	Duration of tx[b] (years)	Endpoint	Effect of beta-carotene supplementation, RR (95% CI)
Alpha-Tocopherol, Beta-Carotene Cancer Prevention Trial (ATBC)	29,133 male smokers aged 50–69 years; Finland	Beta-carotene (20 mg/d), vitamin E (50 mg/d), or both	6	CVD mortality	1.12 (1.00–1.25)
				Fatal ischemic heart disease	1.12 (CI not available)
				Fatal ischemic stroke	1.23 (CI not available)
				Fatal hemorrhagic stroke	1.17 (CI not available)
Skin Cancer Prevention Study	1,805 men and women with history of skin cancer; United States	Beta-carotene (50 mg/d)	4.3[c]	CVD mortality	1.15 (0.81–1.63)
Physicians' Health Study I (PHS I)	22,071 male physicians aged 40–84 years; United States	Beta-carotene (50 mg every other day), aspirin (325 mg every other day), or both	12	CVD mortality	1.09 (0.93–1.27)
				MI	0.96 (0.84–1.09)
				Stroke	0.96 (0.83–1.11)
				CVD mortality + MI + stroke	1.00 (0.91–1.09)
				Nonsmokers:	
				CVD mortality	1.00 (0.78–1.29)
				MI	0.88 (0.72–1.07)
				Stroke	0.92 (0.73–1.16)
				CVD mortality + MI + stroke	1.00 (0.91–1.09)
				Former smokers:	
				CVD mortality	1.16 (0.92–1.48)
				MI	1.00 (0.82–1.22)
				Stroke	0.90 (0.72–1.12)
				CVD mortality + MI + stroke	1.00 (0.87–1.15)

Study	Population		Intervention	Outcome	Result
Women's Health Study (WHS)	39,876 female health professionals aged ≥45 years; United States	2.1	Beta-carotene (50 mg every other day), vitamin E (600 IU every other day), aspirin (100 mg every other day), or a combination (2 × 2 × 2 factorial design)	*Current smokers:*	
				CVD mortality	1.13 (0.80–1.61)
				MI	1.08 (0.80–1.48)
				Stroke	1.18 (0.83–1.67)
				CVD mortality + MI + stroke	1.15 (0.93–1.43)
				CVD mortality	1.17 (0.54–2.53)
				MI	0.84 (0.56–1.27)
				Stroke	1.42 (0.96–2.10)
				CVD mortality + MI + stroke	1.14 (0.87–1.49)
				Smokers:	
				CVD mortality + MI + stroke	1.01 (0.62–1.63)
Physicians' Health Study II (PHS II)	15,000 male physicians aged ≥55 years; United States	8	Beta-carotene (50 mg every other day), vitamin E (400 IU every other day), vitamin C (500 mg/day), multivitamin (daily), or a combination (2 × 2 × 2 × 2 factorial design)	CVD mortality	Ongoing
				MI	
				Stroke	

[a] All trials were placebo controlled.
[b] Except as indicated, duration of treatment equals duration of follow-up.
[c] In Skin Cancer Prevention Study, treatment was for 4.3 years and follow-up was for 8.2 years.

(RR = 1.09; 95% CI, 0.93–1.27), MI (RR = 0.96; 95% CI, 0.84–1.09), stroke (RR = 0.96; 95% CI, 0.83–1.11), or a composite of the three endpoints (RR = 1.00; 95% CI, 0.91–1.09). The beta-carotene group also did not have any significant change in rates of cancer mortality, malignant neoplasms, or lung cancer. In analyses limited to current or former smokers, there were no early or late effects of beta-carotene on any endpoint.

Due to the null results of other studies, the ongoing Physicians' Health Study II (PHS II)[36] terminated its beta-carotene treatment arm (50 mg every other day) early (results not yet published). The Women's Health Study (WHS) also initially had a beta-carotene arm (50 mg every other day)[54] that was stopped early after 2.1 years, at which time participants assigned to active beta-carotene had no benefit with respect to CVD mortality (RR = 1.17; 95% CI, 0.54–2.53), MI (RR = 1.08; 95% CI, 0.56–1.27), stroke (RR = 1.42; 95% CI, 0.96–2.10), or a composite of these endpoints (RR = 1.14; 95% CI 0.87–1.49), as compared with those assigned to placebo. In the WHS, there was no significant benefit or harm from beta-carotene during the shortened follow-up time.

The results of these primary prevention trials of beta-carotene provide strong evidence that this antioxidant taken alone does not have a protective effect on CVD.

Beta-carotene Secondary Prevention Trials

Supplementation with beta-carotene alone has not been well studied in secondary prevention. Two subgroup analyses and an ongoing trial are listed in Table 3.5.

In the ATBC trial, 1,862 men with a history of MI assigned to beta-carotene had a reduction in the risk of nonfatal MI (RR = 0.67; 95% CI, 0.44–1.02) and an increased risk of fatal CHD (RR = 1.58; 95% CI, 1.05–2.40) after 6 years of treatment. In the PHS I, 333 men with a history of chronic stable angina or coronary revascularization who were assigned to beta-carotene had a reduced risk of a major CVD event after 5 years (RR = 0.46; 95% CI, 0.24–0.85), but the effect was attenuated after 12 years (RR = 0.71; 95% CI, 0.47–1.07).[55] In addition, beta-carotene supplementation was associated with a reduced risk of nonfatal MI (RR = 0.76; 95% CI, 0.36–1.60), nonfatal stroke (RR = 0.66; 95% CI, 0.28–1.58), and revascularization (RR = 0.66; 95% CI, 0.34–1.30), but it was also associated with an increased risk of CVD mortality (RR = 1.42; 95% CI, 0.72–2.80). The WACS was the only large trial that evaluated beta-carotene alone in the secondary prevention of CVD,[56] and after 9.4 years, beta-carotene (50 mg every other day) had no effect on CVD outcomes (RR = 1.01; 95%CI, 0.91–1.12).[48]

A meta-analysis of large antioxidant trials that evaluated beta-carotene supplementation alone or in combination with other antioxidants found a small but significant increased risk of CVD death (RR = 1.10; 95% CI, 1.03–1.17) and total mortality

Table 3.5 Completed and ongoing randomized clinical trials of beta-carotene alone in the secondary prevention of cardiovascular disease (CVD)

Study	Population; Country	Agent(s)[a]	Duration of tx[b] (years)	Endpoint	Effect of beta-carotene supplementation, RR (95% CI)
Alpha-Tocopherol, Beta-Carotene Cancer Prevention Trial (ATBC) substudy	1,862 male smokers aged 50–69 years with prior MI; Finland	Beta-carotene (20 mg/d), vitamin E (50 mg/d), or both	6	Major coronary event	1.11 (0.84–1.49)
				Nonfatal MI	0.67 (0.44–1.02)
				CHD mortality	1.75 (1.16–2.64)
Physicians' Health Study (PHS) substudy	333 male physicians aged 40–84 years with angina or coronary revascularization; United States	Beta-carotene (50 mg/d), aspirin (325 mg every other day), or both	12	CVD mortality + MI + stroke	0.71 (0.24–1.07)
Women's Antioxidant Cardiovascular Study (WACS)	8,171 female health professionals aged ≥45 years, with CVD or ≥3 coronary risk factors; United States	Beta-carotene (50 mg every other day), other antioxidant[c], or a combination (2 × 2 × 2 factorial design)	9.4	MI + stroke + revascularization + CVD mortality	1.01 (0.91–1.12)

[a] All trials were placebo controlled.

[b] Duration of treatment equals duration of follow-up.

[c] Vitamin E (600 IU every other day); vitamin C (500 mg daily); or combination of folic acid (2.5 mg daily), vitamin B6 (50 mg daily), and vitamin B12 (1 mg daily).

(RR = 1.07; 95% CI, 1.02–1.11).[49] In summary, beta-carotene supplementation may have more risk than benefit and cannot be routinely recommended for the primary or secondary prevention of CVD.

Vitamin C Trials

For the primary or secondary prevention of CVD, vitamin C has not been well studied in randomized trials. In the Chinese Cancer Prevention Trial, no reduction in cerebrovascular mortality was found among participants assigned a combination of vitamin C (125 mg) and molybdenum (30 μg). The HDL-Atherosclerosis Treatment Study (HATS) and Heart Protection Study (HPS) trials used antioxidant combinations that contained vitamin C, and both studies failed to show a reduction in CVD events. The only large trial of vitamin C alone (500 mg daily) was in one study arm of the WACS, which found no overall effect of vitamin C on CVD outcomes (RR = 1.02; 95% CI, 0.92–1.13).[48] The Physicians' Health Study II (PHS II) is the only other large trial with a study arm analyzing vitamin C (500 mg daily) alone, and this trial is scheduled to end in 2007.[36]

Combination Antioxidant Primary Prevention Trials

Because observational studies of antioxidants found that individuals with a higher intake of vitamin E or beta-carotene also had a higher intake of other antioxidants and micronutrients,[4,21,25,57,58] it is possible that a combination of antioxidants work together as cofactors to confer a beneficial effect. For example, vitamin E alone can be oxidized to a harmful radical, while vitamin C reduces the radical back to alpha-tocopherol. Vitamin E alone can have neutral, pro-, or antioxidant effects under various cellular conditions.[59] As a result, trials of a single antioxidant supplement may lead to a null result, but an appropriate combination of antioxidants may provide a clinical benefit. Several trials have tested combinations of antioxidants, and the primary prevention trials are summarized in Table 3.6.

The Chinese Cancer Prevention Trial randomized 29,584 poorly nourished residents of Linxian, China to one of eight treatment arms testing various combinations of vitamins and minerals.[60] For participants assigned to a combination of a low dose of vitamin E (30 mg daily), beta-carotene (15 mg daily), and selenium (50 μg daily), there was a reduction in total mortality (RR = 0.91; 95% CI, 0.84–0.99) after nearly 6 years of treatment; most of the mortality benefit was due to a reduction in stomach cancer deaths (RR = 0.79; 95% CI, 0.64–0.99). It is unclear which components of the combination treatment led to any benefit, and the findings may not be generalizable to a well-nourished population with different baseline health risks than this study group.

Table 3.6 Completed and ongoing randomized clinical trials of combinations of antioxidants in the primary prevention of cardiovascular disease (CVD)

Study	Population; Country	Agent(s)[a]	Duration (years)	Endpoint	Effect of combination supplementation RR (95% CI)
Chinese Cancer Prevention Trial	29,584 men and women; China	Cocktail of vitamin E (30 mg/d), beta-carotene (15 mg/d), and selenium (50 mg/d)	5	Cerebrovascular mortality	0.90 (0.76–1.07)
Beta-Carotene and Retinol Efficacy Trial (CARET)	18,314 men and women who were smokers or had been exposed to asbestos; United States	Beta-carotene (30 mg/d) and retinol (25,000 IU/d)	4	CVD mortality	1.26 (0.99–1.61)
Supplémentation en Vitamines et Minéraux AntioXydants Study (SU.VI.MAX)	13,017 men and women aged 35–60 years; France	Cocktail of vitamin E (30 mg/d), vitamin C (120 mg/d), beta-carotene (6 mg/d), selenium (100 µg/d), zinc (20 mg/d)	7.5	Major fatal and nonfatal ischemic cardiovascular events	0.97 (0.77–1.20)
Physicians' Health Study II (PHS II)	15,000 male physicians aged ≥55 years; United States	Vitamin E (400 IU alternate days), beta-carotene (50 mg every other day), vitamin C (500 mg/d), multivitamin (daily), or a combination (2 × 2 × 2 × 2 factorial design)	8	CVD mortality + MI + stroke	Ongoing

[a] All trials were placebo controlled.

The Beta-Carotene and Retinol Efficacy Trial (CARET) evaluated a combined treatment of beta-carotene (30 mg daily) and retinol (25,000 IU daily) in 18,314 men and women at elevated risk of lung cancer due to cigarette smoking and/or occupational exposure to asbestos.[61] The trial was stopped early due to lack of benefit and an increased incidence of lung cancer in the active treatment group (RR = 1.28; 95% CI, 1.04–1.57). After 4 years, the group assigned to the antioxidant combination had an increased risk of total mortality (RR = 1.17; 95% CI, 1.03–1.33) and a trend toward increased CVD mortality (RR = 1.26; 95% CI, 0.99–1.61).

The SUpplémentation en VItamines et Minéraux AntioXydants (SU.VI.MAX) Study evaluated the efficacy of a balanced combination of antioxidants and minerals in the primary prevention of cancer and CVD.[62] By using a daily combination of vitamin C (120 mg), vitamin E (30 mg), beta-carotene (6 mg), selenium (100 μg), and zinc (20 mg), nutritional-level doses of supplements were tested in a representative sample of the French population. In this randomized trial, 13,017 participants (7,876 women aged 35–60 years and 5,141 men aged 45–60 years) were followed for a median of 7.5 years and antioxidant supplementation did not reduce ischemic CVD (RR = 0.97; 95% CI, 0.77–1.20).[63]

The ongoing Physicians' Health Study II (PHS II) randomized nearly 15,000 healthy U.S. male physicians aged > 55 years into a 2 × 2 × 2 × 2 factorial design to test beta-carotene (50 mg every other day), vitamin E (400 IU every other day), vitamin C (500 mg daily), and a multivitamin daily.[36] The vitamin C and multivitamin arms will provide the first randomized data on whether these agents can prevent CVD, cancer, or age-related eye disease. The beta-carotene arm was stopped, and the vitamin E, vitamin C, and multivitamin arms are continuing into 2007.

Combination Antioxidant Secondary Prevention Trials

Trials testing combinations of antioxidants in secondary prevention are summarized in Table 3.7. The HDL-Atherosclerosis Treatment Study (HATS) was a trial of 160 patients with CHD, normal LDL cholesterol, and low HDL cholesterol who were randomized to a relatively high-dose combination of four antioxidants (800 IU of vitamin E, 1,000 mg of vitamin C, 25 mg of beta-carotene, and 100 μg of selenium) and/or lipid-modifying therapy (simvastatin to lower LDL and niacin to raise HDL) vs. placebo.[64] After 3 years, simvastatin/niacin therapy decreased both coronary stenosis ($P = 0.004$ vs. placebo) and the event rate for a combined endpoint of death from coronary causes, MI, stroke, or revascularization (3% vs. 24% for placebo, $P = 0.03$). The antioxidant-only group did not show a reduction in coronary stenosis ($P = 0.16$ vs. placebo) or CVD events. While supplemental antioxidants attenuated the angiographic benefits of lipid-modifying therapy (P for interaction = 0.02) and diminished the clinical benefits as well (P for interaction = 0.13), the confidence intervals were wide and some of the interactions may have been due to chance. This small study raised the possibility that adding antioxidants to an effective lipid-modifying regimen may be harmful, but bigger and longer studies were needed.

Table 3.7 Completed and ongoing randomized clinical trials of combinations of antioxidants in the secondary prevention of cardiovascular disease (CVD)

Study	Population; Country	Agent(s)[a]	Duration (years)	Endpoint	Effect of combination supplementation (RR, 95% CI)
HDL-Atherosclerosis Treatment Study (HATS)	142 men and 18 women with CHD, low HDL, and normal LDL levels, mean age = 53 years; United States	Simvastatin and niacin[b]; combination of vitamin E (800 IU/d), vitamin C (1,000 mg/d), beta-carotene (25 mg/d), selenium (100 µg/d); or both	3	MI + stroke + revascularization + death	Simvastatin/niacin alone: 3%[c] Antioxidants alone: 21% Simvastatin/niacin + Antioxidant: 14% Placebo: 24%
Heart Protection Study (HPS)	20,536 men and women aged 40–80 years, with CHD, diabetes or treated hypertension; United Kingdom	Simvastatin (40 mg/d): cocktail of vitamin E (600 mg/d), beta-carotene (20 mg/d), and vitamin C (250 mg/d); or both	>5	Nonfatal MI + CHD mortality Nonfatal MI + CHD mortality + stroke + revascularization	1.02 (0.94–1.11) 1.00 (0.94–1.06)
Women's Angiographic Vitamin and Estrogen (WAVE)	423 postmenopausal women with coronary artery disease	Vitamin E (400 IU twice daily) + vitamin C (500 mg twice daily)	2.8	Nonfatal MI + stroke + death	1.5 (0.80–2.9)
Women's Antioxidant Cardiovascular Study (WACS)	8,171 female health professionals aged ≥45 years, with CVD or ≥3 coronary risk factors; United States	Beta-carotene (50 mg every other day), other antioxidant[d], or a combination (2 × 2 × 2 × 2 factorial design)	9.4	CVD mortality + MI + stroke + revascularization	Completed in 2006; final results for combinations not yet available

[a] All trials were placebo controlled.

[b] Initial simvastatin dose was 10 mg if baseline LDL ≤ 110 mg/dL, and 20 mg if LDL > 110 mg/dL, with subsequent dose adjustment dependent on LDL level. Initial niacin dose was 250 mg twice per day, increasing to 1,000 mg twice per day over a 4-week period.

[c] The comparison between simvastatin/niacin alone with placebo was statistically significant ($p < 0.05$); other comparisons were not.

[d] Beta-carotene (50 mg every other day); vitamin C (500 mg every other day); or combination of folic acid (2.5 mg daily), vitamin B6 (50 mg daily), and vitamin B12 (1 mg daily).

In the much larger Heart Protection Study (HPS), 20,536 participants with CHD, diabetes, or treated hypertension were randomized in a 2 × 2 factorial trial to either a daily antioxidant combination (600 mg of vitamin E, 250 mg of vitamin C, and 20 mg of beta-carotene), simvastatin 40 mg daily, both, or neither. After 5 years, simvastatin proved effective in reducing major vascular events (CVD death, MI, stroke, or revascularization)[65] while the antioxidant combination did not (RR = 1.00; 95% CI, 0.94–1.06).[66] There was no increased harm observed in the antioxidant group, and in contrast to the HATS study, there were no adverse interactions between the study groups. This large study demonstrated neither harm nor benefit to taking large daily doses of antioxidants over a substantial amount of time.

In the Women's Angiographic Vitamin and Estrogen (WAVE) trial, 423 postmenopausal women with coronary artery disease were randomized to a combination of vitamin E (400 IU twice daily) and vitamin C (500 mg twice daily) or placebo.[67] After a mean follow-up of 2.8 years, those assigned to the high-dose antioxidant combination had the suggestion of an increased risk of death, stroke, or nonfatal MI (RR = 1.5; 95% CI, 0.80–2.9), but the confidence intervals were wide. This study suggested that there may be an increased risk associated with antioxidant combination supplements.

In the Antioxidant Supplementation in Atherosclerosis Prevention (ASAP) trial, 520 Finnish men and postmenopausal women with hypercholesterolemia were assigned to one of four treatment arms: vitamin E (136 IU twice daily), slow-release vitamin C (250 mg twice daily), placebo, or both. After 3 years of follow-up, men assigned to both antioxidants had a slowing of the progression of carotid atherosclerosis that was not seen in participants assigned to placebo or a single antioxidant.[68] Three more years of an open-label follow-up comparing the combination therapy and placebo confirmed the initial findings that moderate doses of vitamin E and vitamin C safely slowed atherosclerotic disease, particularly in men.[69]

Because transplant patients are under increased oxidative stress and often have accelerated atherosclerosis, antioxidant supplements may be particularly beneficial in this group. In a small study of 40 patients who had received a heart transplant within the last 2 years, a combination of vitamin E (400 IU twice daily) and vitamin C (500 mg twice daily) was compared to placebo. After 1 year, the progression of transplant-associated coronary atherosclerosis was significantly slowed in the group assigned to the antioxidant combination.[70]

The WACS was a secondary prevention trial that utilized a 2 × 2 × 2 factorial design to evaluate vitamin C (500 mg daily), vitamin E (600 IU every other day), and beta-carotene (50 mg every other day). In this trial, 8,171 U.S. female health professionals at high risk of CVD either because of preexisting CVD or the presence of three or more CVD risk factors were randomized in a study design that allowed for analyses of multiple interactions between antioxidants.[56] In this study of high-risk individuals, supplementation with vitamin E, beta-carotene, or vitamin C did not have a beneficial effect on CVD outcomes, and there were no significant interactions between the antioxidants.[48]

Conclusions

Basic laboratory research findings strongly suggest that oxidative stress may play an important role in the development of atherosclerosis. Basic and animal studies suggest that antioxidant vitamins may delay or prevent various steps in the pathophysiologic process. Several observational studies have demonstrated an association between antioxidant intake either from foods or supplements and subsequent risk of CVD. However, neither basic research nor observational research can provide conclusive evidence. Because of these results and an increasing use of antioxidant supplements despite lack of documented benefit, many large-scale trials of antioxidant supplements have been completed and others are ongoing to test further the efficacy both of single supplements and combinations in varied populations.

Clinical trials of vitamin E alone for primary prevention of CVD have not generally supported the observational results, but the largest trials may have used subtherapeutic doses (ATBC and the Chinese Cancer Prevention Trial) or had inadequate follow-up time (PPP). Secondary prevention trials of vitamin E supplementation have shown minimal or no benefit. One of the first trials (CHAOS) found benefits for vitamin E, but subsequent large trials have not confirmed those results. Patients with high oxidative stress (e.g., hemodialysis patients in the SPACE trial) may benefit more from vitamin E supplementation. Both the CHAOS and SPACE trials demonstrated a risk reduction after less than 2 years of vitamin E supplementation while longer and larger trials (GISSI, HOPE, and HPS) found no benefit. Subsequent larger studies with longer follow-up have not demonstrated an overall CVD benefit to vitamin E supplementation (WHS, WACS), and the PHS II is scheduled to be completed in 2007. There have not been any large randomized trials evaluating antioxidants consumed in natural food sources.

Primary prevention trials of beta-carotene in well-nourished populations have demonstrated no reduction in CVD or cancer (ATBC, Skin Cancer Prevention Study, CARET, PHS, WHS), and some studies have raised the possibility of harm (ATBC, CARET). The few secondary prevention trials have also failed to show any benefit of beta-carotene supplementation. A meta-analysis of major beta-carotene trials found a slight increase in both total and CVD mortality. At this time beta-carotene supplementation cannot be routinely recommended for either the primary or secondary prevention of CVD.

The only completed large trial of vitamin C in primary prevention (Chinese Cancer Prevention Trial) found no effect on cerebrovascular mortality but did not have adequate power to analyze CVD outcomes. In a secondary prevention trial (WACS), vitamin C did not have any beneficial effect on CVD. A large randomized trial of vitamin C in a well-nourished population is scheduled to end in 2007 (PHS II).

Antioxidants may be most effective when taken in particular combinations. A few trials of combinations have shown a CVD benefit (Chinese Cancer Prevention Trial, ASAP), while others show no benefit (SU.VI.MAX) or raise the question of increased risk (CARET, HATS, WAVE). Two large-scale secondary prevention trials have demonstrated no beneficial effect on total CVD from antioxidant combinations (HPS,

WACS), but one these trials found a reduction in stroke with the combination of vitamin E and vitamin C (WACS). One large ongoing primary prevention trial was specifically designed to test the effect of antioxidant supplements both alone and in various combinations in order to identify potential therapeutic interactions (PHS II).

Recommendations

The American Heart Association (AHA) issued its first Science Advisory on antioxidant vitamins in 1999.[71] At that time, the committee concluded that there was insufficient efficacy and safety data from completed randomized trials to justify the establishment of population-wide recommendations regarding the use of vitamin E supplements for CVD prevention; however, the AHA discouraged the use of beta-carotene supplements.[72] Instead, the AHA endorsed dietary guidelines that recommended a balanced diet with an emphasis on antioxidant-rich fruits and vegetables and whole grains.[72] This type of diet is likely to provide a wide range of nutritional benefits beyond any potential antioxidant effects. In 2002, the Institute of Medicine agreed with this recommendation while noting that the relationship between vitamin E supplement use and CVD prevention is "uncertain."[73] In 2003, the U.S. Preventive Services Task Force (USPSTF) concluded that trials of antioxidants have not demonstrated a "consistent or significant effect of any single vitamin or combination of vitamins" on CVD and encouraged the design of better long-term clinical trials.[74] Although the evidence was deemed insufficient to recommend for or against the use of vitamins A, C, or E, multivitamins with folic acid, or antioxidant combinations, the USPSTF did recommend against the routine use of beta-carotene supplementation for the prevention of CVD. In 2004, the AHA Science Advisory committee reviewed completed trials of antioxidants and concluded that the trials failed to demonstrate a beneficial effect on CVD and "the existing scientific database does not justify routine use of antioxidant supplements for the prevention and treatment of CVD."[75]

Even if future clinical trials demonstrate that antioxidant vitamin supplements reduce the risk of CVD, the use of these supplements should be considered an adjunct to other established cardioprotective measures, such as smoking abstention, avoidance of obesity, adequate physical activity, and control of high blood pressure and dyslipidemia.

References

1. Bazzano LA, He J, Ogden LG, et al. Fruit and vegetable intake and risk of cardiovascular disease in US adults: the first National Health and Nutrition Examination Survey Epidemiologic Follow-up Study. Am J Clin Nutr 2002;76:93–99.
2. Joshipura KJ, Hu FB, Manson JE, et al. The effect of fruit and vegetable intake on risk for coronary heart disease. Ann Intern Med 2001;134:1106–1114.

3. Liu S, Manson J, Lee IM, et al. Fruit and vegetable intake and risk of cardiovascular disease: the Women's Health Study. Am J Clin Nutr 2000;72:922–928.

4. Knekt A, Reunanen A, Jarvinen R, Seppanen R, Heliovaara M, Aromaa A. Antioxidant vitamin intake and coronary mortality in a longitudinal population study. Am J Epidemiol 1994;139:1180–1189.

5. Joshipura KJ, Ascherio A, Manson JE, et al. Fruit and vegetable intake in relation to risk of ischemic stroke. JAMA 1999;282:1233–1239.

6. Gillman MW, Cupples LA, Gagnon D, et al. Protective effect of fruits and vegetables on development of stroke in men. JAMA 1995;273:1113–1117.

7. Steinberg D, Parthasarathy S, Carew TE, Khoo JC, Witztum JL. Beyond cholesterol. Modifications of low-density lipoprotein that increase its atherogenicity. N Engl J Med 1989;320:915–924.

8. Hessler JR, Morel DW, Lewis LJ, Chisolm GM. Lipoprotein oxidation and lipoprotein-induced cytotoxicity. Arteriosclerosis 1983;3:215–222.

9. Yagi K. Increased serum lipid peroxides initiate atherogenesis. Bioassays 1984;1:58–60.

10. Gerrity RG. The role of the monocyte in atherogenesis: I. Transition of blood-borne monocytes into foam cells in fatty lesions. Am J Pathol 1981;103:181–190.

11. Quinn MT, Parthasarathy S, Fong LG, Steinberg D. Endothelial cell-derived chemotactic activity for mouse peritoneal macrophages and the effects of modified forms of low density lipoprotein. Proc Natl Acad Sci 1985;82:5949–5953.

12. Schaffner T, Taylor K, Bartucci EJ, et al. Arterial foam cells with distinctive immunomorphologic and histochemical features of macrophages. Am J Pathol 1980;100:57–80.

13. Goldstein JL, Ho YK, Basu SK, Brown MS. Binding site on macrophages that mediates uptake and degradation of acetylated low density lipoprotein, producing massive cholesterol deposition. Proc Natl Acad Sci 1979;76:333–337.

14. Fogelman AM, Shechter I, Seager J, Hokom M, Child JS, Edwards PA. Malondialdehyde alteration of low density lipoproteins leads to cholesteryl ester accumulation in human monocyte-macrophages. Proc Natl Acad Sci 1980;77:2214–2218.

15. Salonen JT, Yla-Herttuala S, Yamamoto R, et al. Autoantibody against oxidised LDL and progression of carotid atherosclerosis. Lancet 1992;339:883–887.

16. Beckman JS, Beckman TW, Chen J, Marshall PA, Freeman BA. Apparent hydroxyl radical production by peroxynitrite: implications for endothelial injury from nitric oxide and superoxide. Proc Natl Acad Sci 1990;87:1620–1624.

17. Marcus AJ, Silk ST, Safier LB, Ullman HL. Superoxide production and reducing activity in human platelets. J Clin Invest 1977;59:149–158.

18. Saran M, Michel C, Bors W. Reaction of NO with $O_2^{\cdot-}$ implications for the action of endothelium-derived relaxing factor (EDRF). Free Radic Res Commun 1990;10:221–226.

19. Gaziano JM, Steinberg D. Natural Antioxidants. New York: Oxford University Press, 1996.

20. Albert CM, Manson JE. Aspirin, antioxidants, and alcohol. In: Charney P (ed). Coronary Artery Disease in Women. Philadelphia: American College of Physicians, 1999: pp. 236–63.

21. Stampfer MJ, Hennekens CH, Manson JE, Colditz GA, Rosner B, Willett WC. Vitamin E consumption and the risk of coronary disease in women. N Engl J Med 1993;328:1444–1449.

22. Rimm EB, Stampfer MJ, Ascherio A, Giovannucci E, Colditz GA, Willett WC. Vitamin E consumption and the risk of coronary heart disease in men. N Engl J Med 1993;328:1450–1456.

23. Kushi LH, Fee RM, Sellers TA, Zheng W, Folsom AR. Intake of vitamins A, C, and E and postmenopausal breast cancer. Am J Epidemiol 1996;144:165–174.

24. Losonczy KG, Harris TB, Havlik RJ. Vitamin E and vitamin C supplement use and risk of all-cause and coronary heart disease mortality in older persons: the established populations for epidemiologic studies of the elderly. Am J Clin Nutr 1996;64:190–196.

25. Klipstein-Grobusch K, Geleijnse JM, den Breeijen JH, et al. Dietary antioxidants and risk of myocardial infarction in the elderly: the Rotterdam Study. Am J Clin Nutr 1999;69:261–266.

26. Evans RW, Shaten BJ, Day BW, Kuller LH. Prospective association between lipid soluble antioxidants and coronary heart disease in men. The multiple risk factor intervention trial. Am J Epidemiol 1998;147:180–186.

27. Steinberg D. Antioxidants in the prevention of human atherosclerosis. Summary of the proceedings of a National Heart, Lung, and Blood Institute Workshop: September 5–6, 1991, Bethesda, Maryland. Circulation 1992;85:2337–2344.

28. Esterbauer H, Gebicki J, Puhl H, Jurgens G. The role of lipid peroxidation and antioxidants in oxidative modification of LDL. Free Radic Biol Med 1992;13:341–390.

29. Alpha-Tocopherol Beta Carotene Cancer Prevention Study Group. The effect of vitamin E and beta carotene on the incidence of lung cancer and other cancers in male smokers. N Engl J Med 1994;330:1029–1035.

30. Rapola JM, Virtamo J, Haukka JK, et al. Effect of vitamin E and beta carotene on the incidence of angina pectoris. A randomized, double-blind, controlled trial. JAMA 1996;275:693–698.

31. ATBC study group. Incidence of cancer and mortality following alpha-tocopherol and beta-carotene supplementation: a postintervention follow-up. JAMA 2003;290:476–485.

32. Collaborative Group of the Primary Prevention Project. Low-dose aspirin and vitamin E in people at cardiovascular risk: a randomised trial in general practice. Collaborative Group of the Primary Prevention Project. Lancet 2001;357:89–95.

33. Hodis HN, Mack WJ, LaBree L, et al. Alpha-tocopherol supplementation in healthy individuals reduces low-density lipoprotein oxidation but not atherosclerosis: the Vitamin E atherosclerosis prevention study (VEAPS). Circulation 2002;106(12):1453–1459.

34. Buring JE, Hennekens CH. The Women's health Study: summary of the study design. J Myocardial Ischemia 1992;4:27–29.

35. Lee IM, Cook NR, Gaziano JM, et al. Vitamin E in the primary prevention of cardiovascular disease and cancer. JAMA 2005;294:56–65.

36. Christen WG, Gaziano JM, Hennekens CH. Design of Physicians' health Study II – a randomized trial of beta-carotene, vitamins E and C, and multivitamins, in prevention of cancer, cardiovascular disease, and eye disease, and review of results of completed trials. Ann Epidemiol 2000;10:125–134.

37. DeMaio SJ, King SB, Lembo NJ, et al. Vitamin E supplementation, plasma lipids and incidence of restenosis after percutaneous transluminal coronary angioplasty (PTCA). J Am Coll Nutr 1992;11:68–73.

38. Leng GC, Lee AJ, Fowkes FG, et al. Randomized controlled trial of antioxidants in intermittent claudication. Vasc Med 1997;2:279–285.

39. Tornwall M, Virtamo J, Haukka JK, et al. Effect of alpha-tocopherol (vitamin E) and beta-carotene supplementation on the incidence of intermittent claudication in male smokers. Vasc Biol 1997;17:3475–3480.

40. Anderson TW, Reid DB. A double-blind trial of vitamin E in angina pectoris. Am J Clin Nutr 1974;27:1174–1178.

41. Gillilan RE, Mondell B, Warbasse JR. Quantitative evaluation of vitamin E in the treatment of angina pectoris. Am Heart J 1977;93:444–449.

42. Rapola JM, Virtamo J, Ripatti S, et al. Effects of alpha tocopherol and beta carotene supplements on symptoms, progression, and prognosis of angina pectoris. Heart 1998;79:454–458.

43. Stephens NG, Parsons A, Schofield PM, Kelly F, Cheeseman K, Mitchinson MJ. Randomised controlled trial of vitamin E in patients with coronary disease: Cambridge Heart Antioxidant Study (CHAOS). Lancet 1996;347:781–786.

44. GISSI-Prevenzione Investigators. Dietary supplementation with n-3 polyunsaturated fatty acids and vitamin E after myocardial infarction: results of the GISSI-Prevenzione trial. Gruppo Italiano per lo Studio della Sopravvivenza nell'Infarto miocardico. Lancet 1999;354:447–455.

45. Yusuf S, Dagenais G, Pogue J, Bosch J, Sleight P. Vitamin E supplementation and cardiovascular events in high-risk patients. The Heart Outcomes Prevention Evaluation Study Investigators. N Engl J Med 2000;342:154–160.

46. HOPE and HOPE-TOO Trial investigators. Effects of long-term vitamin E supplementation on cardiovascular events and cancer. JAMA 2005;293:1338–1347.

47. Boaz M, Smetana S, Weinstein T, et al. Secondary prevention with antioxidants of cardiovascular disease in endstage renal disease (SPACE): randomised placebo-controlled trial. Lancet 2000;356:1213–1218.

48. Cook NR, Albert CM, Gaziano JM, et al. A randomized factorial trial of vitamins C, E and beta-carotene in the secondary prevention of cardiovascular events in women: results from the Women's antioxidant cardiovascular study (WACS). American Heart Association Scientific Sessions 2006, Chicago, IL, 2006.

49. Vivekananthan DP, Penn MS, Sapp SK, Hsu A, Topol EJ. Use of antioxidant vitamins for the prevention of cardiovascular disease: meta-analysis of randomised trials. Lancet 2003;361:2017–2023.

50. Halliwell B. The antioxidant paradox. Lancet 2000;355:1179–1180.

51. Steinberg D. Clinical trials of antioxidants in atherosclerosis: are we doing the right thing? Lancet 1995;346:36–38.

52. Greenberg ER, Baron JA, Karagas MR, et al. Mortality associated with low plasma concentration of beta carotene and the effect of oral supplementation. JAMA 1996;275:699–703.

53. Hennekens CH, Buring JE, Manson JE, et al. Lack of effect of long-term supplementation with beta carotene on the incidence of malignant neoplasms and cardiovascular disease. N Engl J Med 1996;334:1145–1149.

54. Lee IM, Cook NR, Manson JE, Buring JE, Hennekens CH. Beta-carotene supplementation and incidence of cancer and cardiovascular disease: the Women's health Study. J Natl Cancer Inst 1999;91:2102–2106.

55. Gaziano JM, Manson JE, Ridker PM, Buring JE, Hennekens CH. Beta carotene therapy for chronic stable angina (abstract). Circulation 1990;82:III-202.

56. Manson JE, Gaziano JM, Spelsberg A, et al. A secondary prevention trial of antioxidant vitamins and cardiovascular disease in women. Rationale, design, and methods. The WACS Research Group. Ann Epidemiol 1995;5:261–269.

57. Gaziano JM, Manson J, Branch LG, Colditz GA, Willett WC, Buring JE. A prospective study of consumption of carotenoids in fruits and vegetables and decreased cardiovascular mortality in the elderly. Ann Epidemiol 1995;5:255–260.

58. Kushi LH, Folsom AR, Prineas RJ, Mink PJ, Wu Y, Bostick RM. Dietary antioxidant vitamins and death from coronary heart disease in postmenopausal women. N Engl J Med 1996;334:1156–1162.

59. Stocker R. The ambivalence of vitamin E in atherogenesis. Trends Biochem Sci 1999; 24:219–223.

60. Blot WJ, Li JY, Taylor PR, et al. Nutrition intervention trials in Linxian, China: supplementation with specific vitamin/mineral combinations, cancer incidence, and disease- specific mortality in the general population. J Natl Cancer Inst 1993;85:1483–1492.

61. Omenn GS, Goodman GE, Thornquist MD, et al. Effects of a combination of beta carotene and vitamin A on lung cancer and cardiovascular disease. N Engl J Med 1996;334:1150–1155.

62. Hercberg S, Preziosi P, Briancon S, et al. A primary prevention trial using nutritional doses of antioxidant vitamins and minerals in cardiovascular diseases and cancers in a general population: the SU.VI.MAX study – design, methods, and participant characteristics. SUpplementation en VItamines et Mineraux AntioXydants. Control Clin Trials 1998; 19:336–351.

63. Hercberg S, Galan P, Preziosi P, et al. The SU.VI.MAX study: a randomized, placebo-controlled trial of the health effects of antioxidant vitamins and minerals. Arch Intern Med 2004;164:2335–2342.

64. Brown BG, Zhao XQ, Chait A, et al. Simvastatin and niacin, antioxidant vitamins, or the combination for the prevention of coronary disease. N Engl J Med 2001;345:1583–1592.

65. Heart Protection Study Collaborative Group. MRC/BHF Heart Protection Study of cholesterol lowering with simvastatin in 20,536 high-risk individuals: a randomised placebo-controlled trial. Lancet 2002;360:7–22.

66. Heart Protection Study Collaborative Group. MRC/BHF Heart Protection Study of antioxidant vitamin supplementation in 20,536 high-risk individuals: a randomised placebo-controlled trial. Lancet 2002;360:23–33.

67. Waters DD, Alderman EL, Hsia J, et al. Effects of hormone replacement therapy and antioxidant vitamin supplements on coronary atherosclerosis in postmenopausal women: a randomized controlled trial. JAMA 2002;288:2432–2440.

68. Salonen JT, Nyyssonen K, Salonen R, et al. Antioxidant Supplementation in atherosclerosis prevention (ASAP) study: a randomized trial of the effect of vitamins E and C on 3-year progression of carotid atherosclerosis. J Intern Med 2000;248:377–386.

69. Salonen RM, Nyyssonen K, Kaikkonen J, et al. Six-year effect of combined vitamin C and E supplementation on atherosclerotic progression. Circulation 2003;107:947–953.

70. Fang JC, Kinlay S, Beltrame J, et al. Effect of vitamins C and E on progression of transplant-associated arteriosclerosis: a randomised trial. Lancet 2002;359:1108–1113.

71. Tribble DL. AHA Science Advisory. Antioxidant consumption and risk of coronary heart disease: emphasis on vitamin C, vitamin E, and beta-carotene: a statement for healthcare professionals from the American Heart Association. Circulation 1999;99:591–595.

72. Krauss RM, Eckel RH, Howard B, et al. AHA Dietary Guidelines: revision 2000: a statement for healthcare professionals from the Nutrition Committee of the American Heart Association. Circulation 2000;102:2284–2289.

73. Institute of Medicine. Evolution of Evidence for Selected Nutrient and Disease Relationships. Washington, DC: National Academy Press; 2002.

74. Morris CD, Carson S. Routine vitamin supplementation to prevent cardiovascular disease: a summary of the evidence for the U.S. Preventive Services Task Force. Ann Intern Med 2003;139(1):56–71.

75. Kris-Etherton P, Lichtenstein AH, Howard BV, Steinberg D, Witzwum JL. Antioxidant vitamin supplements and cardiovascular disease. Circulation 2004;110:637–641.

Chapter 4
Oxidative stress and Hypertension

Rhian M. Touyz and Ernesto L. Schiffrin

Abstract Oxidative stress is defined as the imbalance between the formation of ROS and antioxidant defense mechanisms. The vasculature is a rich source of ROS, which under pathological conditions, plays an important role in vascular damage. There is growing evidence that increased oxidative stress and associated oxidative damage are mediators of vascular injury in cardiovascular pathologies, including hypertension, atherosclerosis, and ischemia-reperfusion. Increased production of superoxide anion and hydrogen peroxide has been demonstrated in experimental and human hypertension. This development has evoked considerable interest because of the possibilities that therapies targeted against reactive oxygen intermediates by decreasing generation of ROS and/or by increasing availability of antioxidants, may be useful in minimizing vascular injury and hypertensive end organ damage. This chapter focuses on vascular actions of ROS, the role of oxidative stress in vascular damage in hypertension and the therapeutic potential of modulating oxygen radical bioavailability in hypertension.

Introduction

Reactive oxygen species (ROS) and reactive nitrogen species (RNS) are highly reactive byproducts of O_2 metabolism that play an important physiological role in vascular biology and a pathophysiological role in hypertensive vascular disease.[1,2] Under normal conditions, the rate of ROS production is balanced by the rate of elimination. However, a mismatch between ROS formation and the ability to defend against them by antioxidants results in increased bioavailability of ROS leading to a state of oxidative stress.[2,3] The pathogenic outcome of oxidative stress is oxidative damage, a major cause of vascular injury in hypertension. Among the major ROS important in these processes are superoxide anion ($\bullet O_2^-$), hydrogen peroxide (H_2O_2), hydroxyl radical ($\bullet OH$), hypochlorous acid (HOCl) and the RNS, nitric oxide (NO), and peroxynitrite ($ONOO^-$). Under physiological conditions, ROS/RNS are produced in a controlled manner at low concentrations and function

51

J.L. Holtzman (ed.), *Atherosclerosis and Oxidant Stress: A New Perspective.*
© Springer 2008

as signaling molecules to maintain vascular integrity by regulating vascular smooth muscle cell contraction–relaxation and vascular smooth muscle cell growth.[4–7] Under pathological conditions, increased production of ROS leads to endothelial dysfunction, increased contractility, vascular smooth muscle cell growth and apoptosis, monocyte migration, lipid peroxidation, inflammation, and increased deposition of extracellular matrix proteins, major processes contributing to vascular damage in hypertension.[7–9]

In experimental models of hypertension, production of cardiac, renal, neural, and vascular ROS is increased.[10–13] In human hypertension, plasma and urine levels of thiobarbituric acid-reactive substances (TBARS) and 8-epi-isoprostane, markers of systemic oxidative stress, are elevated.[14,15] Treatment with antioxidants or superoxide dismutase (SOD) mimetics improves vascular function and structure and reduces blood pressure in experimental and human hypertension.[12,13,16,17] Mouse models deficient in ROS-generating oxidases have lower blood pressure compared with wild-type counterparts and Ang II infusion in these mice does not increase blood pressure.[18,19] Furthermore, in cultured vascular smooth muscle cells (VSMC) and isolated arteries from hypertensive rats and humans, production of ROS is enhanced and antioxidant capacity is reduced.[12,13,20] Accordingly, evidence at multiple levels supports a role for oxidative stress in the pathogenesis of hypertension.

The cardiovascular, renal, and central nervous systems, all important in the development of hypertension, are major targets for oxidative damage by ROS. The present review focuses on the role of oxidative stress in the vasculature in hypertension. The reader is referred to excellent reviews on the other systems.[21–23] Here, we will discuss recent progress in mechanisms whereby ROS are generated in vascular cells, particularly with respect to NAD(P)H oxidase and NOS uncoupling, how ROS influence vascular function, and what the implications of oxidative stress are in hypertensive vascular injury. Finally strategies to counter oxidative stress-induced vascular damage as a putative therapeutic modality in the management of hypertension are discussed.

The Paradigm of Oxidative Stress: Reduction–Oxidation Concepts

Reactive oxygen species are formed as intermediates in reduction–oxidation (redox) processes, leading from oxygen to water. The fundamental mechanism underlying redox processes in chemico-biologic interactions is that of addition of an oxygen molecule (oxidation) to form an oxidant or removal of oxygen (reduction) to form a reductant[24–26] (Fig. 4.1). Alternative approaches to describe oxidation and reduction are the loss of electrons (or hydrogen) and the gaining of electrons (or hydrogen), respectively.[25] The univalent reduction of oxygen, in the presence of a free electron (e^-), yields $\cdot O_2^-$, H_2O_2 and $\cdot OH$ (Fig. 4.2). Superoxide has an unpaired electron, which imparts high reactivity and renders it unstable and short lived. Superoxide is water soluble and acts either as an oxidizing agent, where it is reduced to H_2O_2, or as a reducing agent, where it donates its extra electron to form $ONOO^-$ with NO.[27] Under

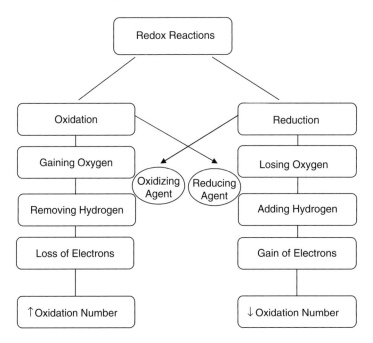

Fig. 4.1 Schematic of the basic mechanisms mediating reduction-oxidation (redox) processe

physiological conditions in aqueous solutions at a neutral pH, its preferred reaction is the dismutation reaction yielding H_2O_2. However, when produced in excess, a significant amount of $\bullet O_2^-$ reacts with NO to produce $ONOO^-$.[27] Superoxide is membrane-impermeable, but can cross cell membranes via anion channels.[28,29] Hydrogen peroxide is produced primarily from dismutation of $\bullet O_2^-$. This reaction can be spontaneous or it can be catalyzed by superoxide dismutase.[24] The SOD-catalyzed dismutation is favored when the concentration of $\bullet O_2^-$ is low and when the concentration of SOD is high, which occurs normally. Hydrogen peroxide is lipid soluble, crosses cell membranes, and is stable under physiological conditions. In biologic systems, it is scavenged by catalase and by glutathione peroxidase.[30] Hydrogen peroxide can also be reduced to generate the highly reactive $\bullet OH$ (Haber–Weiss or Fenton reaction) in the presence of iron-containing molecules such as Fe^{2+}. Hydroxyl radical is extremely reactive and unlike $\bullet O_2^-$ and H_2O_2, which travel some distance from their site of generation, $\bullet OH$ induces local damage where it is formed.

Humans consume $\approx 250\,g$ of oxygen per day, and of this 3–5% is converted to $\bullet O_2^-$ and other ROS.[31] A typical human cell metabolizes about 10^{12} molecules of O_2 daily and generates approximately 3×10^9 molecules of H_2O_2 per hour. Superoxide anion, H_2O_2 NO, $OONO^-$, and $\bullet OH$ are all produced to varying degrees in the vasculature. These pro-oxidants, which are tightly regulated by antioxidants under normal conditions, act as second messengers to control vascular function and structure. An imbalance between oxidant production and antioxidant defenses results in oxidative stress and consequent cell damage.[25,30]

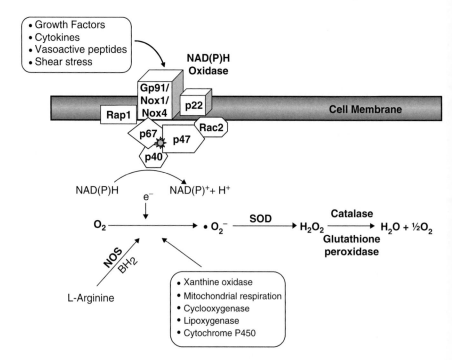

Fig. 4.2 Regulation of reactive oxygen species (ROS) production in vascular smooth muscle cells. The major source of vascular $\cdot O_2^-$ is cell-membrane-associated non-phagocytic NAD(P)H oxidase. NAD(P)H oxidase is a multi-subunit enzyme comprising gp91phox (Nox2)/Nox1/Nox4, p22phox, p47phox, p67phox and p40phox. Many other enzyme systems, including uncoupled nitric oxide synthase (NOS), also produce $\cdot O_2^-$ but their role is minor in vascular cells in hypertension. Extracellular stimuli, such as Ang II, activate NAD(P)H oxidase activity. H_2O_2 but not $\cdot O_2^-$ is lipid soluble and can freely cross the cell membrane SOD, superoxide dismutase; e⁻, electron, BH_2, dihydrobiopterin

Vascular Production of Reactive Oxygen Species

Vascular NAD(P)H Oxidases

The cellular source of vascular ROS varies in different vascular beds and in different species. Studies using dihydroethidium fluorescence reveal marked $\cdot O_2^-$ production from the media and adventitia and a modest proportion from the endothelium.[32] Endothelial $\cdot O_2^-$ generation appears to be predominant in vessels from patients with diabetes and in conditions associated with severe endothelial dysfunction, such as in DOCA-salt hypertensive rats.[33] ROS can be produced from multiple cellular sources in the vessel wall,[34–38] including leakage from the mitochondrial electron transport chain, small molecules, enzymes, including cyclooxygenase, lipoxygenase, heme oxygenase, cytochrome P450 monooxygenase, xanthine oxidase, and NAD(P)H (nicotinamide adenine dinucleotide phosphate, reduced form) oxidase

(Fig. 4.2). However, only a few $\cdot O_2^-$-generating enzymes have been implicated in vascular disease, including xanthine oxidase, which oxidizes xanthine and hypoxanthine to form $\cdot O_2^-$, H_2O_2 and uric acid, cytochrome P450, and NAD(P)H oxidase. In addition it is becoming increasingly evident that $\cdot O_2^-$ can be generated by nitric oxide synthase (NOS) when it is deprived of its critical co-factor tetrahydrobiopterin or its substrate L-arginine.[39,40] This state of NOS uncoupling is usually associated with endothelial dysfunction.[32,41]

Vascular ROS are produced in endothelial, adventitial, and vascular smooth muscle cells and derived predominantly from NAD(P)H oxidase, which is a multisubunit enzyme[38,42-44] that catalyzes the production of $\cdot O_2^-$ by the one electron reduction of oxygen using NAD(P)H as the electron donor: $2O_2 + NAD(P)H \rightarrow 2O_2^- + NAD(P)^+ + H^+$ (Fig. 4.2). The prototypical and best characterized NAD(P)H oxidase is that found in phagocytes.[45-47] Phagocytic NAD(P)H oxidase comprises five components: (phox for *PH*agocyte *OX*idase), p47phox, p67phox, p40phox, p22phox, and gp91phox.[45,46,48] Additional components include the small G proteins Rac 2 (Rac 1 in some cells) and Rap1A. In unstimulated cells, p40phox, p47phox, and p67phox exist in the cytosol, whereas p22phox and gp91phox are located in the membranes, where they occur as a heterodimeric flavoprotein, cytochrome b558. Upon cell stimulation, p47phox becomes phosphorylated, the cytosolic subunits form a complex, which then migrates to the membrane where it associates with cytochrome b558 to assemble the active oxidase, which now transfers electrons from the substrate to O_2 leading to the generation of $\cdot O_2^-$.[45] A defect in any of the genes encoding gp91phox, p22phox, p67phox, or p47phox results in chronic granulomatous disease, a genetic disorder characterized by severe and recurrent infections, illustrating the role of $\cdot O_2^-$ and the derived metabolites H_2O_2 and HOCl in host defense against invading microorganisms.[49]

Growing evidence indicates that NAD(P)H oxidase is also functionally important in nonphagocytic cells. In fact NAD(P)H oxidase is the principal source of $\cdot O_2^-$ in the vasculature[20,32,42,50] and is functionally active in all layers of the vessel wall, in the endothelium,[51] the media,[20] the adventitia,[52] and in cultured VSMCs.[50,53,54] Unlike phagocytic NAD(P)H oxidase, which is activated only upon stimulation and which generates $\cdot O_2^-$ in a burst-like manner extracellulary, vascular oxidases are constitutively active, produce $\cdot O_2^-$ intracellulary in a slow and sustained fashion, and act as intracellular signaling molecules.[42] All of the phagocytic NAD(P)H oxidase subunits are expressed, to varying degrees, in vascular cells. In endothelial and adventitial cells p47phox, p67phox, p22phox, and gp91phox are present.[42,50,55] The situation is more complex in VSMCs, where the major subunits are not always detected. Only p47phox and p22phox seem to be consistently expressed.[42] In rat aortic VSMCs, p22phox, and p47phox, but not gp91phox, are present, whereas in human resistance arteries, all of the major subunits, including gp91phox, are expressed.[35,43,50]

Although NADPH oxidases were originally considered as enzymes expressed only in phagocytic cells involved in host defense and innate immunity, recent evidence indicates that there is an entire family of NADPH oxidases, based on the discovery of gp91phox homologues. The new homologues, along with gp91phox are now designated the Nox family of NADPH oxidases.[56-61] The family comprises

Table 4.1 mRNA expression of Nox isoforms in cardiovascular cells

Enzyme	VSMC	EC	Fibroblasts	Cardiomyocytes
Nox1	+	+	+	–
Nox2	+	+	+	+
Nox3	–	–	–	–
Nox4	+	+	+	+
Nox5	Human	HUVEC	Human cardiac	–
Duox1	+	–	–	–

VSMC, vascular smooth muscle cells; EC, endothelail cells; HUVEC, human umbilical vein endothelial cells.

seven members, including Nox1, Nox2 (formerly termed gp91phox), Nox3, Nox4, Nox5, Duox1, and Duox2. They are expressed in many tissues, including cardiovascular cells, and mediate diverse biological functions (Table 4.1). Nox1 is found in colon and vascular cells and plays a role in host defense and cell growth; Nox2 is the catalytic subunit of the respiratory burst oxidase in phagocytes, but is also expressed in vascular, cardiac, renal, and neural cells; Nox3 is found in fetal tissue and the adult inner ear and is involved in vestibular function; Nox4, originally termed Renox (renal oxidase) because of its abundance in the kidney, is also found in vascular cells and osteoclasts; Nox5 is a Ca^{2+}-dependent homologue, found in testis and lymphoid tissue, but also in vascular cells. Duox1 and 2 are thyroid Noxes involved in thyroid hormone biosynthesis. While all Nox proteins are present in rodents and man, the mouse and rat genome does not contain the *nox5* gene. The regulation and function of each Nox remains unclear, but it is evident that Nox enzymes are critical for normal biological responses and that they contribute to cardiovascular and renal disease, including hypertension and atherosclerosis. Nox1 mRNA is expressed in rat aortic VSMCs and may be a substitute for gp91phox in these cells.[44,50,61] Although initial studies suggested that nox1 is a subunit-independent low capacity $\bullet O_2^-$-generating enzyme involved in the regulation of mitogenesis[62], recent data indicate that nox1 requires p47phox and p67phox and that it is regulated by NOXO1 (Nox organizer 1) and NOXA1 (Nox activator 1).[62,63] The exact role of NoxO1 and NoxA1 in vascular cells is currently unknown.

Nox1 may be important in pathological processes as it is significantly upregulated in vascular injury.[42] Increasing evidence suggests that Nox1 may be important in the pathogenesis of hypertension.[64–66] Nox1-deficient mice have reduced blood pressure and attenuated pressor responses to Ang II[64], whereas Nox1 over-expressing mice exhibit enhanced blood pressure elevating responses to Ang II and exaggerated vascular remodeling.[65] Nox4 appears to be abundantly expressed in all vascular cell types[35,63] and may play an important role in constitutive production of $\bullet O_2^-$ in nonproliferating cells.[60]

How the NADPH subunits interact in cardiovascular cells and how they generate $\bullet O_2^-$ is not fully known. All Noxes appear to have an obligatory need for p22phox. Whereas Nox2 requires p47phox and p67phox for its activity, Nox1 may interact with the recently identified homologues of p47phox and p67phox, NOXO1 and NOXA1.[62,63]

Activity of vascular NAD(P)H oxidase and expression of oxidase subunits are regulated by cytokines, growth factors, and vasoactive agents. Of particular significance, with respect to hypertension, is angiotensin II (Ang II). Ang II induces activation of NAD(P)H oxidase, increases expression of NAD(P)H oxidase subunits, and stimulates ROS production in cultured VSMC and intact arteries.[35,50,53,54] Mechanisms linking Ang II to the enzyme and upstream signaling molecules modulating NAD(P)H oxidase in vascular cells have not been fully elucidated, but PLD, PKC, c-Src, PI3K, and Rac may be important.[54,55] Platelet-derived growth factor (PDGF), transforming growth factor-β (TGF-β), tumor necrosis factor (TNF)-α and thrombin also activate NAD(P)H oxidase in VSMCs,[56,59,67,68] whereas increasing levels of catalase or the antioxidant glutathione prevents agonist-induced ROS generation. Activators of peroxisome proliferator-activated receptors (PPARs), statins and antihypertensive drugs such as β-blockers, Ca^{2+} channel blockers, ACE inhibitors, and AT_1 receptor blockers, downregulate expression of oxidase subunits and decrease NAD(P)H oxidase activity.[69,70] Physical factors, such as stretch, pulsatile strain and shear stress also stimulate NAD(P)H oxidase activation.[42,71]

Uncoupling of NOS

Recent studies indicate that in addition to NAD(P)H oxidase, nitric oxide synthase can produce $\bullet O_2^-$ in conditions of substrate (arginine) or cofactor (tetrahydrobiopterin) (BH_4) deficiency.[32,40] These findings have led to the concept of "NOS uncoupling", where the activity of the enzyme for NO production is decreased in association with an increase in NOS-dependent $\bullet O_2^-$ formation. All NOS isoforms require BH_4 for NOS homodimerization and electron transfer during arginine oxidation.[72] BH_4 influences NOS through multiple mechanisms. It has the ability to shift the heme iron to its high spin state, it promotes arginine binding, and it stabilizes the active dimeric form of the enzyme as well as stabilizes the ferrous heme iron coordination structure.[72] Whereas the structural effects of BH_4 are mimicked by pterin analogues independent of their oxidation state, pterins must be in the tetrahydro state in order to support NO synthesis, suggesting a redox role of BH_4. Thus decreased bioavailability of BH_4 or oxidation of BH_4 to produce cofactor-inactive pterins, mainly dihydropterin and dihydrobiopterin, results in BH_4-deficient NOS that catalyzes formation of $\bullet O_2^-$ and H_2O_2.[40,41] In the uncoupled state, vascular $\bullet O_2^-$ production appears to be partially mediated by BH_4-dependent eNOS uncoupling in various vascular pathologies, including atherosclerosis,[73] diabetes,[74] hyperhomo-cysteinemia,[75] and hypertension.[41,76,77] In experimental models of hypertension, it has been shown that hypertension is associated with increased NAD(P)H oxidase-derived $\bullet O_2^-$, leading to increased ROS bioavailability, which causes oxidation of

BH_4 and consequent uncoupling of eNOS, which further contributes to ROS production.[41] The potential role of uncoupling of NOS as a source of ROS in hypertension is further supported in human studies where increased endothelial $\cdot O_2^-$ production in vessels from diabetic and hypertensive patients is inhibited by sepiapterin, precursor of BH_4.[78,79] The relative importance of NOS- vs. NAD(P)H oxidase-mediated $\cdot O_2^-$ generation in hypertension probably relates, in part, to the magnitude of endothelial dysfunction, since most conditions in which $\cdot O_2^-$ is derived from NOS are associated with marked endothelial dysfunction.[32]

Vascular Antioxidant Defense Systems

Living organisms have evolved a number of antioxidant defense mechanisms, both enzymatic and nonenzymatic, to maintain their survival against oxidative stress.[24,32,80] Major antioxidant enzymes in the vessel wall include SOD, catalase, and glutathione peroxidase, whereas nonenzymatic sources include small molecules and vitamins.[24,80] Three mammalian SODs have been identified: copper/zinc SOD (SOD1), mitochondrial MnSOD (SOD2), and extracellular SOD (SOD3).[24] The concentration of SOD in the extracellular fluid is lower than in the intracellular fluid. Therefore $\cdot O_2^-$ can survive longer and travel further once it gains access to the extracellular space. Arteries contain large amounts of extracellular SOD in the interstitium, suggesting a special role for this SOD isoform within the vessel wall.[81,82] SOD converts $\cdot O_2^-$ to H_2O_2, which is hydrolyzed by catalase and glutathione peroxidase to H_2O and O_2. Glutathione peroxidase is the major enzyme protecting the cell membrane against lipid peroxidation, since reduced glutathione (GSH) donates protons to membrane lipids maintaining them in a reduced state. In addition to endogenous enzyme antioxidants, numerous nonenzymatic antioxidants are found in biological systems. Scavenging antioxidants include ascorbic acid (vitamin C), α-tocopherol (vitamin E), flavonoids, carotenoids, bilirubin, and thiols.[83] Ascorbic acid is water-soluble, whereas α-tocopherol and β-carotene are lipid-soluble. Metal-binding proteins, such as hemoglobin, myoglobin, transferrin, ferritin, and ceruloplasmin are involved in reducing OH^- formation. Decreased bioavailability of antioxidants results in accumulation of oxygen intermediates and consequent increased oxidative stress. Based on this paradigm it has been suggested that antioxidant supplementation may have beneficial therapeutic effects in reducing oxidative stress in disease process.

Molecular Targets of Reactive Oxygen Species in Vascular Cells

ROS play an important role in normal cellular signaling and function.[84-86] Redox-sensitive signaling molecules that have been implicated in cardiovascular disease include transcription factors, protein tyrosine phosphatases, protein

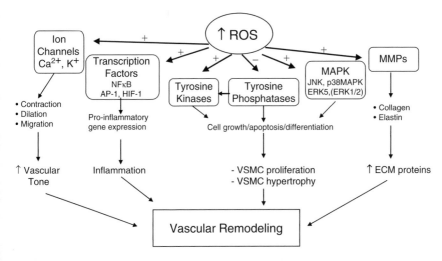

Fig. 4.3 Redox-dependent signaling pathways in vascular cells. Intracellular ROS modify the activity of tyrosine kinases, such as Src, Ras, JAK2, Pyk2, PI3K and EGFR, as well as MAP kinases, particularly p38MAP kinase, JNK and ERK5. ROS may inhibit PTP activity, further contributing to PTK activation. ROS also influence gene and protein expression by activating transcription factors, such as NFκB and AP-1. ROS stimulate ion channels, such as plasma membrane Ca^{2+} and K^+ channels, leading to changes in cation concentration. Activation of these redox-sensitive pathways results in numerous cellular responses, which is uncontrolled, could contribute to altered vascular tone, increased vascular smooth muscle cell (VSMC) growth, inflammation and increased deposition of extracellular matrix protein (EMP), leading to vascular remodeling in hypertension. −, inhibitory effect; +, stimulatory effect

tyrosine kinases, mitogen-activated protein (MAP) kinases, and ion channels (Fig. 4.3). Of these, transcription factors and protein tyrosine phosphatases appear to be directly regulated by ROS,[87–89] whereas the other signaling molecules are probably influenced by ROS through indirect mechanisms.

Transcription Factors

Oxygen intermediates regulate numerous cardiovascular-related genes including adhesion molecules that control inflammatory cell recruitment, antioxidant enzymes that regulate ROS interactions with signaling systems, NOS, and vasoactive agents. Modulation of gene expression by oxidative stress occurs primarily through the redox-regulation of transcription factors, such as NFκB, AP-1 and HIF-1.[87,90] Activation of NFκB, AP-1, and HIF-1 is induced by ROS, probably through redox modification of reactive cysteines.[90] Upstream kinase(s) and or phosphatase(s) prone to thiolation or oxidation of SH groups are at present considered the best candidates mediating the redox regulation of transcription factors. In particular Redox-factor-1

(Ref-1) is an important activator of AP-1, NFκB, and p53 tumor suppressor protein.[91] Thioredoxin, an enzyme involved in the repair of oxidatively damaged proteins, suppresses NFκB, yet activates AP-1.[92] This phenomenon may act as a compensatory, regulatory mechanism in cells predisposed to oxidative stress. Increased activation of vascular NFκB and AP-1 and associated inflammatory and mitogenic responses have been demonstrated in hypertensive rats.[65] These actions have been attributed, in part, to increased oxidative stress.

Protein Tyrosine Phosphatases

The best-established direct targets of ROS signaling are protein tyrosine phosphatases (PTP).[88,89,93] Tyrosine phosphorylation is controlled by the tightly regulated balance between tyrosine kinases and tyrosine phosphatases. All tyrosine phosphatases have a conserved 230-amino acid domain that contains a reactive and redox-regulated cysteine, which catalyzes the hydrolysis of protein phosphotyrosine residues by the formation of a cysteinyl-phosphate intermediate.[94] This cyteine forms thiol phosphate, an intermediate in the dephosphorylation reaction of PTPs. Oxidation of this cyteine residue to sulfenic acid by H_2O_2 renders the tyrosine phosphatase inactive.[94,95] Thus ROS significantly inhibit activity of tyrosine phosphatases, resulting in increased tyrosine phosphorylation.

Inactivation of tyrosine phosphatases is involved in oxidative stress-induced activation of several receptor protein tyrosine kinases such as the EGFR and insulin receptor.[96] This is particularly important with respect to Ang II, which mediates many of its signaling events in vascular cells through EGFR transactivation. H_2O_2 has also been shown to regulate MAP kinases through inhibition of tyrosine phosphatase activity.[97]

Protein Tyrosine Kinases (PTK)

Receptor-and nonreceptor tyrosine kinases are also targets of oxidative stress.[98] Exogenous H_2O_2 induces tyrosine phosphorylation and activation of PDGFR and EGFR, probably due to ROS-mediated inhibition of dephosphorylation of PDGFR and EGFR by inactivation of membrane-associated protein tyrosine phosphatase.[98,99] Oxygen intermediates, which are produced in response to tyrosine kinase receptor activation, are also involved in transactivation of PDGFR and EGFR by Ang II. Under pathological conditions associated with oxidative stress, such as hypertension, ROS may directly activate cell surface receptors, thereby amplifying the process of $\bullet O_2^-$ generation. Nonreceptor tyrosine kinases such as Src, JAK2, Pyk2, and Akt, all of which have been implicated in cardiovascular remodeling and vascular damage, are also regulated by ROS.[3,99–101]

Mitogen-Activated Protein Kinases

MAP kinases participate in signal transduction classically associated with cell proliferation, differentiation, and death.[102] Of the major mammalian MAP kinases, ERK1/2, p38 MAP kinase, and JNK are the best characterized. ERK1/2, phosphorylated by MEK1/2 (MAP/ERK kinase), is a key growth signaling kinase, whereas JNK and p38 MAP kinase, phosphorylated by MEK4/7 and MEK3/6, respectively, influence cell survival, apoptosis, differentiation, and inflammation.[102] ERK5, a recently identified MAP kinase, is regulated by MEK5 and is involved in protein synthesis, cell cycle progression, and cell growth.[102] Enhanced activation of vascular MAP kinases has been demonstrated in hypertension and seems to be a major mechanism contributing to vascular damage in hypertension.[103,104] MAP kinases are regulated by phosphorylation cascades.[102] In addition these kinases are activated by ROS or by a mild oxidative shift of the intracellular thiol/disulfide redox state.[105] In VSMCs intracellular ROS are critical for Ang II-induced activation of p38MAPK, JNK, and ERK5, whereas phosphorylation of ERK1/2 appears to be redox-insensitive.[106,107] However, serotonin-mediated ERK1/2 activation in smooth muscle cells is redox-sensitive, but in fibroblasts, it is not,[108] suggesting that redox-regulation of MAP kinases may be ligand- and cell-specific. Although MAP kinases are influenced by free radicals, they are probably not direct substrates of $\bullet O_2^-$ and H_2O_2. Upstream modulators such as MEKs, tyrosine kinases, and phosphatases may be direct targets.

Cation Transport Systems

In addition to influencing signaling pathways associated with cell growth and inflammation, ROS modulate intracellular Ca^{2+} concentration ($[Ca^{2+}]_i$), a major determinant of vascular contraction. Superoxide and H_2O_2 increase $[Ca^{2+}]_i$ in VSMCs and endothelial cells.[109] These effects have been attributed to redox-dependent inositol-trisphosphate-induced Ca^{2+} mobilization, increased Ca^{2+} influx, and decreased activation of Ca^{2+}-ATPase.[109,110] Plasma membrane K^+ channels in VSMCs that control a hyperpolarization-elicited relaxation are opened by mechanisms associated with thiol oxidation by ROS.[99,100,110] These redox-regulated Ca^{2+} processes may be more important in stress responses than in receptor-mediated signaling by growth factors or cytokines and may play a role in altered vascular contractility in hypertension. In fact contractile responses to H_2O_2 are exaggerated in arteries from SHR compared with normotensive counterparts,[111] suggesting that in addition to impaired endothelium-dependent vasodilation (due to increased quenching of NO by $\bullet O_2^-$), redox-sensitive Ca^{2+} changes could contribute to altered vascular tone in hypertension.

Vascular Mechanisms of Oxidative Stress in Hypertension

Reactive Oxygen Species Influence Vascular Structure and are Pro-inflammatory

In hypertension, oxidative stress promotes vascular smooth muscle cell proliferation and hypertrophy, collagen deposition, and alterations in activity of matrix metalloproteinases (MMP), which lead to arterial remodeling (Fig. 4.3). Superoxide anion and H_2O_2 stimulate growth factor-like cellular responses, such as intracellular alkalinization, MAP kinase phosphorylation, and tyrosine kinase activation. H_2O_2 induces vascular smooth muscle cell DNA synthesis, increases expression of protooncogenes, and promotes cell growth.[7,99] During vascular damage in hypertension when oxidative stress is increased redox-sensitive growth actions may lead to accelerated proliferation and hypertrophy, further contributing to vascular injury and remodeling.[3,7] ROS also modulate vascular structure in hypertension by increasing deposition of extracellular matrix proteins, such as collagen and fibronectin. Superoxide anion and H_2O_2 influence activity of vascular MMP2 and MMP9, which promote degradation of basement membrane and elastin, respectively.[112] Redox-sensitive inflammatory processes, including expression of proinflammatory molecules, such as vascular cell adhesion molecule-1 (VCAM-1) and monocyte chemotactic protein-1 (MCP-1), lipid peroxidation, and cell migration, further contribute to vascular remodeling in hypertension.[113–115]

Reactive Oxygen Species Reduce NO Bioavailability

Impaired endothelium-mediated vasodilatation has been linked to decreased NO bioavailability. This may be secondary to decreased synthesis of NO and/or increased degradation of NO because of its interaction with $\bullet O_2^-$ to form ONOO.[116–118] Peroxynitrite is a weak vasodilator compared with NO and has pro-inflammatory potential.[119] Oxygen radicals also induce endothelial permeability with extravasation of plasma proteins and other macromolecules, and recruitment of inflammatory proteins and cells, which could further impair endothelial function and aggravate vascular damage.[120,121] Peripheral polymorphonuclear leukocytes, which generate $\bullet O_2^-$, participate in oxidative stress and inflammation in patients with hypertension.[112,120,121] The co-existence of an inflammatory reaction with oxidative stress induces endothelial dysfunction. Many of the redox-sensitive vascular changes that occur in hypertension also exist in atherosclerotic vessels. In fact oxidative stress-mediated vascular damage may be a link between hypertension and atherosclerosis.[120]

Reactive Oxygen Species in Hypertension

Oxidative Stress in Experimental Models of Hypertension

Oxidative stress in the vasculature has been associated with genetic and experimental hypertension. Spontaneously hypertensive rats (SHR)[122], and stroke prone SHR (SHRSP)[13], genetic models of hypertension, exhibit increased NAD(P)H-driven generation of $\bullet O_2^-$ in resistance (mesenteric) and conduit (aortic) vessels. These processes are associated with overexpression of NAD(P)H oxidase subunits, particularly p22phox, and enhanced activity of the oxidase.[123] Several polymorphisms in the promoter region of the p22*phox* gene have been identified in SHR, which could contribute to enhanced NAD(P)H oxidase activity in these rats.[124] These findings may have clinical relevance since an association between a p22*phox* gene polymorphism and NAD(P)H oxidase-mediated $\bullet O_2^-$ production in the vascular wall of patients with atherosclerosis has been described.[125] Increased expression of p47phox has been demonstrated in the renal vasculature, macula densa, and distal nephron from young SHR, suggesting that upregulation of renal NAD(P)H precedes development of hypertension.[126] Diminished NO bioavailability as a consequence of enhanced vascular $\bullet O_2^-$ generation has also been suggested to contribute to oxidative stress in SHRSP.[127] Treatment with antioxidant vitamins, NAD(P)H oxidase inhibitors, SOD mimetics, BH_4, and AT_1 receptor blockers decrease vascular $\bullet O_2^-$ production and attenuate, to varying degrees, the development of hypertension in these genetic models of hypertension.[12,13,17,128,129] Taken together, these findings suggest that vascular oxidative stress in SHR and SHR-SP is mediated via enhanced NAD(P)H oxidase activity and dysfunctional eNOS (uncoupled NOS) and regulated, in part, by AT_1 receptors.

Vascular oxidative stress has also been demonstrated in various models of experimental hypertension, including Ang II-induced hypertension,[130] Dahl-salt-sensitive hypertension,[131] lead-induced hypertension,[132] obesity-associated hypertension,[133] mineralocorticoid hypertension,[134,135] and SHR.[136,137] Interestingly, norepinephrine-induced hypertension is not associated with enhanced vascular oxidative stress,[130] suggesting that blood pressure itself may not be the fundamental cause of increased ROS production in hypertension. Increased activation of vascular NAD(P)H oxidase[42,138] and xanthine oxidase[139] and uncoupling of eNOS[39–41] have been implicated in enhanced $\bullet O_2^-$ generation in experimental hypertension. Inhibition of ROS generation with apocynin or allopurinol and scavenging of free radicals with antioxidants or SOD mimetics decrease blood pressure and prevent development of hypertension in most models of experimental hypertension.[17,140–142] These beneficial effects have been attributed to improved endothelial function, regression of vascular remodeling, and reduced vascular inflammation.[23,143]

Oxidative Stress in Human Hypertension

Clinical studies have demonstrated increased ROS production in patients with essential hypertension,[144-146] malignant hypertension,[147] and pre-eclampsia.[148] These findings are based, in large part, on increased levels of plasma and urine TBARS and 8-epi-isoprostanes, systemic markers of lipid peroxidation, and oxidative stress.[144-146] However in never-treated mild-to-moderate hypertension lipid peroxidation is not increased,[149] suggesting that oxidative stress is not implicated in the early stages of human essential hypertension, but may be more important in severe hypertension, such as malignant hypertension and pre-eclampsia.[147,148] Decreased antioxidant activity and reduced levels of ROS scavengers such as vitamin E, glutathione, and SOD,[145] and increased activation of vascular NAD(P)H oxidase may contribute to increased oxidative stress in hypertensive patients.[20,150] Activation of the renin-angiotensin system has been proposed as a major mediator of NAD(P)H oxidase activation and ROS production in human hypertension. In fact some of the therapeutic blood pressure-lowering effects of AT_1 receptor blockers and ACE inhibitors have been attributed to inhibition of NAD(P)H oxidase activity and decreased ROS production.[151] It has also been suggested that p22phox polymorphisms may play a role in altered NAD(P)H oxidase-generated $\cdot O_2^-$ production in human cardiovascular disease.[125,152,153] In particular an association of the C242T p22phox polymorphism with the presence and extent of coronary artery disease was found to be stronger in hypertensive than normotensive subjects.[152,153] However, to confirm that these polymorphisms are indeed markers for hypertensive oxidative stress, studies in large populations are necessary.

Therapeutic Potential of Altering Bioavailability of Reactive Oxygen Species

Based on the evidence that oxidative stress plays a key role in vascular damage, there has been great interest in developing strategies that target ROS in the treatment of hypertension and other cardiovascular diseases. Therapeutic approaches that have been considered include mechanisms to increase antioxidant bioavailability through diet or supplementation and/or to reduce generation of ROS by decreasing activity of $\cdot O_2^-$ -generating enzymes and by increasing levels of BH_4. Gene therapy approaches for cardiovascular disease are also being developed, but will not be discussed here.

The potential value of antioxidants in treating conditions associated with oxidative stress, such as hypertension, is suggested by experimental studies.[154] This is further supported by observational and epidemiological data in humans.[155-158] Evidence from prospective studies suggests that a high intake of antioxidants is protective for hypertension and cardiovascular disease. However findings have not been consistent and clinical trial data have not been conclusive. In the Nurse's Health Study[159] and the Health Professional's Study[160] the relative risk of coronary heart disease was significantly lower in subjects with the highest vitamin E intake. Similar findings were reported in the Iowa Women's Study.[161] Data from the EPIC-Norfolk study[162] demonstrated an inverse association between plasma ascorbic acid concentration and mortality from cardiovascular disease. Data from the Third National Health and Nutrition Examination Survey demonstrated that serum α-carotene, β-carotene, and vitamin C are inversely associated with blood pressure.[163]

To date, at least six large clinical trials and a recent meta-analysis have been published regarding the effects of antioxidant vitamins on the risk of cardiovascular disease (Table 4.2): The Cambridge Heart Antioxidant Study (CHAOS),[164] the

Table 4.2 Clinical trials of antioxidant vitamin supplements and cardiovascular outcomes

Trial (year)	Design	Subject	Antioxidant, daily dose	Duration (years)	Outcome
CHAOS (1996)	p,r,p-c	CHD ($n = 2002$)	800 or 400 IU α-tocopherol or placebo	≈1.5	RR:0.53 for cardiovascular death
ATBC (1996)	p,r,p-c	Healthy ($n = 27{,}271$)	50 mg Vit E, 20 mg α-carotene or placebo	≈6.1	RR: 0.92 for fatal CHD
GISSI Prevenzione (1999)	p,r	Previous MI ($n = 3658$)	300 mg Vit E	≈3.5	RR: 0.88 for combined cardiovascular outcomes RR: 0.80 for cardiovascular death
HOPE (2000)	p,r,p-c	CVD or Diabetes ($n = 9{,}541$)	400 IU Vit E, or placebo	≈4.5	No effect on cardiovascular outcomes
MRC/BHF (2000)	p,r,p-c	CVD ($n = 20{,}536$)	600 mg Vit E, 250 mg Vit C 20 mg β-carotene or placebo	≈5.0	No effect on cardiovascular outcomes
PPP (4495)	R	HT, HC Diabetes, obesity, family history MI, eldery	300 mg Vit E, 100 mg aspirin	≈3.6	No effect of Vit E on cardiovascular outcomes

p,prospective; r,randomized; p-c, placebo-controlled; CHAOS, The Cambridge Heart Antioxidant Study; ATBC, Alpha Tocopherol, Beta-Carotene Cancer Prevention Study; GISSI-Prevenzione, GISSI-Prevenzione trial; HOPE, Heart Outcomes Prevention Evaluation study; MRC/BHF, MRC/BHF Heart Protection Study; PPP, Primary Prevention Project; RR, relative risk; CHD, coronary heart disease; MI, myocardial infarction; HT, hypertension; HC, hypercholesterolemia. 1 IU = 0.67 mg.

Alpha Tocopherol, Beta-Carotene Cancer Prevention Study (ATBC),[165] the GISSI-Prevenzione trial,[166] the Heart Outcomes Prevention Evaluation (HOPE) study,[167] the MRC/BHF Heart Protection Study,[168] and the Primary Prevention Project (PPP).[169] CHAOS enrolled 2,002 patients with documented cardiovascular disease and assessed effects of 400 or 800 IU α-tocopherol. Treatment resulted in a decreased risk primarily due to reduction in nonfatal myocardial infarction. The ATBC trial evaluated daily effects of 50 mg (75 IU) vitamin E, 20 mg β-carotene, or both on cardiovascular outcomes in 27,271 male smokers. This trial reported a nonsignificant, small reduction in the incidence of fatal coronary disease. The GISSI-Prevenzione trial enrolled 3,658 patients with a previous myocardial infarct and tested cardiovascular effects of daily supplementation with 300 mg vitamin E. Although there was no significant effect of treatment on the combined endpoints of cardiovascular death, nonfatal myocardial infarction, and nonfatal stroke, there was a decreased risk of cardiovascular death, including cardiac, coronary, and sudden death. The HOPE study, which included 2,545 females and 6,996 males with a high risk of cardiovascular disease, assessed daily effects of 400 IU vitamin E on cardiovascular outcomes. Results from this study failed to demonstrate any beneficial effect of vitamin E treatment. The MRC/BHF Heart Protection Study, which studied 20,536 adults with cardiovascular disease, assessed effects of daily supplementation of 600 mg vitamin E, 250 mg vitamin C, and 20 mg β-carotene on cardiovascular outcomes. Results demonstrated that these antioxidants were safe, but did not produce any significant reduction in 5-year mortality from any cause. The PPP, which investigated in general practice the efficacy of antiplatelet and antioxidant therapy in primary prevention of cardiovascular events in patients with one or more cardiovascular risk factors. This was a randomized controlled 2×2 factorial trial that investigated low-dose aspirin (100 mg/day) and vitamin E (300 mg/day) in 4,495 subjects. After a mean follow-up of 3.6 years the trial was stopped prematurely on ethical grounds when newly available evidence from other trials on the benefit of aspirin in primary prevention was consistent with results of the second planned interim analysis. Aspirin lowered the frequency of all the endpoints, being significant for cardiovascular death (from 1.4 to 0.8%; relative risk 0.56 [95% CI 0.31–0.99]) and total cardiovascular events (from 8.2 to 6.3%; 0.77 [0.62–0.95]). Vitamin E showed no effect on any pre-specified endpoint. A recent meta-analysis that included more than 200,000 patients investigated vitamin E and β carotene effects on long-term cardiovascular outcomes.[170] Vitamin E failed to have any beneficial effects whereas β-carotene lead to a small, but significant, increase in all-cause mortality and a small increase in cardiovascular death.[170] Consequently, the overall results of clinical trials are disappointing given the consistent and promising findings from experimental studies and epidemiological data. However, many of these trials enrolled patients with significant cardiovascular disease and the choice of antioxidant vitamins used may not have been the best considering the relative poor antioxidant potential of vitamins C and E.

    Numerous smaller clinical studies, which investigated effects of antioxidants specifically on blood pressure, demonstrated, in large part, beneficial actions. Duffy et al.[171] reported in a randomized, double-blind, placebo controlled study that treatment of hypertensive patients with ascorbic acid (500 mg/day) for 30 days, lowers blood pressure. Similar blood pressure-lowering effects of vitamin C were observed in an elderly population when measured by ambulatory blood pressure recording.[172] In patients with type II diabetes, 500 mg ascorbic acid daily for 4 weeks resulted in a significant reduction in blood pressure and reduced arterial stiffening.[173] In newly diagnosed mildly hypertensive patients, 200 IU/day vitamin E for 27 weeks reduced blood pressure by 24/12.5% vs. placebo 1.6/6.2%.[174] Combined oral antioxidant supplementation (200 mg zinc sulphate, 500 mg ascorbic acid, 60 mg α-tocopherol) given for 8 weeks, significantly reduced blood pressure in an adult cohort in the UK.[175] However, in Japanese patients given vitamin C (500 mg/day) for 5 years, blood pressure was not reduced.[176] However these patients also had atrophic gastritis, which may have confounded the results. In a randomized trial in pregnant women, vitamin C (1,000 mg/day) and vitamin E (400 IU/day) were found to significantly reduce the occurrence of pre-eclampsia in women at increased risk.[177] In addition, numerous clinical studies have demonstrated that local infusion of antioxidant vitamins improves endothelial function in hypertensive patients.[178] Taken together, findings from these clinical investigations suggest that antioxidants, particularly vitamin C, may indeed have some beneficial blood pressure-lowering actions. In fact, long-term vitamin C intake has been shown to increase vascular BH_4 levels and NOS activity in experimental animals, which, in addition to the scavenging properties, may contribute to the potentially beneficial actions of vitamin C in vascular disease.[179]

Why then have primary and secondary prevention trials of antioxidant protocols provided such negative results? Possible reasons relate to insufficient dosing regimens or durations of antioxidant therapy, harmful interactions between antioxidant agents, and cellular compartmentalization of antioxidants.[156,180] In addition in large clinical trials, patients had significant cardiovascular disease, in which case damaging effects of oxidative stress may be irreversible. Furthermore, most of the studied patients were taking aspirin prophylactically. Since aspirin has intrinsic antioxidant properties,[181] additional antioxidant therapy with vitamin C or vitamin E may be ineffective. Finally, in patients studied in whom negative results were obtained, it was never proven that these subjects did in fact have increased oxidative stress.[149] In fact, negative results of clinical trials should be interpreted with caution in the absence of verification that antioxidant therapy successfully reduces vascular oxidative stress.

Based on the current data, it is recommended that the general population should consume a balanced diet with emphasis on antioxidant rich fruits and vegetables and whole grains.[182,183] This recommendation, which is consistent with the dietary guidelines of the American Heart Association,[182] considers the role of the total diet in influencing disease risk, and is supported by findings from the Dietary Approaches to Stop Hypertension (DASH) study.[184] To further support this, a recently completed randomized trial from the UK demonstrated that subjects consuming high fruit and vegetable diets had blood pressure reduction of 4/1.5 mmHg.[185] Although this reduction would be expected to produce small clinical effects, effects on cardiovascular disease at the population level would be significant, since a reduction of 2 mmHg diastolic blood pressure results in a decrease of 17% in the incidence of hypertension, 6% in the risk of coronary heart disease, and 15% in the risk of stroke and transient ischemic attack.[155]

Another factor that needs consideration is that antioxidants do not inhibit production of ROS. Theoretically, agents that abrogate oxidant formation should be more efficacious than scavenger agents in ameliorating oxidative stress and vascular damage. This is based on experimental evidence, where it has been shown that inhibition of NAD(P)H oxidase-mediated generation of $\cdot O_2^-$, usingpharmacological and gene-targeted strategies, leads to regression of vascular remodeling, improved endothelial function, and lowering of blood pressure.[67–70] In fact, vascular NAD(P)H oxidase may be a novel therapeutic target for vascular disease. Another strategy that has been shown to be effective in oxidative stress-related hypertension in animals, is BH_4, which prevents NOS uncoupling and decreases NOS-generated ROS.

It has also been suggested that some of the beneficial actions of classical antihypertensive agents such as β-adrenergic blockers (carvedilol), ACE inhibitors, AT_1 receptor antagonists, and Ca^{2+} channel blockers may be mediated, in part, by decreasing vascular oxidative stress. These effects have been attributed to direct inhibition of NAD(P)H oxidase activity, as shown for AT_1 receptor blockers, and to intrinsic antioxidant properties of the agents.[186] The possible role of antihypertensive drugs as modulators of vascular oxidative stress is currently an active area of research.

Conclusions

Until recently it was thought that ROS were toxic byproducts of cellular metabolism, which induced DNA damage, lipid peroxidation, and cell death. However, it has become clear that oxygen free radicals are produced in the vessel wall in a controlled and tightly regulated manner and that they have critical signaling functions that maintain vascular integrity. In hypertension, dysregulation of enzymes such as NAD(P)H oxidase, NOS, xanthine oxidase, or SOD that generate $\cdot O_2^-$, H_2O_2, and $\cdot OH$, or reduced scavenging by endogenous antioxidants, results in increased formation of ROS, which has damaging actions on vascular structure and function. Oxidative stress in hypertension contributes to vascular injury by promoting VSMC growth, endothelial dysfunction, inflammation, increased vascular tone, and MMP activation. These processes lead to altered vascular contractility and structural remodeling, characteristic features of vessels in hypertension. Although inconclusive, clinical data suggest that treatment strategies to alter ROS production may improve vascular damage and reduce blood pressure in hypertensive patients. With a greater insight into the understanding of mechanisms that regulate ROS metabolism and identification of processes that tip the balance to states of oxidative stress which cause vascular damage, it should be possible to target therapies more effectively so that detrimental actions of vascular oxygen free radicals can be reduced and beneficial effects of NO• can be enhanced. Such therapies would be useful in the prevention and treatment of many disease processes associated with vascular damage, including hypertension, atherosclerosis, and diabetes. Novel targets that have been proposed include the nox isoforms, specifically nox1.

References

1. Zalba G, San Jose G, Moreno MU, Fortuno MA, Fortuno A, Beaumont FJ, Diez J. Oxidative stress in arterial hypertension: role of NAD(P)H oxidase. Hypertension 2001;38(6): 1395–1399.
2. Landmesser U, Harrison DG. Oxidative stress and vascular damage in hypertension. Coron Artery Dis 2001;12(6):455–461.
3. Griendling KK, Sorescu D, Lassegue B, Ushio-Fukai M. Modulation of protein kinase activity and gene expression by reactive oxygen species and their role in vascular physiology and pathophysiology. Arterioscler Thromb Vasc Biol 2000;20:2175–2183.
4. Cosentino F, Sill JC, Katusic ZS. Role of superoxide anions in the mediation of endothelium-dependent contractions. Hypertension 1994;23:229–235.
5. Touyz RM, Schiffrin EL. Ang II-stimulated superoxide production is mediated via phospholipase D in human vascular smooth muscle cells. Hypertension 1999;34(4): 976–982.
6. Zafari AM, Ushio-Fukai M, Akers M, Griendling K. Role of NADH/NADPH oxidase-derived H_2O_2 in angiotensin II-induced vascular hypertrophy. Hypertension 1998;32: 488–495.
7. Rao GN, Berk BC. Active oxygen species stimulate vascular smooth muscle cell growth and proto-oncogene expression. Circ Res 1992;70:593–599.
8. Harrison DG. Cellular and molecular mechanisms of endothelial cell dysfunction. J Clin Invest 1997;2153–2157.
9. Chin JH, Azhar S, Hoffman BB. Inactivation of endothelium derived relaxing factor by oxidized lipoproteins. J Clin Invest 1992;89:10–18.
10. Zimmerman MC, Lazartigues E, Lang JA, Sinnayah P, Ahmad IM, Spitz DR, Davisson RL. Superoxide mediates the actions of angiotensin II in the central nervous system. Circ Res 2002;91(11):1038–1045.
11. Kerr S, Brosnan J, McIntyre M, Reid JL, Dominiczak AF, Hamilton CA. Superoxide anion production is increased in a model of genetic hypertension. Role of endothelium. Hypertension 1999;33:1353–1358.
12. Schnackenberg CG, Welch W, Wilcox CS. Normalization of blood pressure and renal vascular resistance in SHR with a membrane-permeable superoxide dismutase mimetic. Role of nitric oxide. Hypertension 1999;32:59–64.
13. Chen X, Touyz RM, Park JB, Schiffrin EL. Antioxidant effects of vitamins C and E are associated with altered activation of vascular NAD(P)H oxidase and superoxide dismutase in stroke-prone SHR. Hypertension 2001;38(2):606–611.
14. Quinones-Galvan A, Pucciarelli A, Fratta-Pasini A, Garbin U, Franzoni F, Galetta F, Natali A, Cominacini L, Ferrannini E. Effective blood pressure treatment improves LDL-cholesterol susceptibility to oxidation in patients with essential hypertension. J Intern Med 2001;250(4):322–326.
15. Romero JC, Reckelhoff JF. Role of angiotensin and oxidative stress in essential hypertension. Hypertension 1999;34(4):943–949.
16. Hoagland KM, Maier KG, Roman RJ. Contributions of 20-HETE to the antihypertensive effects of Tempol in Dahl salt-sensitive rats. Hypertension 2003;41(3 Pt 2):697–702.
17. Sharma RC, Hodis HN, Mack WJ. Probucol suppresses oxidant stress in hypertensive arteries. Immunohistochemical evidence. Am J Hypertens 1996;9:577–590.

18. Bendall JK, Cave AC, Heymes C, Gall N, Shah AM. Pivotal role of a gp91(phox)-containing NADPH oxidase in angiotensin II-induced cardiac hypertrophy in mice. Circulation 2002;105(3):293–296.
19. Li JM, Shah AM. Mechanism of endothelial cell NADPH oxidase activation by angiotensin II. Role of the p47phox subunit. J Biol Chem 2003;278(14):12094–12100.
20. Berry C, Hamilton CA, Brosnan MJ, Magill FG, Berg GA, McMurray JJ, Dominiczak AF. Investigation into the sources of superoxide in human blood vessels: angiotensin II increases superoxide production in human internal mammary arteries. Circulation 2000;101(18): 2206–2212.
21. Cantor EJ, Mancini EV, Seth R, Yao XH, Netticadan T. Oxidative stress and heart disease: cardiac dysfunction, nutrition, and gene therapy. Curr Hypertens Rep 2003;5(3): 215–220.
22. Zanzinger J. Mechanisms of action of nitric oxide in the brain stem: role of oxidative stress. Auton Neurosci 2002;98(1–2):24–27.
23. Wilcox CS. Reactive oxygen species: roles in blood pressure and kidney function. Curr Hypertens Rep 2002;4:160–166.
24. Fridovich I. Superoxide anion radical, superoxide dismutases, and related matters. J Biol Chem 1997;272:18515–18517.
25. Bunn HF, Higgins PJ. Oxygen sensing and molecular adaptation to hypoxia. Physiol Rev 1996;76(3):839–885.
26. Cimino F, Esposito F, Ammendola R, Russo T. Gene regulation by reactive oxygen species. Curr Top Cell Regul 1997;35:123–148.
27. Darley-Usmar V, Wiseman H, Halliwell B. Nitric oxide and oxygen radicals, a question of balance. FEBS Lett 1995;369:13–15.
28. Han D, Antunes F, Canali R, Rettori D, Cadenas E. Voltage-dependent anion channels control the release of the superoxide anion from mitochondria to cytosol. J Biol Chem 2003; 278(8):5557–5563.
29. Decoursey TE, Morgan D, Cherny VV. The voltage dependence of NADPH oxidase reveals why phagocytes need proton channels. Nature 2003;422:531–534.
30. Schafer FQ, Buettner GR. Redox environment of the cell as viewed through the redox state of the glutathione disulfide/glutathione couple. Free Radic Biol Med 2001;30(11): 1191–1212.
31. Rice-Evans CA, Burdon RH. Free Radical Damage and Its Control. Amsterdam: Elsevier, 1994, pp. 25–27.
32. Channon KM, Guzik TJ. Mechanisms of superoxide production in human blood vessels: relationship to endothelial dysfunction, clinical and genetic risk factors. J Physiol Pharmacol 2002;53(4):515–524.
33. Cai H, Harrison DG. Endothelial dysfunction in cardiovascular diseases: the role of oxidant stress. Circ Res 2000;87:840–844.
34. Wang D, Hope S, Du Y. Paracrine role of adventitial superoxide anion in a model of genetic hypertension. Role of endothelium. Hypertension 1999;33:1353–1358.
35. Sorescu D, Weiss D, Lassegue B, Clempus RE, Szocs K, Sorescu GP, Valppu L, Quinn MT, Lambeth JD, Vega JD, Taylor WR, Griendling KK. Superoxide production and expression of nox family proteins in human atherosclerosis. Circulation 2002;105(12): 1429–1435.
36. Abe J-I, Berk BC. Reactive oxygen species of signal transduction in cardiovascular disease. Trends Cardiovasc Med 1998;8:59–64.
37. Rajagopalan S, Kurz S, Munzel T. Angiotensin II mediated hypertension in the rat increases vascular superoxide production via membrane NADH/NADPH oxidase activation: contribution to alterations of vasomotor tone. J Clin Invest 1996;97:1916–1923.
38. Jones SA, O'Donnell VB, Wood JD. Expression of phagocyte NADPH oxidase components in human endothelial cells. Am J Physiol 1996;H1626–H1634.
39. Milstien S, Katusic Z, Oxidation of tetrahydrobiopterin by peroxynitrite: implications for vascular endothelial function. Biochem Biophys Res Commun 1999;263(3):681–684.

40. Cosentino F, Barker JE, Brand MP, Heales SJ, Werner ER, Tippins JR, West N, Channon KM, Volpe M, Luscher TF. Reactive oxygen species mediate endothelium-dependent relaxations in tetrahydrobiopterin-deficient mice. Arterioscler Thromb Vasc Biol 2001;21(4): 496–502.

41. Landmesser U, Dikalov S, Price SR, McCann L, Fukai T, Holland SM, Mitch WE, Harrison DG. Oxidation of tetrahydrobiopterin leads to uncoupling of endothelial cell nitric oxide synthase in hypertension. J Clin Invest 2003;111(8):1201–1209.

42. Lassegue B, Clempus RE. Vascular NAD(P)H oxidases: specific features, expression, and regulation. Am J Physiol Regul Integr Comp Physiol 2003;285(2):R277–R297.

43. Azumimi H, Inoue N, Takeshita S. Expression of NADH/NADPH oxidase p22phox in human coronary arteries. Circulation 1999;100:1494–1498.

44. Griendling KK, Sorescu D, Ushio-Fukai M. NAD(P)H oxidase: role in cardiovascular biology and disease. Circ Res 2000;86:494–501.

45. Babior BM, Lambeth JD, Nauseef W. The neutrophil NADPH oxidase. Arch Biochem Biophys 2002;397:342–344.

46. Vignais PV. The superoxide-generating NADPH oxidase: structural aspects and activation mechanism. Cell Mol Life Sci 2002;59(9):1428–1459.

47. Leusen JHW, Verhoeven AJ, Roos D. Interactions between the components of the human NADPH oxidase: a review about the intrigues in the phox family. Front Biosci 1996;1:72–90.

48. De Leo FR, Ulman KV, Davis AR, Jutila KL, Quinn MT. Assembly of the human neutrophil NADPH oxidase involves binding of p67phox and flavocytochrome b to a common functional domain in p47phox. J Biol Chem 1996;271:17013–17020.

49. Geiszt M, Kapus A, Ligeti E. Chronic granulomatous disease: more than the lack of superoxide? J Leukoc Biol 2001;69(2):191–196.

50. Touyz RM, Chen X, He G, Quinn MT, Schiffrin EL. Expression of a gp91phox-containing leukocyte-type NADPH oxidase in human vascular smooth muscle cells – modulation by Ang II. Circ Res 2002;90:1205–1213.

51. Muzaffar S, Jeremy JY, Angelini GD, Stuart-Smith K, Shukla N. Role of the endothelium and nitric oxide synthases in modulating superoxide formation induced by endotoxin and cytokines in porcine pulmonary arteries. Thorax 2003;58(7):598–604.

52. Rey FE, Pagano PJ. The reactive adventitia: fibroblast oxidase in vascular function. Arterioscler Thromb Vasc Biol 2002;22(12):1962–1971.

53. Griendling KK, Minieri CA, Ollerenshaw JD, Alexander RW. Angiotensin II stimulates NADH and NADPH oxidase activity in cultured vascular smooth muscle cells. Circ Res 1994;74(6):1141–1148.

54. Seshiah PN, Weber DS, Rocic P, Valppu L, Taniyama Y, Griendling KK. Angiotensin II stimulation of NAD(P)H oxidase activity. Upstream mediators. Circ Res 2002;91: 406–413.

55. Touyz RM, Yao G, Schiffrin EL. c-Src induces phosphorylation and translocation of p47phox: role in superoxide generation by angiotensin II in human vascular smooth muscle cells. Arterioscler Thromb Vasc Biol 2003;23(6):981–987.

56. Bedard K, Krause K-H. The NOX family of ROS-generating NADPH oxidases: physiology and pathophysiology. Physiol Rev 2007;87(1);245–313.

57. Geiszt M. NADPH oxidases: new kids on the block. Cardiovasc Res 2006:71:289–299.

58. Sumimoto H, Miyano K, Takeya R. Molecular composition and regulation of the Nox family NAD(P)H oxidases. Biochem Biophys Res Commun 2005;338(1):677–686.

59. Cave AC, Brewer AC, Panicker AN, Ray R, Grieve DJ, Walker S, Shah AM. NADPH oxidases in cardiovascular health and disease. Antioxid Redox Signal 2006;8:691–727.

60. Clempus RE, Sorescu D, Dikalova AE, Pounkova L, Jo P, Sorescu GP, Schmidt HH, Lassegue B, Griendling KK. Nox4 is required for maintenance of the differentiated vascular smooth muscle cell phenotype. Arterioscler Thromb Vasc Biol 2007;27(1):42–48.

61. Suh YA, Arnold RS, Lassegue B. Cell transformation by the superoxide-generating Mox-1. Nature 1999;410:79–82.

62. Banfi B, Clark RA, Steger K, Krause K-H. Two novel proteins activate superoxide generation by the NADPH oxidase Nox1. J Biol Chem 2003;278(6):3510–3513.

63. Ueyama T, Lekstrom K, Tsujibe S, Saito N, Leto TL. Subcellular localization and function of alternatively spliced Noxo1 isoforms. Free Radic Biol Med 2007;42(2): 180–190.

64. Matsuno K, Yamada H, Iwata K, Jin D, Katsuyama M, Matsuki M, Takai S, Yamanishi K, Miyazaki M, Matsubara H, Yabe-Nishimura C. Nox1 is involved in angiotensin II-mediated hypertension: a study in Nox1-deficient mice. Circulation 2005;112(17): 2677–2685.

65. Dikalova A, Clempus R, Lassegue B, Cheng G, McCoy J, Dikalov S, San Martin A, Lyle A, Weber DS, Weiss D, Taylor WR, Schmidt HH, Owens GK, Lambeth JD, Griendling KK. Nox1 overexpression potentiates angiotensin II-induced hypertension and vascular smooth muscle hypertrophy in transgenic mice. Circulation 2005;112(17):2668–2676.

66. Touyz RM, Mercure C, He Y, Javeshghani D, Yao G, Callera GE, Yogi A, Lochard N, Reudelhuber TL. Angiotensin II-dependent chronic hypertension and cardiac hypertrophy are unaffected by gp91phox-containing NADPH oxidase. Hypertension 2005;45(4): 530–537.

67. Brandes RP, Miller FJ, Beer S, Haendeler J, Hoffmann J, Ha T, Holland SM, Gorlach A, Busse R. The vascular NADPH oxidase subunit p47phox is involved in redox-mediated gene expression. Free Radic Biol Med 2002;32(11):1116–1122.

68. Moe KT, Aulia S, Jiang F, Chua YL, Koh TH, Wong MC, Dusting GJ. Differential upregulation of Nox homologues of NADPH oxidase by tumor necrosis factor-alpha in human aortic smooth muscle and embryonic kidney cells. J Cell Mol Med 2006; 10(1):231–239.

69. Diep QN, Amiri F, Touyz RM, Cohn JS, Endemann D, Neves MF, Schiffrin EL. PPARalpha activator effects on Ang II-induced vascular oxidative stress and inflammation. Hypertension 2002;40(6):866–871.

70. Dandona P, Karne R, Ghanim H, Hamouda W, Aljada A, Magsino CH. Carvedilol inhibits reactive oxygen species generation by leukocytes and oxidative damage to amino acids. Circulation 2000;101:122–124.

71. Grote K, Flach I, Luchtefeld M, Akin E, Holland SM, Drexler H, Schieffer B. Mechanical stretch enhances mRNA expression and proenzyme release of matrix metalloproteinase-2 (MMP-2) via NAD(P)H oxidase-derived reactive oxygen species. Circ Res 2003;92(11): e80–e86.

72. Witteveen CF, Giovanelli J, Kaufman S. Reactivity of tetrahydrobiopterin bound to nitric-oxide synthase. J Biol Chem 1999;274(42):29755–29762.

73. Vasquez-Vivar J, Duquaine D, Whitsett J, Kalyanaraman B, Rajagopalan S. Altered tetrahydrobiopterin metabolism in atherosclerosis: implications for use of oxidized tetrahydrobiopterin analogues and thiol antioxidants. Arterioscler Thromb Vasc Biol 2002;22(10): 1655–1661.

74. Bagi Z, Koller A. Lack of nitric oxide mediation of flow-dependent arteriolar dilation in type I diabetes is restored by sepiapterin. J Vasc Res 2003;40(1):47–57.

75. Virdis A, Iglarz M, Neves MF, Amiri F, Touyz RM, Rozen R, Schiffrin EL. Effect of hyperhomocystinemia and hypertension on endothelial function in methylenetetrahydrofolate reductase-deficient mice. Arterioscler Thromb Vasc Biol (Jun 26 2003) [Epub ahead of print].

76. Podjarny E, Benchetrit S, Rathaus M, Pomeranz A, Rashid G, Shapira J, Bernheim J. Effect of tetrahydrobiopterin on blood pressure in rats after subtotal nephrectomy. Nephron Physiol 2003;94(1):6–9.

77. Yang D, Levens N, Zhang JN, Vanhoutte PM, Feletou M. Specific potentiation of endothelium-dependent contractions in SHR by tetrahydrobiopterin. Hypertension 2003;41(1):136–142.

78. Guzik TJ, Mussa S, Gastaldi D, Sadowski J, Ratnatunga C, Pillai R, Channon KM. Mechanisms of increased vascular superoxide production in human diabetes mellitus: role of NAD(P)H oxidase and endothelial nitric oxide synthase. Circulation 2002; 105(14):1656–1562.

79. Higashi Y, Sasaki S, Nakagawa K, Fukuda Y, Matsuura H, Oshima T, Chayama K. Tetrahydrobiopterin enhances forearm vascular response to acetylcholine in both normotensive and hypertensive individuals. Am J Hypertens 2002;15(4):326–332.

80. Finkel T. Oxygen radicals and signaling. Curr Opin Cell Biol 1998;10:248–253.

81. Stralin P, Karlsson K, Johannson BO, Marklund SL. The interstitium of the human arterial wall contains very large amounts of extracellular superoxide dismutase. Arterioscler Thromb Vasc Biol 1995;15:2032–2036.

82. McIntyre M, Bohr DF, Dominiczak AF. Endothelial function in hypertension. The role of superoxide anion. Hypertension 1999;34:539–545.

83. Schafer FQ, Wang HP, Kelley EE, Cueno KL, Martin SM, Buettner GR. Comparing beta-carotene, vitamin E and nitric oxide as membrane antioxidants. Biol Chem 2002;383(3–4):671–681.

84. Forman HJ, Torres M, Redox signaling in macrophages. Mol Aspects Med 2001; 22:189–216.

85. Touyz RM. Recent advances in intracellular signalling in hypertension. Curr Opin Nephrol Hypertens 2003;12(2):165–174.

86. Griendling KK, Harrison DG. Dual role of reactive oxygen species in vascular growth. Circ Res 1999;85:562–563.

87. Turpaev KT. Reactive oxygen species and regulation of gene expression. Biochemistry 2002;67(3):281–292.

88. Lee SR, Kwon KS, Kim SR, Rhee SG. Reversible inactivation of protein-tyrosine phosphatase 1B in A431 cells stimulated with epidermal growth factor. J Biol Chem 1998; 273(25):15366–153372.

89. Meng TC, Fukada T, Tonks NK. Reversible oxidation and inactivation of protein tyrosine phosphatases in vivo. Mol Cell 2002;9(2):387–399.

90. Haddad JJ. Antioxidant and prooxidant mechanisms in the regulation of redox(y)-sensitive transcription factors. Cell Signal 2002;14(11):879–897.

91. Seo YR, Kelley MR, Smith ML. Selenomethionine regulation of p53 by a ref1-dependent redox mechanism. Proc Natl Acad Sci USA 2002;99(22):14548–14553.

92. Fritz G, Human APE/Ref-1 protein. Int J Biochem Cell Biol 2000;32(9):925–929.

93. Anderson JN, Mortensen OH, Peters GH, Drake PG, Iversen LF, Olsen OH, Jansen PG, Andersen HS, Tonks NK, Moller NP. Structural and evolutionary relationships among protein tyrosine phosphatase domains. Mol Cell Biol 2001;21:7117–7136.

94. Denu JM, Tanner KG. Specific and reversible inactivation of protein tyrosine phosphatases by hydrogen peroxide: evidence for a sulfenic acid intermediate and implications for redox regulation. Biochemistry 1998;7:5633–5642.

95. Blanchetot C, Tertoolen LGJ, Hertog JD. Regulation of receptor protein tyrosine phosphatase α by oxidative stress. EMBO J 2002;21(4):493–503.

96. Kamata H, Shibukawa Y, Oka S-I, Hirata H. Epidermal growth factor receptor is modulated by redox through multiple mechanisms. Effects of reductants and H_2O_2. Eur J Biochem 2000;267:1933–1944.

97. Lee K, Esselman WJ. Inhibition of PTPS by H_2O_2 regulates the activation of distinct MAPK pathways. Free Radic Biol Med 2002;33(8):1121–1132.

98. Yang S, Hardaway M, Sun G, Ries WL, Key Jr L. Superoxide generation and tyrosine kinase. Biochem Cell Biol 2000;78:11–17.

99. Droge W. Free radicals in the physiological control of cell function. Physiol Rev 2001;82:47–95.

100. Touyz RM, Wu XH, He G, Salomon S, Schiffrin EL. Increased angiotensin II-mediated Src signaling via epidermal growth factor receptor transactivation is associated with decreased

C-terminal Src kinase activity in vascular smooth muscle cells from spontaneously hypertensive rats. Hypertension 2002;39(2 Pt 2):479–485.

101. Touyz RM, Schiffrin EL. Signal transduction mechanisms mediating the physiological and pathophysiological actions of angiotensin II in vascular smooth muscle cells. Pharmacol Rev 2000;52(4):639–672.

102. Pearson G, Robinson F, Beers Gibson T. Mitogen-activated protein kinase pathways: regulation and physiological functions. Endoc Rev 2001;22(2):153–183.

103. Xu Q, Liu Y, Gorospe M. Acute hypertension activates mitogen-activated protein kinases in arterial wall. J Clin Invest 1996;97(2):508–514.

104. Touyz RM, Deschepper C, Park JB, Schiffrin EL. Inhibition of mitogen-activated protein/ extracellular signal-regulated kinase improves endothelial function and attenuates Ang II-induced contractility of mesenteric resistance arteries from spontaneously hypertensive rats. J Hypertens 2002;20(6):1127–1134.

105. Torres M. Mitogen-activated protein kinase pathway in redox signaling. Front Biosc 2003;8:369–391.

106. Ushio-Fukai M, Alexander RW, Akers M, Griendling KK. p38 Mitogen-activated protein kinase is a critical component of the redox-sensitive signaling pathways activated by angiotensin II. Role in vascular smooth muscle cell hypertrophy. J Biol Chem 1998; 273(24):15022–15029.

107. Touyz RM, Cruzado M, Tabet F, Yao G, Salomon S, Schiffrin EL. Redox-dependent MAP kinase signaling by Ang II in vascular smooth muscle cells – role of receptor tyrosine kinase transactivation. Can J Physiol Pharmacol 2003;81:159–167.

108. Lee SL, Wang WW, Finlay GA, Fanburg BL. Serotonin stimulates MAP kinase activity through the formation of superoxide anion. Am J Physiol Lung Cell Mol Physiol 1999;277: L282–L291.

109. Lounsbury KM, Hu Q, Ziegelstein RC. Calcium signaling and oxidant stress in the vasculature. Free Radic Biol Med 2000;28(9):1362–1369.

110. Ermak G, Davies KJA, Calcium and oxidative stress: from cell signaling to cell death. Mol Immunol 2001;38:713–721.

111. Gao YJ, Lee RM. Hydrogen peroxide induces a greater contraction in mesenteric arteries of spontaneously hypertensive rats through thromboxane A(2) production. Br J Pharmacol 2001;134(8):1639–1646.

112. Rajagopalan S, Meng XP, Ramasamy S, Harrison DG, Galis ZS. Reactive oxygen species produced by macrophage-derived foam cells regulate the activity of vascular matrix metalloproteinases in vitro. J Clin Invest 1996;98:2572–2579.

113. Muller DN, Dechend R, Mervaala EMA, Park JK, Schmidt F, Fiebeler A, et al. NFκB inhibition ameliorates angiotensin II-induced inflammatory damage in rats. Hypertension 2000; 35:193–201.

114. Suematsu M, Suzuki H, Delano FA, Schmid-Schonbein GW. The inflammatory aspect of the microcirculation in hypertension: oxidative stress, leukocytes/endothelial interaction, apoptosis. Microcirculation 2002;9(4):259–276.

115. Luft FC, Mechanisms and cardiovascular damage in hypertension. Hypertension 2001;37: 594–598.

116. List BM, Klosch B, Volker C, Gorren AC, Sessa WC, Werner ER, Kukovetz WR, Schmidt K, Mayer B. Characterization of bovine endothelial nitric oxide synthase as a homodimer with down-regulated uncoupled NADPH oxidase activity: tetrahydrobiopterin binding kinetics and role of haem in dimerization. Biochem J 1997;323(Pt 1): 159–165.

117. Somers MJ, Harrison DG. Reactive oxygen species and the control of vasomotor tone. Curr Hypertens Rep 1999;1:102–108.

118. Tschudi M, Mesaros S, Luscher TF, Malinski T. Direct in situ measurement of nitric oxide in mesenteric reistance arteries: increased decomposition by superoxide in hypertension. Hypertension 1996;27:32–35.

119. Szabo C. Multiple pathways of peroxynitrite cytotoxicity. Toxicol Lett 2003;140:105–112.

120. Alexander RW. Hypertension and the pathogenesis of atherosclerosis. Oxidative stress and the mediation of arterial inflammatory response: a new perspective. Hypertension 1995; 25:155–161.

121. Kristal B, Shurta-Swirrski R, Chezar J. Participation of peripheral polymorphonuclear leukocytes in the oxidative stress and inflammation in patiemnts with essential hypertension. Am J Hypertens 1998;11:921–928.

122. Welch WJ, Wilcox CS. AT1 receptor antagonist combats oxidative stress and restores nitric oxide signaling in the SHR. Kidney Int 2001;59:1257–1263.

123. Zalba G, Beaumont FJ, San Jose G, Fortuno A, Fortuno MA, Etayo JC, Diez J. Vascular NADH/NADPH oxidase is involved in enhanced superoxide production in spontaneously hypertensive rats. Hypertension 2000;35(5):1055–1061.

124. Zalba G, San Jose G, Beaumont FJ, Fortuno MA, Fortuno A, Diez J. Polymorphisms and promoter overactivity of the p22(phox) gene in vascular smooth muscle cells from spontaneously hypertensive rats. Circ Res 2001;88(2):217–222.

125. Guzik TJ, West NE, Black E, McDonald D, Ratnatunga C, Pillai R, Chanon KM. Functional effect of the C242T polymorphism in the NAD(P)H oxidase p22^{phox} gene on vascular superoxide production in atherosclerosis. Circulation 2000;102:1744–1747.

126. Chabrashvili T, Tojo A, Onozato ML, Kitiyakara C, Quinn MT, Fujita T, Welch WJ, Wilcox CS. Expression and cellular localization of classic NADPH oxidase subunits in the spontaneously hypertensive rat kidney. Hypertension 2002;39(2):269–274.

127. Hamilton CA, Brosnan MJ, McIntyre M, Graham D, Dominiczak AF. Superoxide excess in hypertension and aging: a common cause of endothelial dysfunction. Hypertension 2001; 37(2):529–534.

128. Brosnan MJ, Hamilton CA, Graham D, Lygate CA, Jardine E, Dominiczak AF. Irbesartan lowers superoxide levels and increases nitric oxide bioavailability in blood vessels from spontaneously hypertensive stroke-prone rats. J Hypertens 2002;20(2):281–286.

129. Hong HJ, Hsiao G, Cheng TH, Yen MH. Supplemention with tetrahydrobiopterin suppresses the development of hypertension in spontaneously hypertensive rats. Hypertension 2001;38(5):1044–1048.

130. Laursen JB, Rajagopalan S, Galis Z, Tarpey M, Freeman BA, Harrison DG. Role of superoxide in angiotensin II-induced but not catecholamine-induced hypertension. Circulation 1997;95:588–593.

131. Rodriguez-Iturbe B, Zhan CD, Quiroz Y, Sindhu RK, Vaziri ND. Antioxidant-rich diet relieves hypertension and reduces renal immune infiltration in spontaneously hypertensive rats. Hypertension 2003;41(2):341–346.

132. Tojo A, Onozato ML, Kobayashi N, Goto A, Matsuoka H, Fujita T. Angiotensin II and oxidative stress in Dahl Salt-sensitive rat with heart failure. Hypertension 2002;40(6):834–839.

133. Ding Y, Gonick HC, Vaziri ND, Liang K, Wei L. Lead-induced hypertension. III. Increased hydroxyl radical production. Am J Hypertens 2001;14:169–173.

134. Dobrian AD, Davies MJ, Schriver SD, Lauterio TJ, Prewitt RL. Oxidative stress in a rat model of obesity-induced hypertension. Hypertension 2001;37:554–560.

135. Wu R, Millette E, Wu L, de Champlain J. Enhanced superoxide anion formation in vascular tissues from spontaneously hypertensive and desoxycorticosterone acetate-salt hypertensive rats. J Hypertens 2001;19(4):741–748.

136. Virdis A, Fritsch Neves M, Amiri F, Viel E, Touyz RM, Schiffrin EL. Spironolactone improves angiotensin-induced vascular changes and oxidative stress. Hypertension 2002; 40(4):504–510.

137. Girouard H, Chulak C, LeJossec M, Lamontagne D, de Champlain J. Chronic antioxidant treatment improves sympathetic function and beta-adrenergic pathway in the SHR. J Hypertens 2003;21(10):179–188.

138. Reckelhoff JF, Romero JC. Role of oxidative stress in angiotensin-induced hypertension. Am J Physiol Regul Integr Comp Physiol 2003;284(4):R893–R912.

139. Wallwork CJ, Parks DA, Schmid-Schonbein GW. Xanthine oxidase activity in the dexamethasone-induced hypertensive rat. Microvasc Res 2003;66(1):30–37.

140. Schnackenberg CS. Oxygen radicals in cardiovascular-renal disease. Curr Opin Pharmacol 2002;2:121–125.
141. Frenoux JM, Noirot B, Prost ED, Madani S, Blond JP, Belleville JL, Prost JL. Very high alpha-tocopherol diet diminishes oxidative stress and hypercoagulation in hypertensive rats but not in normotensive rats. Med Sci Monit 2002;8(10):BR401–BR407.
142. Park JB, Touyz RM, Chen X, Schiffrin EL. Chronic treatment with a superoxide dismutase mimetic prevents vascular remodeling and progression of hypertension in salt-loaded stroke-prone spontaneously hypertensive rats. Am J Hypertens 2002;15:78–84.
143. Touyz RM. Oxidative stress and vascular damage in hypertension. Curr Hypertens Rep 2000;2:98–105.
144. Minuz P, Patrignani P, Gaino S, Degan M, Menapace L, Tommasoli R, et al. Increased oxidative stress and platelet activation in patients with hypertension and renovascular disease. Circulation 2002;106:2800–2805.
145. Sagar S, Kallo IJ, Kaul N, Ganguly NK, Sharma BK. Oxygen free radicals in essential hypertension. Mol Cell Biochem 1992;111:103–108.
146. Stojiljkovic MP, Lopes HF, Zhang D, Morrow JD, Goodfriend TL, Egan BM. Increasing plasma fatty acids elevates F2-isoprostanes in humans: implications for the cardiovascular risk factor cluster. J Hypertens 2002;20(6):1215–1221.
147. Lip GY, Edmunds E, Nuttall SL, Landray MJ, Blann AD, Beevers DG. Oxidative stress in malignant and non-malignant phase hypertension. J Hum Hypertens 2002; 16(5):333–336.
148. Lee VM, Quinn PA, Jennings SC, Ng LL. Neutrophil activation and production of reactive oxygen species in pre-eclampsia. J Hypertens 2003;21(2):395–402.
149. Cracowski JL, Baguet JP, Ormezzano O, Bessard J, Stanke-Labesque F, Bessard G, Mallion JM. Lipid peroxidation is not increased in patients with untreated mild-to-moderate hypertension. Hypertension 2003;41(2):286–288.
150. Touyz RM, Schiffrin EL. Increased generation of superoxide by angiotensin II in smooth muscle cells from resistance arteries of hypertensive patients: role of phospholipase D-dependent NAD(P)H oxidase-sensitive pathways. J Hypertens 2001;19(7):1245–1254.
151. Ghiadoni L, Magagna A, Versari D, Kardasz I, Huang Y, Taddei S, Salvetti A. Different effect of antihypertensive drugs on conduit artery endothelial function. Hypertension 2003; 41(6):1281–1286.
152. Schachinger V, Britten MB, Dimmeler S, Zeiher AM. NADH/NADPH oxidase p22 phox gene polymorphism is associated with improved coronary endothelial vasodilator function. Eur Heart J 2001;22(1):96–101.
153. Gardemann A, Mages P, Katz N, Tillmanns H, Haberbosch W. The p22 phox A640G gene polymorphism but not the C242T gene variation is associated with coronary heart disease in younger individuals. Atherosclerosis 1999;145(2):315–323.
154. Rey FE, Pagano PJ. The reactive adventitia: fibroblast oxidase in vascular function. Arterioscler Thromb Vasc Biol 2002;22(12):1962–1971.
155. Brown AA, Hu FB. Dietary modulation of endothelial function: implications for cardiovascular disease. Am J Clin Nutr 2001;73:673–686.
156. Shihabi A, Li W-G, Miller FJ, Weintraub NL. Antioxidant therapy for atherosclerotic vascular disease: the promise and the pitfalls. Am J Physiol 2002;282:H797–H802.
157. Salvemini D, Cuzzocrea S. Therapeutic potential of superoxide dismutase mimetics as therapeutic agents in critical care medicine. Crit Care Med 2003;31(1):S29–S38.
158. Digiesi D, Lenuzza M, Digiese G. Prospects for the use of antioxidant therapy in hypertension. Ann Ital Med Int 2001;16(20): 93–100.
159. Stampfer MJ, Hennekens CH, Manson JE, Colditz GA, Rosner B, Willett WC. Vitamin E consumption and the risk of coronary heart disease in women. N Engl J Med 1993; 328(20):1444–1449.
160. Rimm EB, Stampfer MJ, Ascherio A, Giovannucci E, Colditz GA, Willett WC. Vitamin E consumption and the risk of coronary heart disease in men. N Engl J Med 1993; 328(20):1450–1456.

161. Kushi LH, Folsom AR, Prineas RJ, Mink PJ, Wu Y, Bostick RM. Dietary antioxidant vitamins and death from coronary heart disease in postmenopausal women. N Engl J Med 1996; 334(18):1156–1162.

162. Khaw K-T, Bingham S, Welch A, Luben R, Wareham N, Oakes S, et al. Relation between plasma ascorbic acid and mortality in men and women in EPIC-Norfolk prospective study: a prospective population study. Lancet 2001;357:657–663.

163. Chen J, He J, Hamm L, Batuman V, Whelton PK. Serum antioxidant vitamins and blood pressure in the United States population. Hypertension 2002;40(60):810–816.

164. Stephens NG, Parsons A, Schofield PM, Kelly F, Cheeseman K, Mitchinson MJ. Randomised controlled trial of vitamin E in patients with coronary disease: Cambridge Heart Antioxidant Study (CHAOS). Lancet 1996;347(9004):781–786.

165. Virtamo J, Rapola JM, Ripatti S, Heinonen OP, Taylor PR, AlbanesD, Huttunen JK. Effect of vitamin E and beta carotene on the incidence of primary nonfatal myocardial infarction and fatal coronary heart disease. Arch Intern Med 1998;158(6):668–675.

166. GISSI-Prevenzione Investigators. Dietary supplementation with n-3 polyunsaturated fatty acids and vitamin E after myocardial infarction: results of the GISSI-Prevenzione trial, Gruppo Italiano per lo Studio della Sopravvivenza nell'Infarto miocardico. Lancet 1999; 354(9177):447–455.

167. HOPE Investigators. Vitamin E supplementation and cardiovascular events in high risk patients. N Engl J Med 2000;342:154–160.

168. MRC/BHF Heart protection study of antioxidant vitamin supplementation in 20 536 high-risk individuals: a randomized placebo-controlled trial. Lancet 2002;360:23–33.

169. de Gaetano G. Collaborative Group of the Primary Prevention Project, Low-dose aspirin and vitamin E in people at cardiovascular risk: a randomised trial in general practice, Collaborative Group of the Primary Prevention Project. Lancet 2001;357(9250):89–95.

170. Vivekananthan DP, Penn MS, Sapp SK, Hsu A, Topol EJ. Use of antioxidant vitamins for the prevention of cardiovascular disease: meta-analysis of randomised trials. Lancet 2003; 361(9374):2017–2023.

171. Duffy SJ, Gokce N, Holbrook M, Huang A, Frei B, Keaney JF, Vita JA. Treatment of hypertension with ascorbic acid. Lancet 1999;354:2048–2049.

172. Fotheby MD, Williams JC, Forster LA, Craner P, Ferns GA. Effect of vitamin C on ambulatory blood pressure and plasma lipids in older patients. J Hypertens 2000;18:411–415.

173. Mullan B, Young IS, Fee H, McCance DR. Ascorbic acid reduces blood pressure and arterial stiffness in type 2 diabetes. Hypertension 2002;40:804–809.

174. Boshtam M, Rafiei M, Sadeghi K, Sarraf-Zadegan N. Vitamin E can reduce blood pressure in mild hypertensives. Int J Vitam Nutr Res 2002;72(5):309–314.

175. Galley HF, Thornton J, Howdle PD, Walker BE, Webster NR. Combination oral antioxidant supplementation reduces blood pressure. Clin Sci (Lond) 1997;92(4):361–365.

176. Kim MY, Sasaki S, Sasazuki S, Okubo S, Hayashi M, Tsugane S. Lack of long-term effect of vitamin C supplementation on blood pressure. Hypertension 2002;40:797–803.

177. Chappell LC, Seed PT, Briley AL, Kelly FJ, Lee R, et al. Effect of antioxidants on the occurrence of pre-eclampsia in women at increased risk: a randomized trial. Lancet 1999;354: 810–815.

178. Taddei S, Virdis A, Ghiadoni L, Magagna A, Salvetti A. Vitamin C improves endothelium-dependent vasodilation by restoring nitric oxide activity in essential hypertension. Circulation 1998;97:2222–2229.

179. d'Uscio LV, Milstein S, Rischardson D, Smith L, Katusic ZS. Long-term vitamin C treatment increases vascular tetrahydrobiopterin levels and nitric oxide synthase activity. Circ Res 2003;92:88–95.

180. Maxwell S, Greig L. Antioxidants – a protective role in cardiovascular disease? Expert Opin Pharmacother 2001;2(11):1737–1750.

181. Wu R, Lamontagne D, de Champlain J. Antioxidative properties of acetylsalicylic acid on vascular tissues from normotensive and spontaneously hypertensive rats. Circulation 2002;105(3):387–392.

182. Tribble DL. Antioxidant consumption and risk of coronary heart disease: emphasis on vitamin C, vitamin E and β-carotene, A statement for the healthcare professionals from the American Heart Association. Circulation 1999;99:591–595.

183. Carr A, Frei B. The role of natural antioxidants in preserving the biological activity of endothelium-derived nitric oxide. Free Rad Biol Med 2000;28:1806–1814.

184. Sacks FM, Svetkey LP, Vollmer WM, Appel LJ, Bray GA, Harsha D, Obarzanek E, Conlin PR, Miller III ER. Simons-Morton DG, Karanja N, Lin PH. DASH-Sodium Collaborative Research Group. Effects on blood pressure of reduced dietary sodium and the Dietary Approaches to Stop Hypertension (DASH) diet. DASH-Sodium Collaborative Research Group. N Engl J Med 2001;344(1):3–10.

185. John JH, Ziebland S, Yudkin P, Roe LS, Neil HAW. Effects of fruit and vegetable consumption on plasma antioxidant concentrations and blood pressure: a randomized controlled trial. Lancet 2002;359:1969–1973.

186. Schiffrin EL, Touyz RM. Multiple actions of angiotensin II in hypertension: benefits of AT_1 receptor blockade. J Am Coll Cardiol 2003;42(5):911–913.

Chapter 5
Lipids, Oxidation, and Cardiovascular Disease

Myron D. Gross

Abstract Blood cholesterol and LDL levels are well-established risk factors for cardiovascular disease and, in particular, coronary heart disease. In recent years, the role of LDL in the pathogenesis of atherosclerosis, the underlying cause of coronary heart disease, has been studied extensively. These studies have highlighted the complexity of atherosclerotic processes and identified oxidative damage and inflammation as important components of the process. In addition, the formation and possible involvement of various oxidized lipids in atherosclerosis have been identified by the studies. The oxidized lipids include the products of oxidative enzymes, located in the vasculature, as well as nonspecific oxidation products. Many of these lipids have been found in atherosclerotic plaque and have potent bioactivities. Moreover, these oxidation products and, reactive oxygen and nitrogen species, have been linked with cellular signaling pathways that can influence the development of atherosclerosis.

The Impact of Cardiovascular Disease and Its Major Component, Coronary Heart Disease on Human Health

Cardiovascular disease is the most prevalent threat to life and health in the United States.[1,2] It is the major cause of mortality, with 44% of deaths, and it is a major cause of morbidity.[3] A major cardiovascular disease develops in 1/3 of men and 1/10 of women before the age of 60.[4] The incidence of major cardiovascular events in men increases dramatically with age, from 7 events/1,000 people at age 35–44 to 68 events/1,000 people at age 85–94; comparable rates occur for women about 10 years later in life, but the difference narrows with age.[5] In the United States, the cost of medical care is higher for cardiovascular disease than for any other diagnostic group.[3] This diagnostic group includes the major forms of cardiovascular disease, which are coronary heart disease, stroke, congestive heart failure, pulmonary embolism, cardiac dysrhythmias, hypertensive disease, and peripheral artery disease. Together, these diseases are a massive burden on our health care system.

J.L. Holtzman (ed.), *Atherosclerosis and Oxidant Stress: A New Perspective.*
© Springer 2008

Coronary heart disease accounts for approximately two-thirds of all cardiovascular disease and approximately 50% of the coronary heart disease patients have had myocardial infarctions.[1,5] Coronary heart disease alone is the major cause of death in men over 40 years and women older than 64 years.[6] It is the leading cause of death in adults over the age of 35 and accounts for greater than 25% of all deaths.[6] In 1998 there were approximately one-half million deaths attributable to coronary heart diseases and a lower, but similar number of deaths has continued to occur in recent years.[5] Approximately, 800,000 new cardiovascular events and 450,000 recurrent events occur each year.[3] The lifetime risk of coronary heart disease, at age 40, is about 1 in 2 for men and 1 in 3 for women.[7] The lifetime risk remains high with a 35% chance for men and a 25% chance for women at age 70. Coronary heart disease is the third most frequent cause of short stay hospitalizations and ranks among the greatest cost per hospital admission and is also the leading cause of premature permanent disability.[8] The cost of medical care for coronary heart disease has been estimated at $53 billion in direct costs plus 47 billion in indirect costs per year.[1]

The incidence of cardiovascular disease is disproportionate across gender and ethnic groups. The most pronounced difference is in the incidence of CHD in men vs. women. The mortality rate is 4.5 times greater in men than women aged 25–34 years old.[2] This ratio declines to about 1.5 for the age group from 75 to 84 years. Regarding ethnic groups, the incidence of coronary heart disease is higher in African-Americans as compared to Caucasians;[2] the lowest rates of these three groups occur in Hispanics.[9]

Blood Lipids and Coronary Heart Disease

The major risk factors for coronary heart disease are well known and include smoking, high blood pressure, and blood cholesterol levels. In addition, obesity, diabetes, and family history are recognized as important factors. While each of these factors is important, the predominant factor may be blood cholesterol levels. Serum total cholesterol and lipoproteins are well-established risk factors for coronary artery disease. Numerous studies have confirmed the relationship between serum total cholesterol and coronary heart disease.[10–13] A rule of thumb from epidemiologic studies suggest that for every 1% increase in total cholesterol, the risk of CHD increases by 2%.[14,15] The National Cholesterol Education Program defines three categories of serum total cholesterol. These are desirable (<200 mg/dL), borderline high (200–239 mg/dL) and high (>240 mg/dL). These classifications have been used as a basis for prescribing preventive treatments including dietary changes and pharmaceutical drugs.[14] NCEP guidelines have changed with the development of methods for the measurement of subclasses of serum lipoproteins and recognition that the distribution of cholesterol among lipoproteins improved the prediction of coronary artery disease risk.[16] The informative lipoproteins included low-density lipoprotein, high-density lipoprotein, and very low-density lipoproteins. Most of the attention has focused on low-density lipoproteins, which are very atherogenic.

In early studies, low-density lipoprotein cholesterol concentrations have been associated with coronary artery disease[17] and this finding was confirmed in numerous subsequent studies. For clinical purposes, LDL levels have been defined as optimal (<100 mg/dL), near optimal (100–129 mg/dL), borderline high (130–159 mg/dL), high (160–189 mg/dL) and very high (>190 mg/dL). Another lipoprotein, HDL is associated inversely with the risk of coronary heart disease. HDL is involved in reverse cholesterol transport, which reduces tissue cholesterol levels and may provide a protective effect. Low HDL cholesterol levels are recognized as a common and powerful risk factor for coronary artery disease.[18] The AHA guidelines suggest that levels of HDL lower than 40 mg/dL result in an elevated risk for coronary artery disease. Two additional forms of LDL may be atherogenic particles and should be given consideration for their association with elevated risk. These are LP(a) and small dense low-density lipoproteins. The association of LP(a) with coronary disease is independent of serum LDL cholesterol levels.[19] Structural studies have found that this apolipoprotein has a structure similar to plasminogen.[20] These structural studies have provided a basis for a possible mechanism of LP(a) action as it could block the binding of plasminogen and prevent the lysis of clots. Risk factor studies have been mixed, sometimes showing LP(a) and isoforms to be a risk factor, but only in the presence of other risk factors and other times showing it to be an independent risk factor for clinical coronary heart disease.[21] Thus, definition of its role remains unclear. Small dense LDL is associated with the risk for coronary artery disease. However, this association is complicated by a simultaneous association with components of the metabolic syndrome. It is unclear whether small dense LDL is a primary risk factor or it is only associated with other atherogenic factors.[22,23] Very low density lipoproteins are a primary source of circulating triglycerides which has been identified as an independent risk factor for coronary artery disease. The association has been frequent, but inconsistent and may reflect an association with the metabolic syndrome.[24] This association was recognized recently and requires further study to define the relationship. More recently, the measurement of nonhigh density lipoprotein cholesterol has been shown to be a simpler or and perhaps equally effective predictor of coronary artery disease as LDL.[13] Nonhigh density lipoprotein cholesterol contains all the known and potential atherogenic lipoproteins and is easier to measure than each subclass. Further studies are needed to define the predictive value of nonhigh density lipoprotein cholesterol.

The Influence of Dietary Fats on Blood Cholesterol Levels and Distribution of Fatty Acids

Blood cholesterol levels and risk of cardiovascular disease are influenced by dietary intakes of fats. The intake of red meats and saturated fats are a primary cause of elevated blood cholesterol levels.[25] Monounsaturated fats generally have a neutral effect on cholesterol, whereas polyunsaturated fats decrease cholesterol levels.[26] Dietary cholesterol can increase blood cholesterol levels, but contributes less to blood cholesterol levels than saturated fats.[13] Specific fatty acids within each major class, saturated, monounsaturated, and polyunsaturated, often have unique effects on blood cholesterol levels and should be considered on an individual basis. Palmitic acid, a 16-carbon saturated fatty acid, is a major contributor of saturated fat intake in the United States diet, accounting for greater than 60% of the saturated fat intake. It is associated with an elevation in LDL levels[27] and may cause these elevated levels by inhibiting the expression of LDL receptors on cell surfaces.[28] Its effect is very specific for LDL and does not increase HDL or VLDL levels. Meats, coconut oil, palm oil, and dairy fats are the primary sources of palmitic acid. Myristic acid, a 14-carbon saturated fatty acid, occurs in much lower amounts in the diet than palmitic, but has similar effects on LDL levels as palmitic acid.[29] Its primary sources are butter fat and tropical oils. Lauric acid, the shortest of the long-chain saturated fatty acids, 12 carbons, also increases cholesterol levels. The effect per gram of lauric acid is approximately two-thirds of the effect of palmitic acid.[30] Dietary medium chain saturated fatty acids (8 and 10 carbon fats) increase cholesterol levels.[31] Their contribution is a small portion of the overall effect of dietary fats. The longest of the saturated fatty acids, stearic acid, is 18 carbons long. Interestingly, it does not increase blood cholesterol levels. This lack of an effect may be the result of its rapid metabolism to oleic acid, a monounsaturated fatty acid.[32,33] Several studies have confirmed that stearic acid has a short half-life. The most common monounsaturated fatty acid, oleic, has a "neutral" effect on blood cholesterol levels.[27,29,34] Oleic is an 18-carbon fatty acid with a single double bond in a cis conformation. This fatty acid is a significant component of dietary fat, being the most prevalent fatty acid and the major monounsaturated fatty acid in the United States diet. Oleic acid is found in both plant and animal food sources. More importantly, it is well known as the major source of fat in the Mediterranean diet. The cardioprotective effects of the Mediterranean diet have been attributed to its high content of monounsaturated fatty acids. The mechanism of action may involve the enzyme, acyl cholesterol acyl transferase. It catalyzes the esterification of cholesterol. Oleic acid is a preferred substrate for the enzyme, which lowers unesterified cholesterol concentrations and thereby allows more expression of the LDL receptor and removal of LDL from blood. Another monounsaturated fat is trans fat, which consists of several fatty acids of 18 carbons and a double bond in a trans configuration. It is a product of hydrogenation of oleic acid, with the most common product being elaidic acid. This fatty acid increases blood cholesterol levels.[35] Hydrogenation is used in food processing and has been commonly used in the manufacture of margarines, oils, and shortening. The trans fat content of common food sources generally ranges from several percent to as high as 35% of total fat. Beginning in 2006, the trans fat content of foods was listed on the food labels. Many manufacturers changed their processes and eliminated the formation of trans fats in foods in recent years. Trans fat levels should be less than 1% of total fat. Polyunsaturated fatty acids generally lower blood cholesterol levels relative to saturated fatty acids, but the effect differs depending on the particular PUFA, polyunsaturated fatty acid. PUFAs can be divided into classes according to the position of double bonds in the fatty acid, as omega-3 or omega-6. Omega-3 fatty acids include linoleic, which is the most common form of PUFA. Linoleic acid is effective in reducing blood cholesterol concentrations and has been evaluated in numerous studies.[29,34] While some reduction occurs in LDL-cholesterol, most of the reduction occurs in HDL-cholesterol and VLDL-cholesterol. The United States diet has increased its linoleic content from 4 to about 7% in recent years and it has been associated with a decreased risk of cardiovascular disease. However, there are concerns about raising the levels further. Linoleic intakes have been associated with several possible detrimental effects. These include suppression of immune responses, promotion of carcinogenesis, increased susceptibility of LDL to oxidation, decreases in HDL levels, and formation of gallstones.[36-40] The omega-6 category of PUFA includes fatty acids in fish oils which are eicosopentaenoic acid, EPA, and docosahexanoic acid, DHA. These fatty acids constitute approximately 25% of the total fatty acids in fish oils. The intake of these fatty acids has a slight effect on blood cholesterol levels, in the absence of high triglyceride levels, and more pronounced effect on blood triglyceride levels.[41] The effect on LDL-cholesterol is similar to that of oleic acid, but is not specific for LDL-cholesterol.

It is apparent that dietary intakes of lipids, especially particular fatty acids, can alter lipoprotein levels, especially those of LDL in blood. Thus, vasculature exposure to lipids, especially LDL and its activity as a substrate for oxidation and uptake can be altered by dietary practices, which often increase blood lipid concentrations. In addition, the dietary intake of fatty acids can influence the composition of LDL and some cell membranes, especially red blood cell membranes. Their content of PUFA, MUFA, and saturated fats readily reflects dietary intakes of these fatty acids. Changes in the fatty acid composition of cellular membranes may influence the formation of particular oxidized and bioactive lipids, when lipids are exposed to oxidative and inflammatory activity from free radicals and/or oxidative enzymes. This area should be explored further as it holds considerable promise for better preventive efforts.

The Pathogenesis of Coronary Heart Disease

The underlying cause of coronary heart disease is atherosclerosis, which from a clinical view leads to the formation of plaque, degeneration of vessel intima, thromobosis, and ultimately vessel occlusion and ischemia. An interesting aspect of atherosclerosis is that it occurs more frequently at certain locations than others in the vasculature, albeit throughout the body. Atherosclerosis is commonly located at bifurcations and areas of vessel stress. These areas often have a low oscillating shear stress. Presumably, this stress facilitates the accumulation of lipid and initiation of atherosclerosis.[42] In recent years, oxidation and inflammation have been viewed as primary mechanisms in the initiation and progression of atherosclerosis. Oxidative damage and inflammation have been linked with the risk of coronary heart disease in several instances.[43,44] Together, these observations suggest that factors other than hypercholesterolemia alone are important in the generation of atherosclerosis and vessel damage. The "oxidation hypothesis" was developed and states that non-specific oxidative damage induces the formation of oxidized LDL and the initial stages of atherosclerosis.[45] This hypothesis also is consistent with the idea of a "response-to-injury" model,[46] wherein inflammation is a response to an initial injury of the vasculature; in this case, possibly due to oxidative damage.

Oxidative damage and inflammation may be tightly linked in the developmental atherosclerosis and subsequently cardiovascular disease. Oxidative stress can be elevated as a result of lifestyle factors and subject characteristics, such as an elevated BMI.[43] It may initiate vascular damage that precedes inflammation. Inflammation is a response to the oxidative vascular damage, which also precipitates further oxidative damage. Oxidative damage, in turn, leads to the generation of oxidized lipids, which are bioactive and induce inflammation. Both oxidative damage and inflammation have been associated with several stages in the pathogenesis of atherosclerosis. While the exact order of events is not well established, we could envision a sequence of reactions involving an increase in oxidative stress which leads to vessel damage, accompanied by the production of bioactive lipids and consequently an inflammatory response, which generates further oxidative damage and atherosclerosis.

Pioneering research in the 1980s found that cellular uptake of cholesterol in the form of LDL particles was a very tightly controlled process. It did not allow accumulation of excess unesterified (free) cholesterol by cells; several control mechanisms maintained cellular unesterified cholesterol levels at a constant level.[47] This observation was inconsistent with observation of foam cell formation, which was characterized by excessive uptakes of LDL particles and cholesterol by macrophages and smooth muscle cells. Then a fundamental set of experiments found that modifications of LDL led to an uncontrolled uptake of LDL particles by macrophages.[48] Modifications, which induced LDL uptake, included acetylation and oxidation as well as several modifications generally considered unphysiological. Modification allowed for identification of the LDL particle by a scavenger receptor (CD36).[49] This receptor was not controlled by cellular cholesterol levels and provided for the accumulation of cellular cholesterol and formation of foam cells, and subsequently the squeale leading to the formation of advanced atherosclerotic plaque. These studies induced a massive expansion of vascular biology research and identification of the mechanisms involved in the development of atherosclerosis. Oxidative stress and damage produced vascular damage in the form of oxidized LDL particles.[50] The damaged particles induced a "response-to-injury", which was an inflammatory response. Thus, an interaction between lipids, oxidative stress, and inflammation may provide an environment for the development of atherosclerosis.

The pathogenesis of atherosclerosis can be divided into three stages consisting of fatty streak formation, development of advanced (fibrous) plaque, and thrombosis.[51] In the initial stage, there may be an increase in vessel permeability and a movement of LDL particles into the subendothelial space of vessels. LDL becomes oxidized forming an oxidized particle and bioactive oxidized lipids; some of which induce an inflammatory response. These activities induce the expression of chemotactic factors (MCP-1, Fractalkine and Rantes) and adhesion molecules

(P-selectin, ICAM, VCAM-1, Cs-1, and fibronectin) by endothelial cells, which facilitate monocyte migration and uptake. Under these conditions, there is also an elevation in monocyte differentiation factors (M-CSF, IL-8, GM-CSF). Simultaneously, lymphocyte activity is enhanced by chemotactic factors. The macro phages and lymphocytes produce reactive oxygen species, which cause further oxidative damage and macrophage uptake of oxidized LDL via scavenger receptors (CD36, SRA-1, and LOX-1). Foam cell formation occurs and ultimately leads to the development of fatty streaks. This activity is facilitated by a decrease in the release of cholesterol from macrophages via ABCA-1 and ABCG-1. Together these activities may be regarded as an initial "response to injury."

The development of advanced plaque is a complex process, which involves several distinct activities and cell types. These include an increase in smooth muscle proliferation, which is induced by FGF-1, HBEGF, and PDGF, and the movement of smooth muscle cells into plaque. It is facilitated by the smooth muscle cell chemotactic factor, PDGF. Smooth muscle cells can participate in the uptake of oxidized LDL and matrix synthesis, which is stimulated by TGF_{beta}. Also, basement membranes around the plaque can be remodeled through the actions of metalloproteinases. During this phase, there can be development of a necrotic core, which is formed from the death of foam cells through necrosis or apoptosis. Necrosis and apoptosis also cause the formation of oxidized bioactive lipids, some of which have thrombotic activities.

The final stage of atherosclerosis is the induction of thromobosis. This includes changes in the release or expression of prothromobotic molecules from endothelial cells, many of which are oxidized lipids, including tissue factor, plasminogen activator, and plasminogen activator inhibitor. It includes increased smooth muscle and macrophage expression of tissue factor and other prothromobotic molecules. Also, the weakening and possibly the rupture of the vessel wall through activities of metalloproteinase's and their inhibitors. These activities promote the development of cardiac events.

Oxidized Lipids and Atherosclerosis

Each stage of atherosclerosis involves the formation of oxidized lipids, many of which are bioactive. The lipids in lipoprotein particles and cell membranes provide the substrates for the formation of these bioactive molecules. The oxidized lipids can be a product of interactions with reactive oxygen species or reactive nitrogen species (ROS/RNS), or oxidative enzymes and lipids in the vasculature.[52-54] The oxidative enzymes include: myeloperoxidase, 12/15 lipooxygenase, NADPH oxidase, NADH oxidase, cyclooxygenase, P-450 enzymes, and nitric oxide synthase. Products include oxidized phospholipids, fatty acids, and cholesterol as well as specific products of enzymatic reactions, such as prostaglandins and leukotrienes. The oxidized phospholipids include products such as hexadecyl azelaoyl phosphatidyl choline, palmitoyl epoxyisoprostane phosphatidyl choline, palmitoyl oxovalerol phosphatidyl choline, palmitolyl glutaroyl phosphatidyl choline, and palmitoyl cyclopentenone phosphatidyl choline.[51] Oxidized fatty acids are derived from arachidonic acid and include HETE, HNE, and isoprostanes. This category also includes prostaglandins, well-known products of cyclooxygenase and leukotrienes, well-known products of lipooxygenase. Products of cholesterol oxidation include 7-hydroperoxycholesterol and 22-hydroxycholesterol.

Many of these oxidized lipids have been found in atherosclerotic lesions[55–57] and cells,[58,59] at all stages of atherosclerosis. In addition, apoptotic bodies in atherosclerosis and IL-1 treated cells also contain oxidized lipids.[59–61]

Indications that oxidized lipids, found in atherosclerosis, have bioactivity, come from several types of studies. Polymorphisms, which alter the activity of oxidative enzymes, have been associated with low amounts of atherosclerosis.[62,63] Knockout mice for lipooxygenase and cyclooxygenase have shown lower levels of atherosclerosis, indicating a significant role of these enzymes in atherosclerosis.[64–66] Their products, prostaglandins and leukotrienes, have well-known effects on the vasculature.[67–69] Low amounts of atherosclerosis also are found in knockout mice for the CD 36 receptor, toll-like 2 and 4 receptors, PAF receptors, P-selectin, VCAM-1, IL-8, Fractalkine, MCP-1, and M-CSF.[65,66,70–72] Oxidized, but not native, phospholipids bind to receptors and induce activities associated with atherosclerosis.[73] Oxidized phospholipids activate endothelial cells to bind monocytes. These bioactive lipids also induce production of MCP-1 and MCF by smooth muscle and endothelial cells.[60,74,75] The formation of protein adducts by oxidation products, in particular, with apolipoprotein B can alter the activity of proteins. Some oxidized lipids induce immune responses by creating new epitopes.[65] Also, several oxidized lipid products are potent inflammatory mediators such as platelet activating factor (PAF), PAF-like lipids, certain oxidized phospholipids, and lysophosphotidylcholine (LYSO-PC).[76] The induction of inflammation promotes several activities, but in particular, further oxidative damage. Oxidized lipids can modify the expression of various cytokines and transcription factors that are involved in atherosclerosis[77,78] and may enhance platelet activation. In contrast, oxidized lipids also apparently signal oxidative stress and act in the induction of antioxidative and cytoprotective activities.[61] Thus, the oxidized lipids have a wide range of biological activities; some related to the pathogenesis of atherosclerosis and others to the protection of the vasculature.

Some of the bioactive oxidized lipids can be removed by protective enzymes such as phospholipase A2 and paraoxonase, which cleave phospholipid hydroperoxides of various carbon lengths.[79,80] This activity accounts for a portion of the protective effect of HDL. It is important to remember that there are two phospholipases, which may have a role in atherogenesis, the nonpancreatic type of secretory phospholipids A2 and the lipoprotein-associated PLA2. The secretory form of phospholipase A2 is relatively nonspecific, calcium-dependent, and of less current interest in the risk of coronary heart disease. The lipoprotein-associated PLA2 is under intense research as a risk factor for CVD. Other protective enzymes may include ACAT and aldose reductase. Thus, the extent of oxidized lipid exposure is dependent upon a balance between their formation and enzymes which hydrolyze these oxidized products.

Oxidized phospholipids, associated with LDL, have been linked with the risk of coronary heart disease. A study of coronary artery disease patients found an association between the ratio of oxidized phospholipid:apo B-100 and the presence of vessel stenosis, greater than 50%. Since LP(a) binds proinflammatory oxidized phospholipids and was also related to the presence of stenosis, the atherogenicity of LP(a) may be mediated by an association with oxidized lipids.[81,82]

Mitochondria, Oxidative Stress, and Bioactive Lipids: A New Concept

The formation and bioactivity of oxidized lipids may be influenced by several activities associated with mitochondria. In recent years, a new concept of mitochondria involvement in coronary heart disease has been evolving, wherein mitochondria have a central role in the pathogenesis of atherosclerosis. The cellular organelle is a major source of reactive oxygen species and oxidized lipids. The formation of mitochondrial ROS and oxidized lipids are linked with each other and both products are active in the induction of the early stages of atherosclerosis. In addition, reactive oxygen species may have a dual role of causing nonspecific oxidative damage of lipids, proteins, and DNA, and participating in a "redox cell signaling" system. The original oxidative hypothesis held that excessive oxidative damage was responsible for the causation of atherosclerosis; the oxidation of LDL and its subsequent uptake by macrophages. This concept is still applicable and provides the foundation for many of the concepts in the initiation of early steps in atherosclerosis. However, another relatively recently developed concept may explain additional aspects of the relationship between oxidation and atherosclerosis. Mitochondrial reactive oxygen species may be active in a "redox cell signaling" system, wherein reactive oxygen species induce additional vascular cell activities. These activities include the induction of apoptosis and cytoprotective effects, superficially contradictory effects. In fact, the effect of ROS may be biphasic with high levels of ROS inducing apoptosis and low levels of ROS inducing antioxidative enzyme activity and cytoprotective effects. In these scenarios, oxidized bioactive lipids are formed and may be the mediators of many of the biological effects. Also, the formation of ROS is highly controlled, rather than being "leakage of electrons" as suggested previously for mitochondrial oxidative stress. Both of these concepts of mitochondrial activities are described in more detail below.

Nonspecific oxidative damage can occur as a result of excessive reactive oxygen species formation and their release from the respiratory chain in mitochondria. These species, especially, superoxide anions, are produced primarily by complex I and complex III. This production of the superoxide anions by the respiratory chain may be a by-product, an "electron leak," or part of a well-orchestrated signaling mechanism. Regardless of the mechanism, a high level of superoxide production has been associated with damage to mitochondria DNA and mitochondrial dysfunction, leading to further cellular oxidative damage. Mitochondria can inflict nonspecific oxidative damage upon themselves and thereby induce further oxidative stress and damage in a vicious cycle.

In this regard, an important aspect of mitochondrial metabolism is the concept that a threshold effect exists, wherein the bioenergetic function of mitochondria is compromised following the attainment of mitochondrial DNA damage at a particular threshold level. Beyond this threshold level, mitochondria cannot produce sufficient energy for the cell and there is an increase in reactive oxygen species. This causes extensive damage of surrounding cells, lipid peroxidation, and further elevation above the threshold levels. Mitochondrial DNA encodes 13 proteins which have important roles in the respiratory chain. Maintenance of bioenergetic capacity is dependent on the synthesis of these proteins. As the level of mitochondrial DNA damage increases, the likelihood of dysfunction also increases. When the threshold for DNA damage is reached, there is low synthesis of the critical proteins and a low bioenergetic capacity, relative to needs. Mitochondrial DNA damage is associated with several of the common risk factors for cardiovascular disease, including age, hypercholesterolemia, and smoking. These factors are associated with an accumulation of mitochondrial DNA damage and may lower the threshold level for mitochondrial dysfunction.

Controlled Release of Reactive Oxygen Species for Mitochondria and Cellular Redox Signaling Pathways

Another possible role of mitochondrial involvement in atherosclerosis is the release of reactive oxygen species in a highly controlled process, at least under nonpathologic conditions, and its linkage with a well-orchestrated signal transduction system, the "redox cell signaling" system. In support of this concept, the release of reactive oxygen species from mitochondria appears regulated by specific mechanisms. Superoxide formation by complex I in the respiratory chain is influenced by a thiol switching mechanism. The glutaredoxin system controls the redox couples of a 70-kDa subunit of complex I. S-glutathionylation of the protein increases superoxide release.[83] Another mechanism involves uncoupling protein 2. This protein reduces the proton potential across the mitochondrial membranes. It also reduces the formation of superoxide anion and oxidative damage with increases in its expression.[84,85] This effect is dependent on the particular isoform of UCP, as UCP1 has the opposite effect. These observations suggest a system of controls for the release of reactive oxygen species, which requires further exploration. Efforts have just begun in this area and confirmation of these mechanisms is necessary.

Regarding possible ROS signaling mechanisms within mitochondria, superoxide anions can bind to aconitase, an iron-sulfur protein in the respiratory chain, and cause the release of iron.[86] The released iron can cause lipid peroxidation with the formation of oxidized (electrophilic) lipids. The electrophilic lipids are bioactive. They can react with protein thiols and induce a range of signals. Another possible pathway involves peroxynitrite, which is formed from nitric oxide and superoxide and has been linked with signal transduction systems.[87] It is also a potent oxidant and can induce lipid peroxidation and formation of bioactive lipids.

Hydrogen peroxide may act in two additional pathways, superoxide dismutase produces hydrogen peroxide from superoxide anion and it is ready diffusible through membranes. It can interact with cytosolic redox sensitive proteins and pathways.[88] Hydrogen peroxide also can react with peroxidases, such as myeloperoxidase, and reactive nitrogen species with the production of nitrated proteins.[89]

Pathways Influenced by Mitochondrial ROS and Oxidized Lipids

Reactive oxygen species and possibly oxidized lipids, as described above, may have a central role in numerous mitochondria-related signaling pathways. Growth factors, inflammation-related factors, and reactive oxygen species can induce the production of ROS by mitochondria and the mechanisms described above, which in turn, induces subsequent steps in signaling pathways. These pathways induce responses which promote either cellular protection or cell death. Several cellular signaling pathways, which may be involved, include those activated by the vasoactive agents such as transforming growth factor (TGF)-[beta],[90] epidermal growth factor (EGF),[91] angiotensin II,[92] and tumor necrosis factor (TNF)-[alpha].[19,93,94] These pathways induce the production of ROS, which acts in the "transactivation" of growth factor receptors. The "transactivated" receptors induce protection against oxidative stress.[95] The downstream ROS-activated pathways may involve the MAPK proteins, which includes several kinases such as p38 MAPK, c-jun N-terminal kinase, and extracellular signal-regulated kinases 1 and 2. Activation of these pathways by ROS can be cytoprotective, but the effect is dependent on cell type and conditions. Another cytoprotective pathway is a stimulation of ROS through angiotensin II activation of K channels in smooth muscle cells, which in turn activates MAPKs. Also, reactive oxygen species can react with RNS and form peroxynitrite, which can induce AMPK, a central regulator of energy metabolism. Alternatively, mitochondrial ROS can promote cell proliferation and enhance DNA damage and angiogenesis, the later through decreased expression of MnSOD activity. ROS also can alter the regulation of MAPKs and matrix metalloproteinases and decrease cell survival. Thus, ROS can promote cellular damage and induce cellular apoptosis under certain circumstances. The mechanisms involved in the selection of the specific activity, cell death or protection, are unknown at this time.

Oxidized LDL, Signal Transduction Pathways, and Protection of Vascular Cells

It is becoming increasing clear that cells can respond to oxidative stress in a variety of ways. While most of our attention has focused on responses to high levels of oxidative stress, especially of oxidized LDL, and its promotion of a proinflammatory response, recruitment of macrophages, and the development of atherosclerotic lesions,[96] oxidative stress may also have a protective effect. Vascular cells have the capacity to adapt to oxidative stress and this has been shown at low levels of oxidative stress. Low levels of oxidized LDLs (oxLDLs) were cytoprotective in early studies. The protective effect occurred through mechanisms involving an increase in levels of glutathione (GSH), an intracellular antioxidant.[97–99] Regulation occurs through cell signaling mechanisms. Recent studies have found that the protective response was mediated by the transcriptional control of genes regulated by the electrophile response element, such as hemeoxygenase-1.[100]

Many of the activities of oxidized LDL may be mediated through specific electrophilic lipid products of lipid peroxidation. The following observations support this hypothesis: (1) electrophilic lipids regulate GSH levels, and polymorphisms in proteins involved in GSH synthesis are associated with inflammatory disease in human populations;[101,102] (2) depletion of GSH or loss of hemeoxygenase in animal models enhances susceptibility to the cardiovascular disease process;[103,104] (3) electrophilic lipids derived from both enzymatic and nonenzymatic lipid peroxidation are found in the vasculature of both humans and animal models.

Summary

Cardiovascular disease has placed a huge burden on public health systems and continues to do so, in spite of a dramatic decrease in this burden since the 1950s. It is a complex disease with numerous risk factors and a complex pathogenesis. The primary risk factor is hypercholesterolemia, which is readily influenced by dietary intakes of fats. While fats supply the substrate for atherosclerosis, it is clear that additional factors are essential for the development of plaque and ultimately the precipitation of cardiovascular disease events. Oxidation and inflammation may be the primary mechanisms for initiation and progression of atherosclerosis. Oxidative damage is associated with several CVD risk factors and could initiate vessel damage, which in turn, could induce inflammation and numerous cellular activities of atherogenesis. A primary mediator of these activities may be oxidized lipids. Oxidized lipids are formed readily in a prooxidative environment and consist of a wide variety of molecular species. Many of these species have been found in atherosclerotic plaque. In addition, several mechanisms have been identified for the regulation of reactive oxygen species and formation of oxidized lipids. Recent efforts have found that the oxidized lipids have potent biological activities. Interactions of oxidized lipids with receptors and signaling pathways have been defined and linked with the regulation of cell proliferation and apoptosis. The balance between these activities may have a significant impact on plaque development. A key regulatory factor may be mitochondria and its interaction with various redox cell signaling pathways. Mitochondria may participate in several pathways involving the formation of ROS and oxidized lipids. Subtle changes in the balance of lipid oxidation products, such as may have been induced by inhibitors of cyclooxygenase, could have a large impact on the incidence of CVD. Understanding these mechanisms and their modulation may be of key importance for the prevention of cardiovascular disease.

References

1. Association AH. 1999 Heart and Stroke: Statistical Update. American Heart Association, 1999.
2. Institute NHLaB. Morbidity and Mortality Chartbook on Cardiovascular, Lung, and Blood Diseases. Washington: US Department of Health and Human Services, 1998.
3. National Heart LaBI. NHLBI Fact Book, Fiscal Year 1990. Washington: US Department of Health and Human Services, 1991.
4. Gordon T, Kannel WB. Premature Mortality from Coronary Heart Disease. The Framingham Study. JAMA 1971;215(10):1617–1625.
5. Thom T, Kannel WB, Silbershatz H, et al. Cardiovascular diseases in the U.S. and preventive approaches. In: Fuster V, O'Rourke RA (Eds). Hurst's the Heart. New York: McGraw-Hill, 2001;pp. 3–17.
6. Statistics NCfH. Vital Statistics of the United States. Vol. II, Mortality Part A, 1991. Hyattsville, MD: Center for Disease Control and Prevention, 1988.
7. Lloyd-Jones DM, et al. Lifetime risk of developing coronary heart disease. Lancet, 1999;353(9147):89–92.
8. Kannel WB, Prevalence, incidence, and mortality of coronary heart disease. In: Fuster EJTV, Nabel EG (Eds). Atherothrombosis and Coronary Artery Disease, Chapter 2, 2nd edn. Philadelphia, PA: Lippincott Williams & Wilkins, 2005.
9. Statistics, NCH. Deaths of Hispanic Origin, 15 Reporting States, 1979–1981. Vital and Health Statistics, Series 20 No. 18, DHHS Publication No. (PHS), 1990;pp. 91–1855.
10. Windaus A, Ober. den gehalt normaler und atheromatoser aorten an cholesterjn und cholesterinestern. Zeitschr Physiol Chem 1910;67:174–176.
11. Vartiainen I, Kanerva K. Arteriosclerosis and wartime. Ann Med Inntern Fenn 1947;36: 748–758.
12. Malmros H. The relation of nutrition to health: a statistical study of the effect of the wartime on arteriosclerosis, cardiosclerosis, tuberculosis. Acta Med Scand Suppl 1950;246:137–153.
13. Cui Y, et al. Non-high-density lipoprotein cholesterol level as a predictor of cardiovascular disease mortality. Arch Intern Med 2001;161(11):1413–1419.
14. Third Report of the National Cholesterol Education Program (NCEP) Expert Panel on Detection, Evaluation, and Treatment of High Blood Cholesterol in Adults (Adult Treatment Panel III) final report. Circulation 2002;106(25):3143–3421.
15. Carleton RA. et al. Report of the expert panel on population strategies for blood cholesterol reduction. A statement from the National Cholesterol Education Program, National Heart, Lung, and Blood Institute, National Institutes of Health. Circulation 1991;83(6): 2154–2232.
16. Rosenfeld L. Lipoprotein analysis. Early methods in the diagnosis of atherosclerosis. Arch Pathol Lab Med 1989;113(10):1101–1110.
17. EVALUATION of serum lipoprotein and cholesterol measurements as predictors of clinical complications of atherosclerosis; report of a cooperative study of lipoproteins and atherosclerosis. Circulation 1956;14(4 Part 2):691–742.
18. Sharrett AR. et al. Coronary heart disease prediction from lipoprotein cholesterol levels, triglycerides, lipoprotein(a), apolipoproteins A-I and B, and HDL density subfractions: the Atherosclerosis Risk in Communities (ARIC) Study. Circulation 2001;104(10):1108–1113.

19. Dahlen G, Berg K, Frick MH. Lp(a) lipoprotein/pre-beta1-lipoprotein, serum lipids and atherosclerotic disease. Clin Genet 1976;9(6):558–566.
20. McLean JW, et al. cDNA sequence of human apolipoprotein(a) is homologous to plasminogen. Nature 1987;330(6144):132–137.
21. Howard GC, Pizzo SV. Lipoprotein(a) and its role in atherothrombotic disease. Lab Invest 1993;69(4):373–386.
22. Grundy SM, Small LDL. atherogenic dyslipidemia, and the metabolic syndrome. Circulation 1997;95(1):1–4.
23. Coresh J, Kwiterovich PO. Jr, Small dense low-density lipoprotein particles and coronary heart disease risk: A clear association with uncertain implications. JAMA 1996;276(11): 914–915.
24. Hokanson JE, Austin MA. Plasma triglyceride level is a risk factor for cardiovascular disease independent of high-density lipoprotein cholesterol level: a meta-analysis of population-based prospective studies. J Cardiovasc Risk 1996;3(2):213–219.
25. Mensink RP. Effects of the individual saturated fatty acids on serum lipids and lipoprotein concentrations. Am J Clin Nutr 1993;57(5 Suppl):711S–714S.
26. Katan MB, Zock PL, Mensink RP. Effects of fats and fatty acids on blood lipids in humans: an overview. Am J Clin Nutr 1994;60(6 Suppl):1017S–1022S.
27. Mattson FH, Grundy SM. Comparison of effects of dietary saturated, monounsaturated, and polyunsaturated fatty acids on plasma lipids and lipoproteins in man. J Lipid Res 1985;26(2):194–202.
28. Spady DK, Dietschy JM. Dietary saturated triacylglycerols suppress hepatic low density lipoprotein receptor activity in the hamster. Proc Natl Acad Sci USA 1985;82(13): 4526–4530.
29. Keys A, Parlin RW. Serum cholesterol response to changes in dietary lipids. Am J Clin Nutr 1966;19(3):175–181.
30. Denke MA, Grundy SM. Comparison of effects of lauric acid and palmitic acid on plasma lipids and lipoproteins. Am J Clin Nutr 1992;56(5):895–898.
31. Cater NB, Heller HJ, Denke MA. Comparison of the effects of medium-chain triacylglycerols, palm oil, and high oleic acid sunflower oil on plasma triacylglycerol fatty acids and lipid and lipoprotein concentrations in humans. Am J Clin Nutr 1997;65(1):41–45.
32. Bonanome A, Grundy SM. Effect of dietary stearic acid on plasma cholesterol and lipoprotein levels. N Engl J Med 1988;318(19):1244–1248.
33. Denke MA, Grundy SM. Effects of fats high in stearic acid on lipid and lipoprotein concentrations in men. Am J Clin Nutr 1991;54(6):1036–1040.
34. Hegsted DM. et al. Quantitative effects of dietary fat on serum cholesterol in man. Am J Clin Nutr 1965;17(5):281–295.
35. Mensink RP, Katan MB. Effect of dietary trans fatty acids on high-density and low-density lipoprotein cholesterol levels in healthy subjects. N Engl J Med 1990;323(7):439–445.
36. Carroll KK, Khor HT. Effects of level and type of dietary fat on incidence of mammary tumors induced in female Sprague-Dawley rats by 7,12-dimethylbenz(α)anthracene. Lipids 1971;6(6):415–420.
37. Weyman C, et al. Letter: linoleic acid as an immunosuppressive agent. Lancet 1975; 2(7923):33.
38. Jackson RL, et al. Influence of polyunsaturated and saturated fats on plasma lipids and lipoproteins in man. Am J Clin Nutr 1984;39(4):589–597.
39. Grundy SM. Effects of polyunsaturated fats on lipid metabolism in patients with hypertriglyceridemia. J Clin Invest 1975;55(2):269–282.
40. Parthasarathy S, et al. Low density lipoprotein rich in oleic acid is protected against oxidative modification: implications for dietary prevention of atherosclerosis. Proc Natl Acad Sci USA 1990;87(10):3894–3898.
41. Sanders TA, et al. Triglyceride-lowering effect of marine polyunsaturates in patients with hypertriglyceridemia. Arteriosclerosis 1985;5(5):459–465.

42. Williams KJ, Tabas I. The response-to-retention hypothesis of early atherogenesis. Arterioscler Thromb Vasc Biol 1995;15(5):551–561.
43. Gross M, et al. Plasma F2-isoprostanes and coronary artery calcification: the CARDIA Study. Clin Chem 2005;51(1):125–131.
44. Ridker PM, Glynn RJ, Hennekens CH. C-reactive protein adds to the predictive value of total and HDL cholesterol in determining risk of first myocardial infarction. Circulation 1998;97(20):2007–2011.
45. Steinberg D, et al. Beyond cholesterol. Modifications of low-density lipoprotein that increase its atherogenicity. N Engl J Med 1989;320(14):915–924.
46. Ross R. Atherosclerosis – an inflammatory disease. N Engl J Med 1999;340(2):115–126.
47. Goldstein JL. Familial hypercholesterolemia. In: CS Scriver. (Ed). The Metabolic and Molecular Basis of Inherited Disease, 7th edn. New York: McGraw-Hill Health Profession Division, 1995.
48. Steinberg D, Lewis A. Conner memorial lecture. oxidative modification of LDL and atherogenesis. Circulation 1997;95(4):1062–1071.
49. Parthasarathy S, et al. Macrophage oxidation of low density lipoprotein generates a modified form recognized by the scavenger receptor. Arteriosclerosis 1986;6(5):505–510.
50. Parthasarathy S, et al. Oxidative modification of beta-very low density lipoprotein. Potential role in monocyte recruitment and foam cell formation. Arteriosclerosis 1989;9(3):398–404.
51. Berliner J. Introduction. Lipid oxidation products and atherosclerosis. Vascul Pharmacol 2002;38(4):187–191.
52. Gaut JP, Heinecke JW. Mechanisms for oxidizing low-density lipoprotein. Insights from patterns of oxidation products in the artery wall and from mouse models of atherosclerosis. Trends Cardiovasc Med 2001;11(3–4):103–112.
53. Bey EA, Cathcart MK. In vitro knockout of human p47phox blocks superoxide anion production and LDL oxidation by activated human monocytes. J Lipid Res 2000;41(3):489–495.
54. Schultz D, Harrison DG. Quest for fire: seeking the source of pathogenic oxygen radicals in atherosclerosis. Arterioscler Thromb Vasc Biol 2000;20(6):1412–1413.
55. Bjorkhem I, Diczfalusy U, Lutjohann D. Removal of cholesterol from extrahepatic sources by oxidative mechanisms. Curr Opin Lipidol 1999;10(2):161–165.
56. Hulten LM, et al. Oxysterols present in atherosclerotic tissue decrease the expression of lipoprotein lipase messenger RNA in human monocyte-derived macrophages. J Clin Invest 1996;97(2):461–468.
57. Pratico D, et al. Localization of distinct F2-isoprostanes in human atherosclerotic lesions. J Clin Invest 1997;100(8):2028–2034.
58. Huber J, et al. Oxidized membrane vesicles and blebs from apoptotic cells contain biologically active oxidized phospholipids that induce monocyte-endothelial interactions. Arterioscler Thromb Vasc Biol 2002;22(1):101–107.
59. Subbanagounder G, et al. Epoxyisoprostane and epoxycyclopentenone phospholipids regulate monocyte chemotactic protein-1 and interleukin-8 synthesis. Formation of these oxidized phospholipids in response to interleukin-1beta. J Biol Chem 2002;277(9): 7271–7281.
60. Berliner JA, et al. Evidence for a role of phospholipid oxidation products in atherogenesis. Trends Cardiovasc Med 2001;11(3–4):142–147.
61. Leitinger N. Oxidized phospholipids as modulators of inflammation in atherosclerosis. Curr Opin Lipidol 2003;14(5):421–430.
62. Mackness MI, et al. Paraoxonase and coronary heart disease. Curr Opin Lipidol 1998;9(4): 319–324.
63. Yamada Y, et al. Correlations between plasma platelet-activating factor acetylhydrolase (PAF-AH) activity and PAF-AH genotype, age, and atherosclerosis in a Japanese population. Atherosclerosis 2000;150(1):209–216.
64. Camitta MG, et al. Cyclooxygenase-1 and −2 knockout mice demonstrate increased cardiac ischemia/reperfusion injury but are protected by acute preconditioning. Circulation 2001;104(20):2453–2458.

65. Berliner JA, Watson AD. A role for oxidized phospholipids in atherosclerosis. N Engl J Med 2005;353(1):9–11.
66. Pratico D, et al. Acceleration of atherogenesis by COX-1-dependent prostanoid formation in low density lipoprotein receptor knockout mice. Proc Natl Acad Sci USA 2001;98(6):3358–3363.
67. Miller SB. Prostaglandins in health and disease: an overview. Semin Arthritis Rheum 2006;36(1):37–49.
68. Jala VR, Haribabu B. Leukotrienes and atherosclerosis: new roles for old mediators. Trends Immunol 2004;25(6):315–322.
69. Khan Z, Tripathi CD. Leukotrienes and atherosclerosis. Indian Heart J 2005;57(2):175–180.
70. Reape TJ, Groot PH. Chemokines and atherosclerosis. Atherosclerosis 1999;147(2):213–225.
71. Suzuki H, et al. A role for macrophage scavenger receptors in atherosclerosis and suscepti-bility to infection. Nature 1997;386(6622):292–296.
72. Febbraio M, et al. Targeted disruption of the class B scavenger receptor CD36 protects against atherosclerotic lesion development in mice. J Clin Invest 2000;105(8):1049–1056.
73. Podrez EA, et al. Identification of a novel family of oxidized phospholipids that serve as ligands for the macrophage scavenger receptor CD36. J Biol Chem 2002;277(41): 38503–38516.
74. Chai YC, et al. Smooth muscle cell proliferation induced by oxidized LDL-borne lysophos-phatidylcholine. Evidence for FGF-2 release from cells not extracellular matrix. Vascul Pharmacol 2002;38(4):229–237.
75. Kadl A, et al. Analysis of inflammatory gene induction by oxidized phospholipids in vivo by quantitative real-time RT-PCR in comparison with effects of LPS. Vascul Pharmacol 2002;38(4):219–227.
76. Tselepis AD, John Chapman M. Inflammation, bioactive lipids and atherosclerosis: poten-tial roles of a lipoprotein-associated phospholipase A2, platelet activating factor-acetylhy-drolase. Atheroscler Suppl 2002;3(4):57–68.
77. Ares MP, et al. Oxidized LDL induces transcription factor activator protein-1 but inhibits activation of nuclear factor-kappa B in human vascular smooth muscle cells. Arterioscler Thromb Vasc Biol 1995;15(10):1584–1590.
78. Nagy L, et al. Oxidized LDL regulates macrophage gene expression through ligand activation of PPARgamma. Cell 1998;93(2):229–240.
79. Stafforini DM, et al. Platelet-activating factor acetylhydrolases. J Biol Chem 1997;272(29):17895–17898.
80. Ahmed Z, et al. Apolipoprotein A-I promotes the formation of phosphatidylcholine core aldehydes that are hydrolyzed by paraoxonase (PON-1) during high density lipoprotein oxidation with a peroxynitrite donor. J Biol Chem 2001;276(27):24473–24481.
81. Tsimikas S, et al. Oxidized phospholipids, Lp(a) lipoprotein, and coronary artery disease. N Engl J Med 2005;353(1):46–57.
82. Tsimikas S, et al. Increased plasma oxidized phospholipid:apolipoprotein B-100 ratio with concomitant depletion of oxidized phospholipids from atherosclerotic lesions after dietary lipid-lowering: a potential biomarker of early atherosclerosis regression. Arterioscler Thromb Vasc Biol 2007;27(1):175–181.
83. Beer SM, et al. Glutaredoxin 2 catalyzes the reversible oxidation and glutathionylation of mitochondrial membrane thiol proteins: implications for mitochondrial redox regulation and antioxidant DEFENSE. J Biol Chem 2004;279(46):47939–47951.
84. Teshima Y, et al. Uncoupling protein-2 overexpression inhibits mitochondrial death pathway in cardiomyocytes. Circ Res 2003;93(3):192–200.
85. Blanc J, et al. Protective role of uncoupling protein 2 in atherosclerosis. Circulation 2003;107(3):388–390.
86. Echtay KS, et al. Superoxide activates mitochondrial uncoupling protein 2 from the matrix side. Studies using targeted antioxidants. J Biol Chem 2002;277(49):47129–47135.
87. Go YM, et al. Evidence for peroxynitrite as a signaling molecule in flow-dependent activa-tion of c-Jun NH(2)-terminal kinase. Am J Physiol 1999;277(4 Pt 2):H1647–H1653.

88. Nelson KK, Melendez JA. Mitochondrial redox control of matrix metalloproteinases. Free Radic Biol Med 2004;37(6):768–784.
89. Fries DM, et al. Expression of inducible nitric-oxide synthase and intracellular protein tyrosine nitration in vascular smooth muscle cells: role of reactive oxygen species. J Biol Chem 2003;278(25):22901–22907.
90. Herrera B, et al. Reactive oxygen species (ROS) mediates the mitochondrial-dependent apoptosis induced by transforming growth factor (beta) in fetal hepatocytes. FASEB J 2001;15(3):741–751.
91. Krieg T, et al. Mitochondrial ROS generation following acetylcholine-induced EGF receptor transactivation requires metalloproteinase cleavage of proHB-EGF. J Mol Cell Cardiol 2004;36(3):435–443.
92. Kimura S, et al. Role of NAD(P)H oxidase- and mitochondria-derived reactive oxygen species in cardioprotection of ischemic reperfusion injury by angiotensin II. Hypertension 2005;45(5):860–866.
93. Goossens V, et al. Redox regulation of TNF signaling. Biofactors 1999;10(2–3):145–156.
94. Gurgul E, et al. Mitochondrial catalase overexpression protects insulin-producing cells against toxicity of reactive oxygen species and proinflammatory cytokines. Diabetes 2004;53(9):2271–2280.
95. Chen K, et al. Mitochondrial function is required for hydrogen peroxide-induced growth factor receptor transactivation and downstream signaling. J Biol Chem 2004;279(33):35079–35086.
96. Stocker R, Keaney JF, Jr. Role of oxidative modifications in atherosclerosis. Physiol Rev 2004;84(4):1381–1478.
97. Ishikawa K, Maruyama Y. Heme oxygenase as an intrinsic defense system in vascular wall: implication against atherogenesis. J Atheroscler Thromb 2001;8(3):63–70.
98. Moellering DR, et al. Induction of glutathione synthesis by oxidized low-density lipoprotein and 1-palmitoyl-2-arachidonyl phosphatidylcholine: protection against quinone-mediated oxidative stress. Biochem J 2002;362(Pt 1):51–59.
99. Levonen AL, et al. Biphasic effects of 15-deoxy-delta(12,14)-prostaglandin J(2) on glutathione induction and apoptosis in human endothelial cells. Arterioscler Thromb Vasc Biol 2001;21(11):1846–1851.
100. Bea F, et al. Induction of glutathione synthesis in macrophages by oxidized low-density lipoproteins is mediated by consensus antioxidant response elements. Circ Res 2003;92(4):386–393.
101. Izzotti A, et al. Increased DNA alterations in atherosclerotic lesions of individuals lacking the GSTM1 genotype. FASEB J 2001;15(3):752–757.
102. Koide S, et al. Association of polymorphism in glutamate-cysteine ligase catalytic subunit gene with coronary vasomotor dysfunction and myocardial infarction. J Am Coll Cardiol 2003;41(4):539–545.
103. Dedoussis GV, et al. Antiatherogenic effect of Pistacia lentiscus via GSH restoration and downregulation of CD36 mRNA expression. Atherosclerosis 2004;174(2):293–303.
104. Lapenna D, et al. Aortic glutathione metabolic status: time-dependent alterations in fat-fed rabbits. Atherosclerosis 2004;173(1):19–25.

Chapter 6
Nuclear Receptors in the Control of Lipid Metabolism

Shannon M. Reilly and Chih-Hao Lee

Nuclear hormone receptors are found at the heart of virtually every biological process. In addition to their functions in mediating steroid hormone effects, the role of this superfamily in maintaining metabolic homeostasis has been illuminated by the identification of dietary fats and their metabolites as ligands for several subfamilies. These receptors, in response to derivatives of fatty acids, cholesterol, and bile acids, constitute a transcriptional network controlling glucose and lipid metabolism as well as inflammation, all of which are key determinants of metabolic diseases, including dyslipidemia, insulin resistance, and atherosclerosis. In line with this, synthetic, high-affinity ligands developed to target these receptors have either been used or shown promise in the treatment of metabolic syndrome. For instance, the thiazolidinedione (TZD) class of drugs, one of the leading drug treatments of diabetes, specifically targets PPARgamma. This chapter discusses the metabolic roles and potential therapeutic applications of nuclear receptors, with an emphasis on receptors that sense and are activated by dietary lipids.

The Nuclear Receptor Superfamily

Evidence for the physiological importance of the nuclear hormone receptors lies in the ancient evolutionary origin of the superfamily. The high degree of sequence similarity between vertebrate and invertebrate receptors indicates that these receptors evolved before this branch in the evolutionary tree.[85] The 48 members of the nuclear hormone receptor family found in humans are shown in Table 6.1. With a few exceptions (see below), nuclear receptors share a common structural organization (Fig. 6.1). A ligand-independent activation function (AF-1) is located in the amino terminal region of most receptors. The core DNA binding domain contains two highly conserved zinc finger motifs responsible for the recognition of DNA sequences known as hormone response elements (HRE).[15,84] The nuclear localization signal of receptors that mostly localize in the nucleus can be found in this region. The DNA binding domain is connected to the ligand binding domain by a hinge region, which provides flexibility

J.L. Holtzman (ed.), *Atherosclerosis and Oxidant Stress: A New Perspective.*
© Springer 2008

Table 6.1 Nuclear hormone receptor superfamily

Orphan receptors	Adopted receptors	Identified ligands
SF-1	ER alpha, beta	Estrogen
SHP	AR	Testosterone
TLX	PR	Progesterone
PNR	GR	Glucocorticoid
LRH-1	MR	Mineralocorticoid
DAX-1	VDR	Vitamin D
GCNF	RAR alpha, beta, gamma	Retinoic acid
HNF-4 alpha, gamma	TR alpha, beta	Thyroid hormone
TR 2,4	FXR	Bile acids
ERR alpha, beta, gamma	CAR	Xenobiotics
Rev-erb alpha, beta	LXR alpha, beta	Oxysterols
ROR alpha, beta, gamma	PXR	Xenobiotics
NGFI-B alpha, beta, gamma	RXR	9-*cis*-retinoic acid
COUP-TF alpha, beta, gamma	PPAR alpha, delta/beta, gamma	Fatty acids

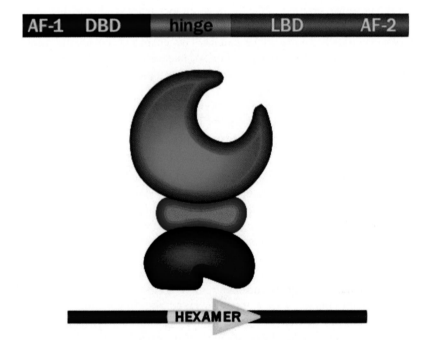

Fig. 6.1 Nuclear hormone receptor structure. Top: schematic of NHR gene depicting different domains. Bottom: Schematic of NHR protein and the hexamer of DNA that it recognizes

between these two domains. The ligand binding domain encompasses a large portion of the c-terminal region of the protein and is responsible for many functions other than ligand binding. The ligand-dependent activation function (AF-2) is at the carboxyl terminus; also contained with- in this domain is the dimerization interface and the nuclear localization signal, for receptors that localize to the cytoplasm in the inactive state.

The first nuclear hormone receptors were identified by endocrinologists searching for the receptors through which steroid hormones elicit their effects. Due to the homology within the receptor superfamily, sequencing the glucocorticoid receptor and estrogen receptor opened the door for discovery of other classic steroid and nonsteroid hormone receptors. The rest of the family members were subsequently identified using the highly conserved DNA binding domain in low stringency hybridization screenings of cDNA libraries, without prior knowledge of the receptors' functions or ligands. Receptors that could not be assigned hormones were called orphan receptors. Over the past two decades since the primary sequences were first discovered, some of the receptors have been "adopted" by ligands. The identified ligands were not novel hormones as was originally assumed, but metabolites of nutrients such as cholesterol and fatty acids, leading to the classification of these adopted receptors as metabolic sensors.[26] Many receptors remain orphans; although they all contain a ligand binding domain it is possible that some of these receptors may be regulated in a solely ligand-independent manner.[19,186]

The subfamilies of nuclear hormone receptors can be classified based on their dimerization partners and specific HRE recognized by the receptors.[112,163] This classification method groups the steroid hormones in class I and the metabolic sensors in class II, while the orphans are in classes III and IV (Table 6.2). As metabolic sensors, the class II receptors are involved in metabolic pathways relevant to metabolic diseases and will be discussed in the most detail. However members of the other classes also regulate metabolism and will be discussed as examples for their class. In this text the common receptor names are used. However all the receptors have been given official names, which split the receptors into seven groups, NR0 through NR6 based on their DNA binding domain sequence.[126] The receptors are then further divided into subfamilies denoted by a letter and isotype denoted by a number; for example, the official name of peroxisome proliferator activated receptor (PPAR) gamma is NR1B3, where B refers to the PPAR subfamily, and 3 refers to the gamma isotype.

Class I Receptors – the Classic Nuclear Hormone Receptors

The class I nuclear hormone receptors comprise the receptors that are activated by steroid hormones, such as estrogen, androgen, and glucocorticoids. The class I receptors, by definition, form homodimers that bind to inverted repeats (IR) of the HREs. These receptors mediate the numerous physiological responses to steroid hormones, not only

Table 6.2 Nuclear hormone receptor classes

Class I	Class II	Class III	Class IV
Response element			
5'-AGAACA Almost always inverted repeats, IR-3	5'-AGGTCA Mostly direct repeat DR-1, DR-2, DR-3, DR-4, DR-5 or IR-0, IR-1	5'-AGGTCA Mostly direct repeat, bind inverted repeats	5'-A $^{T}_{A}$ C $^{T}_{A}$ AGGTCA Extended half-site also with flanking AT rich sequences
Dimerization			
Homodimer	Heterodimer	Homodimer	Monomer
Ligand			
Steroid Hormones	Non-Steroid hormones and other Lipid Metabolites	Unknown	Unknown
Structure			

by the direct transcriptional activation of target genes and the indirect downstream effects of the gene products, but also by modulation of other transcription factors. The glucocorticoid receptor was the first receptor to be identified, followed quickly by the estrogen receptor.[65,115,181,188] Due to its essential role in glucose metabolism, the glucocorticoid receptor will be discussed as an example of this class.

The glucocorticoid receptor (GR) regulates enzymes involved in glucose metabolism and protects from glucose deficiency during the fasted state. Activation of GR by glucocorticoids, such as cortisol, results in a myriad of responses in many different tissues all geared toward ensuring that the plasma glucose levels remain sufficient to support brain function. Glucose is spared in the peripheral tissues, which preferentially use alternative energy sources such as amino acids and triglycerides (TGs). Increased protein degradation and lipolysis in peripheral tissues lead to increased release of gluconeogenic substrates, such as glycerol and amino acids, from these tissues. These gluconeogenic substrates are then taken up by the liver, in which the rate of gluconeogensis and glycogen storage are increased in response to GR activation.

In the basal inactive state, GR resides in the cytosol bound to heat shock proteins.[77] Ligand binding induces a conformational change that causes the receptor to disassociate from the heat shock proteins and form a homodimer. This conformational change also exposes a nuclear localization signal in the ligand binding domain, facilitating the transport of the homodimer into the nucleus, where it binds to glucocorticoid response elements (GRE) in GR target gene promoters. Once in the nucleus, GR can bind DNA and mediate the transcription of its target genes, such as the gluconeogenic enzyme phosphoenolpyruvate carboxykinase (PEPCK).[77]

The anti-inflammatory effects of glucocorticoids, which have proven to be therapeutically valuable, are also mediated by GR. In addition to directly inducing transcription of anti-inflammatory genes, such as lipocortin-1 and secretory leukocyte protease inhibitor (SLPI), GR also inhibits pro-inflammatory transcription factors such as nuclear factor-kappaB (NF-kappaB) and activator protein-1 (AP-1).[12] This so-called transrepression by GR does not involve its DNA binding or dimerization, as mutant receptors deficient in these functions retain their transrepression abilities.[140] Although GR is a much stronger inmmunosuppressor compared to other receptors, it is not a drug candidate for metabolic diseases due to adverse effects, such as induction of hepatic gluconeogenesis.

Class II – the Metabolic Sensors

The discovery of the nuclear hormone receptor superfamily was celebrated as a break through in endocrinology. However, the subsequent adoption of orphan receptors by metabolites of fats and other nutrients made it increasingly obvious that this superfamily also plays a crucial role in the field of metabolism. The nuclear hormone receptors that are stimulated by metabolites mostly fall into the second class of the superfamily. Class II receptors form heterodimers with retinoid X receptor (RXR), also a class II receptor.[163] There are two types of heterodimers, permissive and nonpermissive, which are, respectively, responsive and nonresponsive to RXR ligand activation.[50] The response elements for class II receptors are mostly direct repeats (DR) which create directionality of the heterodimer on the promoter. IRs have also been identified in class II response elements. This section introduces seven class II subfamilies and illustrates the role they play in metabolism.

The first nuclear hormone receptors to be identified as metabolic sensors were members of the PPAR subfamily. Although the PPARs were named based on their activation in response to molecules that promote peroxisome proliferation in rodents, the PPARs are potently activated by fatty acids, especially polyunsaturated fatty acids such as specific ecosanoids derived from aracadonic acid.[46,48,81,83,86] The PPAR response element is a direct repeat separated by one nucleotide (DR-1). There are three forms of PPAR: PPARalpha, PPARbeta-delta, and PPARgamma.[36] PPARalpha coordinates fat mobilization by enhancing the genes involved in beta oxidation.[35,138] PPARgamma promotes fat storage by promoting adipocyte differentiation and fatty acid uptake.[11,38,145] PPARbeta was discovered in Xenopus.[36] The third form of PPAR identified in the mouse was named PPARdelta due to insufficient homology to Xenopus PPARbeta.[72] However, the third PPAR isotype in chickens shares substantial homology with both PPAR beta and PPAR delta suggesting that the two isoforms are in fact homologous.[34] We will refer only to PPARdelta, whose role is less well defined than that of the alpha and gamma isotypes.

PPARalpha is expressed in the liver, heart, muscle, and kidney, where it regulates fat catabolism, especially in the fasted state.[35] In the liver, PPARalpha regulates the expression genes involved in multiple steps in fatty acid utilization. Direct targets of PPARalpha include fatty acid binding protein (FABP), acyl-CoA oxidase, and cytochrome p450s (e.g., cytochrome p450 4a (cyp 4a)), the enzymes, respectively, responsible for fatty acid uptake, the first committed step of beta-oxidation and omega-oxidation.[2,119,148,190] In addition, through its effects on apolipoprotein B (apoB) containing lipoprotein particle assembly in the liver, PPARalpha indirectly regulates fatty acid utilization in tissues where it is not expressed. Apolipoprotein CIII (apoCIII) is down regulated by PPARalpha, which relieves the inhibition apoCIII exerts on lipoprotein lipase (LPL), thereby increasing fatty acid uptake in peripheral tissues.[89,93] Although PPARalpha knockout mice have no obvious phenotype on a normal diet, when fasted they develop sever hypoglycermia and hypoketonemia accompanied by elevated plasma levels of nonesterified fatty acids.[80,100] The inability of PPARalpha knockout mice to increase fatty acid uptake and oxidation in the liver reflects the importance of this receptor in increasing the utilization of fats during the fasted state.

Although the adaptive response of the liver and heart to fasting is severely compromised in PPARalpha knockout mice, the adaptive response of muscle remains intact.[120] PPARdelta, which is expressed at higher levels in the muscle than PPARalpha, may be responsible for the adaptive response in muscle.[120,149] PPARdelta also targets genes involved in fatty acid oxidation such as medium-chain acyl-CoA dehydrogenase (MCAD).[57] PPARdelta appears to be an important regulator of hepatic metabolism, muscle endurance, and reverse cholesterol transport. Elucidating the pathways and genes regulated by PPARdelta has been difficult due to its ubiquitous expression[21] and activities in both repression and activation of target genes. In the absence of ligand, PPARdelta binds to its response element on target genes and represses their expression.[95] Upon ligand binding, PPARdelta changes conformation and recruits co-activators resulting in increased target gene expression. The importance of PPARdelta regulated repression confuses the results of PPARdelta knockout and over expression experiments. Knockout of PPARdelta not only prevents PPARdelta-mediated stimulation of target gene expression, but also removes the effects of PPARdelta-mediated target gene repression. Thus the net effect of PPARdelta knockout depends on the relative repression and activation mediated by PPARdelta under normal conditions. Therefore, PPARdelta knockout leads to decreased expression of some PPARdelta target genes, while other target genes exhibit increased expression.[95] For instance, both PPARdelta knockout[10,139] and ligand treatment result in reduced adipose tissue mass.[163,186] Similarly, ligand intervention and macrophage-specific knockout generated by bone marrow transplant in low density lipoprotein (LDL) receptor (LDLR) knockout mice result in reduced atherosclerotic lesion size, both of which were mediated, in part, by suppression of inflammation.[53,94] The importance of PPARdelta in muscle fatty acid metabolism is revealed by muscle specific over expression of an active form of PPARdelta, which is devoid of the repressive activity and results in an increase in oxidative myofibrils and increased fatty acid catabolism.[107,187]

Many synthetic PPARdelta specific ligands have been developed, providing the opportunity to study PPARdelta targets via ligand activation. PPARdelta specific synthetic ligand GW501516 has been shown to protect mice from obesity.[168,186] Treatment of the obese db/db mouse with synthetic ligand results in improved insulin sensitivity accompanied by lowered fasting glucose, hepatic glucose output, and free fatty acid (FFA) release from adipocytes.[96] PPARdelta specific synthetic ligand treatment in primates results in increased high density lipoprotein (HDL) but has not been show to protect from obesity.[128,180] In both the obese rhesus monkey and the vervet monkey model of atherosclerosis, ligand treatment increases HDL-cholesterol (HDL-c) and apolipoprotein AI (apoAI) levels. These results in primates are especially promising for human studies, as the cholesterol transport system in monkeys more closely resembles that of humans. Studies of human population genetics also indicate that PPARdelta may be an important target for treating metabolic disease. PPARdelta haplotype has been associated with body mass index (BMI). A specific single nucleotide polymorphism (SNP) has been associated with plasma glucose levels in addition to BMI.[154] A different SNP has been associated with increased LDL-cholesterol and total ApoB levels.[156]

PPARgamma is expressed most highly in adipocytes and macrophages and controls adipocyte differentiation, fat storage, and insulin sensitivity.[21,99,171] In vitro over expression of PPARgamma is sufficient to drive adipocyte differentiation.[145] PPARgamma activation plays an important role in adipocyte differentiation and maintenance in vivo.[11,59,88,145,167] Target genes of PPARgamma include the adipocyte P2 (Ap2), FABP, and other genes involved in fatty acid uptake by adipocytes.[94,171] However, it is PPARgamma's role in glucose metabolism that has made it famous. TZDs are synthetic PPARgamma ligands and have proven to be a very effective treatment for insulin resistance in type II diabetes.[159] As discussed above, PPARgamma activation results in fatty acid storage and reduced plasma levels of fatty acids and glucose. However, these effects alone do not explain the robust increase in insulin sensitivity seen with the TZD drugs. Since the muscle is the major site of glucose utilization, PPARgamma is suspected of having a direct or possibly indirect role in glucose uptake in muscle cells. In fact, muscle-specific PPARgamma knock out mice developed insulin resistance supporting its role in muscle glucose metabolism.[62]

PPARgamma is also known to play a role in macrophage lipid metabolism and inflammatory response.[143] When the PPARgamma gene is deleted, macrophages exhibit defects in cholesterol efflux.[26] The underlying mechanism is believed to be mediated by a transcriptional cascade. When macrophages take up oxidized LDL particles, the oxidized lipids act as ligands for PPARgamma.[102,121,173] PPARgamma then stimulates the transcription of the liver X receptor alpha (LXRalpha), which in turn increases the transcription of ATP-binding cassette A1 (ABCA1) and ABCG1, which catalyze the export of cholesterol from the macrophage to lipid poor apoAI and HDL particles, respectively.[29,143,176] The importance of PPARgamma in macrophage lipid handling has been demonstrated in the LDLR$^{-/-}$ mouse model of atheroscelerosis. When the bone marrow of an LDLR$^{-/-}$ mouse is replaced with bone marrow from a PPARgamma$^{-/-}$ mouse, an increase in the lesion size is observed.[26] Conversely, when LDLR$^{-/-}$ are treated with PPARgamma specific ligands, TZDs, a decrease in the lesion size is observed.[102]

The LXRs are master regulators of cholesterol homeostasis, effecting cholesterol conversion into bile acids and direct export from the liver into bile acids, as well as cholesterol efflux in peripheral tissues.[136,172] Oxysterols, metabolites of cholesterol, act as LXR ligands, activating LXR when intracellular cholesterol levels are high.[75,97] The LXR response element (LXRE) is a direct repeat separated by four nucleotides (DR-4). There are two forms of LXR: alpha and beta. LXRalpha is predominantly expressed in the liver, adipose tissue, and macrophages, while LXRbeta is ubiquitously expressed.[141] When challenged with a cholesterol rich diet, LXRalpha knockout mice accumulate cholesterol esters in their liver and have an increased rate of plaque formation.[136,169] The LXRbeta knockout mice have a normal phenotype indicating that LXRalpha is the dominant player in the liver.[1] LXRalpha and LXRbeta macrophage specific double knockout, developed by bone marrow transplantation, displays increased rates of lesion formation, highlighting the importance of LXR regulation of cholesterol homeostasis within macrophages.[169] In addition to increasing cholesterol export, LXR also appears to play an important role in mitigating macrophage inflammation. Although the mechanism remains elusive, in vitro studies of macrophages exposed to LXR ligands show down regulation of inflammatory proteins such as interleukin-6 (IL-6), inducible nitric oxide synthase (iNOS), and cyclooxygenase-2 (COX-2).[76]

In the liver, through oxysterols LXR senses cholesterol status and protects the liver from cholesterol overload by increasing the transcription of genes involved in pathways that reduce hepatic cholesterol, such as cholesterol degradation through bile acid synthesis. The first and rate limiting step in the classical bile acid synthesis pathway is catalyzed by Cyp7a. When an LXRE was discovered in the murine Cyp7a promoter, much excitement was generated about targeting LXR with agonists to increase cholesterol excretion through bile acids.[136] However, the LXRE is not contained within the human Cyp7a promoter, perhaps one of the reasons mice have a higher tolerance than humans for diets rich in cholesterol.[27] Many of the ABC proteins involved in cholesterol metabolism contain LXREs in their promoters in humans as well as mice. As mentioned earlier, the ABCG1 transporter of cholesterol to HDL is induced by LXR in the liver as well as in macrophages.[122] Expression of both ABCG5 and ABCG8 is induced in the liver and intestine by LXR.[194] The functional heterodimer formed by ABCG5 and ABCG8 functions to export indigestible plant sterols from enterocytes in order to prevent their absorption. This heterodimer also exports cholesterol in the intestine resulting in reduced cholesterol absorption. In the liver this heterodimer directly exports cholesterol into bile.

Multiple apolipoproteins and lipoprotein remodeling enzymes are regulated by LXR. Apolipoprotein E (apoE) is a direct LXR target in macrophages and adipose tissue but not in the liver.[153] Clearance of apoB containing apolipoproteins (e.g., LDL and chylomicron) is mediated in part by apoE which binds to LDLR with higher affinity than apoB.[31] The other apolipoproteins regulated by LXR, apoCI, apoCII, and apoCIV, are contained within a gene cluster with apoE.[109] The major lipoprotein remodeling enzymes LPL, phospholipid transfer protein (PLTP), and cholesteryl ester transfer protein (CETP) are all regulated by LXR.[22,91,106,109] The expression of LPL is stimulated by LXR in the liver and macrophages, but not in adipose tissue.[196] LPL catalyzes the hydrolysis of fatty acids in TGs from the glycerol backbone, assisting in the uptake of fatty acids from lipoprotein particles.[51] PLTP assists in the formation of HDL particles by transferring phospholipids from apoB containing lipoprotein particles to apoAI containing apolipoproteins.[44,74] Lipid transfer between HDL particles is also mediated by PLTP. CETP is also an important mediator of HDL metabolism. Secreted from the liver, CETP circulates bound to HDL and catalyzes the transfer of cholesterol from HDL to very low density lipoprotein (VLDL) in exchange for TGs.[13,27]

In addition to its effects on cholesterol metabolism, LXR also effects fatty acid and glucose metabolism. LXR down regulates genes involved in gluconeogenesis, such as PEPCK and glucose-6-phosphatase (G6Pase), while concurrently increasing glucose utilization by increasing transcription of glucokinase.[41,55,162] Recently, LXR has been shown to bind glucose, however, more studies are required to determine the biological significance of this glucose sensing activity.[117] Stimulation of LXR activity results in a profound increase in hepatic lipogenesis through increased expression of sterol-regulatory element-binding protein (SREBP)-1c, fatty acid synthase (FAS), acetyl-CoA carboxylase (ACC), and stearoyl-CoA desaturase 1 (SCD1).[131,136,193] It is possible that increased lipogenesis increases the availability of fatty acids with which cholesterol can form an ester. Cholesteryl esters are highly lipophilic and can be exported in lipoprotein cores. Nevertheless, this unwanted side effect has raised the concern that LXR agonists may reduce cholesterol levels at the expense of steatosis.

While LXR senses the cholesterol status of the liver and protects it from cholesterol overload, farnesoid X receptor (FXR) is a sensor for bile acid status and protects the liver from bile acid toxicity. Bile acid products such as chenodeoxycholic acid and lithocholic acid stimulate FXR, thus linking its activation to bile acid status.[111,135,183] The FXR response element (FXRE) has been characterized to consist of IRs separated by a single nucleotide (IR-1). When put on a high cholic acid diet, FXR null mice develop hepatotoxicity from excess bile acids and suffer 30% mortality within the first week.[155] The expression of FXR in the liver and intestine is consistent with its role as a major regulator of bile acid homeostasis. However, the role of FXR in the kidney and adrenal gland, where it is also expressed is unknown. [47,151] There is an additional isoform, FXRbeta, identified in mice and rats. Human FXRbeta is a nonfunctional pseudogene. Mouse FXRbeta has been shown to be weakly activated by lanosterol.[130] However, the physiological function of this isoform is unclear.

FXR activation reduces bile acid synthesis in the liver by indirectly down regulating Cyp7a. The FXR target gene, short heterodimerization partner (SHP), a nuclear receptor that lacks a DNA binding domain, forms inactive heterodimers with many of the nuclear hormone receptors.[52,105] One of the receptors SHP dimerizes with is liver receptor homolog-1 (LRH-1), a class III nuclear receptor believed to act as a competence factor for LXR, increasing the transcription of Cyp7a. However, LRH-1 transcriptional activation of Cyp7a is called in the question by data from LRH-1 heterozygous knockout mice.[134] Expression of Cyp7a increased in these animals instead of decreasing, as would be expected to result from knockout of an activator. The importance of SHP in FXR-mediated repression of Cyp7a is confirmed in SHP knockout mice, which have higher Cyp7a expression.[79,184] However, these mice retain some ability to repress Cyp7a in response to bile acids, indicating that FXR also has SHP-independent mechanisms of action.

The first clue to SHP-independent FXR repression of bile acids came from studies of primary cultures of human hepatocytes. After stimulation of these cells with synthetic FXR agonist, GW4064, the most highly induced gene was Fibroblast growth factor-19 (FGF-19), which when over expressed resulted in Cyp7a repression without effecting SHP expression.[66] Analysis of the FGF-19 gene revealed an FXRE in the second intron, which when mutated caused loss of FGF-19 responsiveness to FXR. FGF-19 is a secreted protein that elicits its effect through binding FGF receptor-4 (FGFR-4) at the plasma membrane.[191] Stimulation of FGFR-4, a receptor tyrosine kinase, leads to activation of the Jun N-terminal kinase pathway and repression of Cyp7a.[32] However, the in vivo significance of FGF-19 is called into question by the fact that quantitative-polymerase chain reaction (Q-PCR) analysis of human liver samples has failed to detect FGF-19 messenger RNA.[123] Work done in mice with the FGF-19 ortholog, FGF-15, has prompted the generation of a hypothesis where FGF-19 expression is increased in the intestine after FXR stimulation by bile acids, and then FGF-19 acts as an endocrine signal binding to FGFR-4 receptors in the liver thereby reducing Cyp7a expression.[71] In support of this hypothesis FGF-19 expression has been detected in fetal intestine by in situ hybridization.[191]

In addition to reducing bile acid synthesis, FXR increases bile acid export from the liver into the lymphatic intestinal cycle. Bile is exported from the liver by the bile salt export pump (BSEP) which is a direct target gene of FXR.[7,155] In addition, the down regulation of taurocholate cotransporting polypeptide (NTCP) reduces the uptake of bile acids returning from the intestine, keeping bile acids cycling between the lymph and intestine.[33] In the intestine, FXR increases transcription of ileal bile acid binding protein (IBABP), which is responsible for bile acid reuptake and therefore reduces the excretion of bile acids.[56] It has been hypothesized that the reuptake of bile acids reduces micelle formation and therefore reduces cholesterol absorption. Although most cholesterol is believed to be absorbed in the jejunum, reduced cholesterol absorption in patients with ileal pouch-anal anastomosis indicates that the ileum does play an important role in cholesterol absorption, bolstering the reduced cholesterol absorption hypothesis.[124]

In addition to being an important regulator of bile acid metabolism, FXR also plays an important role in the regulation of fatty acid and glucose homeostasis, as indicated by the dysregulation of these systems in FXR knockout mice.[23,108,195] FXR knockout mice develop fatty liver with increased TG content accompanied by increased expression of lipogenic genes including SREBP-1c, FAS, and SCD1[108]. In this regard, FXR appears to exhibit opposing effects to those of LXR. The increase in liver TG corresponds to increased plasma TG and FFA. In addition, fasting plasma glucose levels increase with age, starting at normal levels in young mice.[108] As indicated by the rising fasting glucose levels and by glucose and insulin tolerance tests, FXR knockout mice have impaired glucose metabolism. FXR knockout mice display hepatic insulin resistance and fail to decrease glucose production in response to insulin.[195] Correspondingly, genes involved in gluconeogenesis, such as G6Pase and PEPCK, are up regulated in the knockout liver.[108,195] Insulin resistance is also observed in the peripheral tissues such as muscle and adipose tissues.[108] However, FXR is not normally expressed in muscle and only low levels of expression have been detected in adipose tissue.[108] Thus the peripheral insulin resistance observed in FXR knockout mice has been attributed to the increase in plasma FFA, which is known-cause insulin resistance.

The three subfamilies of nuclear hormone receptors discussed above, PPAR, LXR, and FXR, all form permissive heterodimers with RXR and can be activated by the RXR ligand 9-*cis* retinoic acid (9-*cis* RA).[112] The vitamin D receptor (VDR), however, forms a nonpermissive heterodimer with RXR. Although the RXR ligand does not affect the VDR:RXR heterodimer, the AF-2 domain of RXR is required, indicating that RXR activation plays an integral role in the activity of this complex.[18,170] When VDR is activated by ligand binding, the conformational change in the VDR receptor allosterically modifies RXR, converting it into that active conformation in the absence of ligand.[16] This "phantom ligand effect" allows RXR to recruit co-activators and play an active role in the heterodimer.

VDR is best known for its role in calcium homeostasis. However, this receptor is also involved in immunity and metabolism. The importance of VDR in the immune system is reflected not only in the expression of VDR in immune cells, but also the production of the active form of vitamin D, 1,25(OH)D3, by macrophages.[132,175] VDR affects immune response via its effects on T-helper cells, which direct the nature of the immune response. There are two distinct pathways of T-helper (Th) cell development: Th1 and Th2. Th1 cells produce IL-2, tumor necrosis factor-alpha (TNF-alpha), and interferon-gamma (INF-gamma), which activate cellular immunity. Th2 cells, on the other hand, secrete IL-4 and IL-10, which in addition to activating B-cell antibody production, inhibit Th1 lymphocyte development. Overactive Th1 lymphocyte development has been associated with diseases such as atherosclerosis which involves macrophage-mediated pathogenesis.[8] Activation of VDR inhibits Th1 lymphocyte development via inhibition of INF-gamma and IL-2 transcription, thereby favoring Th2 cell development.[3,28,166]

Vitamin D is derived from cholesterol and is structurally similar to many bile acids. It is therefore not surprising that some of the more hydrophobic bile acids bind to VDR.[110] In response to bile acid stimulation, VDR promotes the transcription of genes involved in bile acid detoxification (Cyp3a4 and Sult2ai) and export (Mrp3).[37,39,113] Cyp3a4 catalyzes the hydroxylation of bile acids, making them more hydrophilic and less toxic.[4] The sulfation reaction catalyzed by Sult2a1 also increases bile acid hydrophilicity and decreases toxicity.[189] These divalent, relatively hydrophilic bile acids are preferred by Mrp3, which is a basolateral bile acid transporter expressed in hepatocytes and enterocytes.[64] VDR is not unique in its effect on bile acid detoxification. Two other nuclear hormone receptors, pregnane X receptor (PXR) and constitutive androstane receptor (CAR), regulate many of the same genes and have similar effects on bile acid detoxification.[197] Like VDR, PXR can be activated by cholesterol-derived bile acids, while CAR has been shown to be stimulated by bilirubin, a component of bile, which is a breakdown product of hemoglobin.[69,161,192] Both PXR and CAR can be activated by xenobiotics and regulate the expression of genes within the Cytochrome P450 (cyp) family, which is responsible for not only detoxification of exogenous compounds, but also drug–drug interaction. The hydroxylation reactions carried out by the Cyps are also important for the metabolism of endogenous compounds, including steroid hormone degradation.

The regulation of CAR is unusual for the NRH family. CAR originally stood for constitutively active receptor.[6] When androstanes were found to be ligands, the name was changed to constitutive androstanes receptor.[49] CAR is constitutively active and androstane binding inhibits its activity, although the in vivo significance of this interaction is questionable due to the extremely low concentration of androstanes in tissues other than the testis. Due to its constitutively active nature, CAR is basally maintained in the cytosol in an inhibited state.[78] CAR activation involves two steps: translocation to the nucleus and release from inhibition. Phenobarbital induces the nuclear translocation of CAR, resulting in the up regulation of Cyp2b genes and metabolism of barbiturates and testosterone. The Phenobarbital-responsive enhancer module (PBREM) contains two nuclear receptor (NR) binding sites, NR1 and NR2.[67] CAR in a heterodimer with RXR binds to NR1 with high affinity and NR2 with lower affinity.[68] NR1 appears to be the key regulatory site, making CAR the key regulator of Phenobarbital responsiveness. Unlike CAR, PXR is localized in the nucleus and is activated by ligand binding.[165] PXR transcriptionally activates Cyp3a genes, which catalyze the hydroxylation of compounds such as glucocorticoids and macrolide antibiotics (rifampicin) in addition to bile acids.[82]

RXR is arguably the most important of the class II nuclear hormone receptor subfamilies. Permissive heterodimers are stimulated by 9-*cis* RA, which binds the RXR ligand binding pocket.[63,101] Although dietary retinal is in the all trans form, two 9-*cis*-retinol dehydrogenases have been identified which may participate in in vivo synthesis of 9-*cis*-RA.[114,144] The 9-*cis* RA isoform can also be derived from dietary 9-*cis* beta-carotene.[60,185] As the heterodimer partner, RXR is required for the functionality of all class II receptors. Since RXR is essential for so many different functions, isolating its effects has proven difficult. Liver-specific RXRalpha knock out mice show a severe metabolic phenotype, suggesting that this is the predominant isoform that heterdimerizes with other class II metabolic sensors in the liver.[182] RXRalpha null mice are embryonic lethal.[164] However, the pinkie mouse line, which harbors a single nucleotide mutation in RXRalpha, has been shown to have an exaggerated Th1 response, indicating RXRalpha involvement in the suppression of Th1 differentiation.[38,160] This effect is likely mediated by the repression of VDR and RAR, a class II nuclear hormone receptor known to suppress Th1 lymphocyte development.[3,28,73,166]

As is especially clear in the case of RXR, the nuclear hormone receptors do not function in isolation but form a complex regulatory network. Receptors may work cooperatively, as occurs in the control of macrophage cholesterol efflux, where PPARgamma activation stimulates LXR transcription.[26] Alternatively, receptors may exert opposing effects. For example, activation of LXR increases bile acid production, which will lead to the activation of FXR and suppression of cholesterol degradation/ bile acid synthesis. Based on studies in various knockout mice mentioned above, this complex regulatory network appears to be essential to maintain metabolic homeostasis of the body.

Class III and Class IV – the Orphans

Class III receptors form homodimers like class I receptors, but bind direct repeats like Class II receptors. Class IV receptors act as monomers and bind extended core sties. While Class I receptors bind steroid hormones, and Class II receptors bind metabolites of nutrients, no pattern has yet emerged for the ligands of Class III or Class IV nuclear receptors. In fact, most of these receptors are orphans with no potential ligands identified. The strictest definition of an endogenous ligand requires not only high affinity binding, but also appropriate in vivo concentrations for dynamic regulation of activity. The molecules that have been proposed to bind Class III and Class IV receptors fall short of the definition of an endogenous ligand. These molecules may play an important endogenous role other than activation. One possibility is that these molecules stabilize the receptor. This seems most plausible for the Class IV receptors, which function as monomers, and therefore are not stabilized by dimerization. Another possibility that cannot be excluded is that Class III and Class IV receptors are regulated by means other than ligand binding and have no endogenous ligand. It has been suggested that ancient orphan receptors may have evolved to acquire ligand-mediated activation.[42,43]

Hepatic nuclear factor-4 (HNF-4) is a Class III nuclear hormone receptor.[158] There are two isotypes: HNF-4alpha and HNF-4gamma.[20,25] However, HNF-4alpha has been studied more extensively. HNF-4alpha is expressed in the liver, small intestine and pancreatic beta-cells where it regulates both lipid and glucose metabolism.[158] In the liver, HNF-4alpha transcriptionally up regulates apoA1, the most abundant apolipoprotein in HDL, and an important player in reverse cholesterol transport.[58] HNF-4alpha also regulates other apolipoproteins, including apoCIII and apoAIV[5,90] and genes involved in bile acid formation (cyp7a, cyp8b),[30,32] lipid homeostasis, and glucose production.[98]

Mutations in HNF-4alpha result in type 1 mature onset diabetes of the young (MODY1) due to the importance of HNF-4alpha in the regulation of insulin transcription in pancreatic beta-cells.[147] MODY is characterized by impaired insulin production with normal insulin sensitivity and is usually noninsulin requiring at the time of diagnosis.[133] HNF-4alpha does not directly bind the insulin promoter but interacts with other transcription factors such as HNF-1alpha, which binds the insulin promoter directly[40] HNF-4alpha acts as a co-activator of HNF-1alpha increasing the transcription of HNF-1alpha target genes upon binding. MODY has also been attributed to mutations in HNF-1alpha.[147] The importance of the HNF-4apha/HNF-1alpha interaction has been illuminated by the investigation of HNF-4alpha mutations that cause MODY1. One such mutant, HNF-4alpha R127W, retains its ability to directly activate gene transcription and bind HNF-1alpha, but is unable to act as a co-activator for HNF-1alpha.[146]

In vitro binding assays show fatty acyl-CoA thioesters binding to HNF-4alpha, although the in vivo significance of this interaction is questionable.[19,61,157] Conversely, there is strong evidence that phospholipids bind to and stimulate the Class IV nuclear hormone receptor, LRH-1.[87,103,129] The phospholipid concentration in the nucleus is far higher than the K_m, which although consistent with the constitutive activity of LRH-1, falls short of the definition of an endogenous ligand, because there is no dynamic regulation.[45,70] The importance of phospholipid binding in vivo may be stabilization and not activation. LRH-1 is constitutively active, but is regulated by the dynamic availability of inactivating heterodimer partners such as SHP. Thus, it is plausible that LRH-1 is stabilized by phospholipid binding to the ligand pocket, but achieves dynamic regulation via dimerization.

Nuclear Receptors as Potential Therapeutic Targets for Metabolic Diseases

Metabolic syndrome is a collection of obesity-related metabolic dysfunctions, including hyperlipidemia, decreased HDL-c, insulin resistance, hypertension, and atherosclerosis. Given their roles in regulating key metabolic pathways, nuclear hormone receptors are current and prospective drug targets to treat these diseases. One reason for the success of nuclear receptor targeted drugs is their ability to have a robust effect on a pathway due to the regulation of multiple target genes within that pathway. Of course the multifaceted effects of nuclear hormone receptors can also be a drawback, when undesirable side effects are the result.

Cholesterol has earned a reputation as the malefactor of atherosclerosis and is a central target of many atherosclerosis reducing drugs, such as statins which inhibit HMG-CoA reductace, the enzyme that catalyzes the rate limiting step in cholesterol synthesis. In addition to reducing total cholesterol, it is desirable to increase the number of HDL particles, which serve as cholesterol janitors removing excess cholesterol from peripheral tissues. The most important class of cholesterol to reduce is LDL cholesterol, especially, smaller LDL particles, which enter to intima more easily and are more susceptible to oxidation.[17,125,174] An attractive target for reducing cholesterol is LXR, a receptor that has evolved to protect the liver from cholesterol overload. An LXR agonist could increase bile acid export from the liver and reduce cholesterol absorption in the gut, thereby reducing total cholesterol.[172,194] LXR also suppresses macrophage foam cell formation through increased cholesterol efflux and HDL-c (discussed below).[169] One of the concerns over using LXR agonists in humans is the differential regulation of Cyp7a and CETP. In humans, LXR does not suppress Cyp7a while inducing the expression of CETP, which removes cholesterol from the anti-atherogenic HDL and transfers it to the pro-atherogenic VLDL.[27,106,127] The greatest disadvantage of LXR agonism is increased lipogenesis, which may result in steatosis and increased TG levels.[136] Since LXRbeta plays a minor role in the liver, a selective LXRbeta agonist may not cause steatosis. Alternatively, an intestinal selective agonist may reduce cholesterol absorption and protect from atherosclerosis.

Both FXR agonists and antagonists have been proposed as potential cholesterol lowering drugs. An FXR antagonist is desirable to increase the conversion of cholesterol into bile acids, a pathway that is inhibited by FXR.[52,105] However, FXR stimulation by an agonist would increase bile acid export and excretion, thereby reducing total cholesterol.[7] The FXR knockout mouse indicates that FXR antagonism may have undesirable side effects, such as development of fatty liver and insulin resistance, while FXR agonism may have the opposite desirable affects: lowering circulating lipid levels and increasing insulin sensitivity.[23,195]

Lowering TG and fatty acids is an important factor in treating the dyslipidemia that often leads to insulin resistance.[24] The PPARs are master regulators of fatty acid metabolism and are therefore very attractive therapeutic targets for treating hypertriglyceridemia. Fibrates, drugs that are already in use for the treatment of dislipidemia, stimulate PPARalpha, which results in increased fatty acid oxidation and reduced fatty acid synthesis.[179]

Fatty acid oxidation, especially in muscle may also be increased by PPARdelta.[120] Results in mice indicate that activation of PPARdelta protects from obesity.[107] Although this effect has not been observed in primate studies, epidemiological studies have shown a correlation between obesity and certain nucleotide polymorphisms in PPARdelta.[154,156] A robust increase in HDL-c has been seen in primate studies, indicating that PPARdelta activation may also have beneficial effects on improving lipoprotein profile and suppressing atherosclerotic lesion progression.[128,180] Synthetic PPARdelta agonists are currently in clinical trials for treatment of dislipidemia. If there is an effect on body weight in humans, it should become evident in these trials. Weight loss stimulated by PPARdelta synthetic ligand treatment is likely mediated by increased peripheral fatty acid oxidation, which also contributes to improvement in insulin sensitivity.

Due to its essential role in adipocyte differentiation and maintenance, PPARgamma antagonist are alluring anti-obesity drugs. However, if fatty acids are not stored in adipocytes, they will accumulate elsewhere. Increased plasma FFAs in addition to other mechanisms will most likely lead to insulin resistance upon PPARgamma inhibition. In addition to increasing insulin sensitivity, PPARgamma agonism has other desirable effects, such as suppression of inflammatory response and stimulation of LXR transcription in macrophages, both of which reduce the risk of developing atherosclerosis.[26,143] Activation of LXR via synthetic ligand increases the expression of the cholesterol transporters ABCA1 and ABCG1, thereby increasing cholesterol efflux to HDL.[29,142,150,176,177] In addition, LXR stimulates expression of apoE in the macrophage.[92] The importance of apoE-mediated lipoprotein uptake is highlighted in the apoE knockout mouse which spontaneously develops atherosclerosis, even on normal chow.[31] Reintroduction of apoE into only macrophages protects from atherosclerosis, indicating the importance of macrophage apoE expression.[14,104]

In addition to effects on cholesterol metabolism, LXR ligand stimulation reduces inflammation, further protecting from the development of foam cells.[76] The VDR is also a potential target for reducing atherogenic inflammation. Activation of VDR has been shown to promote the development of lymphocytes into Th2 cells over Th1 cells.[3,28,166] Since the cytokines released by Th1 cells are especially atherogenic, VDR activation may reduce atherogensis. Although the immunological effects of VDR are relatively weak, epidemiological evidence support the importance of vitamin D. Risk of coronary heart disease is decreased in southern Europe and at higher altitude in America, areas where sunlight exposure is higher.[55,118,178]

Vitamin A may also be an important nutrient due to the stimulation of RXR by the vitamin A metabolite 9-*cis* RA. Stimulation of many of the permissive class II subfamilies (PPAR, LXR and FXR) through RXR would have a beneficial effect on reducing the metabolic syndrome. Beta-carotene (BC) compounds naturally occurring in the 9-*cis* conformation are hydrolyzed to 9-*cis* RA and have been shown to increase the effectiveness of fibrates.[152] In one study, 22 subjects on fibrates treatment were divided into a placebo and 9-*cis* BC treatment group.[152] A statistically significant increase in HDL and decrease in TG in subjects receiving 9-*cis* BC relative to those receiving placebo was observed.[152]

Conclusion

The discovery of dietary lipids as ligands for some of the nuclear receptors has provided a unique opportunity to study metabolic regulation at the transcriptional level and a molecular basis for developing drugs to treat metabolic diseases. Agonists of PPARs have already been used to control levels of circulating lipids and insulin sensitivity. Other potential therapeutic benefits include weight loss, increased HDL-c, and suppression of inflammation. LXR and FXR are novel targets to modulate blood cholesterol and glucose homeostasis. Other orphan receptors such as estrogen receptor-related receptors (ERRs), which regulate oxidative phosphorylation in muscle and whose activities can be modulated by synthetic compounds, also show promise in treating metabolic diseases. Recently, the NURR subfamily has been shown to play an important role in the hepatic glucogenic pathway.[137] Although no ligand has been found for members of this subfamily, their expression is under the control of hormonal regulation. Lastly, about half of the nuclear receptor family members still lack endogenous or synthetic agonists. There is no doubt that the continuation of ligand search combined with studies in knockout mice will lead to discoveries of new roles for the receptors in metabolism and likely many other important biological processes.

References

1. Alberti S, Schuster G, Parini P, Feltkamp D, Diczfalusy U, Rudling M, Angelin B, Bjorkhem I, Pettersson S, Gustafsson JA. Hepatic cholesterol metabolism and resistance to dietary cholesterol in LXRbeta-deficient mice. J Clin Invest 2001;107(5):565–573.
2. Aldridge TC, Tugwood JD, Green S. Identification and characterization of DNA elements implicated in the regulation of CYP4A1 transcription. Biochem J 1995;306(Pt 2):473–479.
3. Alroy I, Towers TL, Freedman LP. Transcriptional repression of the interleukin-2 gene by vitamin D3: direct inhibition of NFATp/AP-1 complex formation by a nuclear hormone receptor. Mol Cell Biol 1995;15(10):5789–5799.
4. Araya Z, Wikvall K. 6alpha-hydroxylation of taurochenodeoxycholic acid and lithocholic acid by CYP3A4 in human liver microsomes. Biochim Biophys Acta 1999;1438(1):47–54.
5. Archer A, Sauvaget D, Chauffeton V, Bouchet PE, Chambaz J, Pincon-Raymond M, Cardot P, Ribeiro A, Lacasa M. Intestinal apolipoprotein A-IV gene transcription is controlled by two hormone-responsive elements: a role for hepatic nuclear factor-4 isoforms. Mol Endocrinol 2005;19(9):2320–2334.

6. Baes M, Gulick T, Choi HS, Martinoli MG, Simha D, Moore DD. A new orphan member of the nuclear hormone receptor superfamily that interacts with a subset of retinoic acid response elements. Mol Cell Biol 1994;14(3):1544–1552.
7. Bahar RJ, Stolz A. Bile acid transport. Gastroenterol Clin North Am 1999;28(1):27–58.
8. Baidya SG, Zeng QT. Helper T cells and atherosclerosis: the cytokine web. Postgrad Med J 2005;81(962):746–752.
9. Baker KD, Shewchuk LM, Kozlova T, Makishima M, Hassell A, Wisely B, Caravella JA, Lambert MH, Reinking JL, Krause H, Thummel CS, Willson TM, Mangelsdort DJ. The Drosophila orphan nuclear receptor DHR38 mediates an a typical ecdysteriod signalling pathway. Cell 2003;113(6):731–742.
10. Barak Y, Liao D, He W, Ong ES, Nelson MC, Olefsky JM, Boland R, Evans RM. Effects of peroxisome proliferator-activated receptor delta on placentation, adiposity, and colorectal cancer. Proc Natl Acad Sci USA 2002;99(1):303–308.
11. Barak Y, Nelson MC, Ong ES, Jones YZ, Ruiz-Lozano P, Chien KR, Koder A, Evans RM. PPAR gamma is required for placental, cardiac, and adipose tissue development. Mol Cell 1999;4(4):585–595.
12. Barnes PJ, Karin M. Nuclear factor-kappaB: a pivotal transcription factor in chronic inflammatory diseases. N Engl J Med 1997;336(15):1066–1071.
13. Barter, P. CETP and atherosclerosis. Arterioscler Thromb Vasc Biol 2000;20(9):2029–2031.
14. Bellosta S, Mahley RW, Sanan DA, Murata J, Newland DL, Taylor JM, Pitas RE. Macrophage-specific expression of human apolipoprotein E reduces atherosclerosis in hypercholesterolemic apolipoprotein E-null mice. J Clin Invest 1995;96(5):2170–2179.
15. Berg JM. DNA binding specificity of steroid receptors. Cell 1989;57(7):1065–1068.
16. Bettoun DJ, Burris TP, Houck KA, Buck 2nd, DW, Stayrook KR, Khalifa B, Lu J, Chin WW, Nagpal S. Retinoid X receptor is a nonsilent major contributor to vitamin D receptor-mediated transcriptional activation. Mol Endocrinol 2003;17(11):2320–2328.
17. Bjornheden T, Babyi A, Bondjers G, Wiklund O. Accumulation of lipoprotein fractions and subfractions in the arterial wall, determined in an in vitro perfusion system. Atherosclerosis 1996;123(1-2):43–56.
18. Blanco JC, Dey A, Leid M, Minucci S, Park BK, Jurutka PW, Haussler MR, Ozato K. Inhibition of ligand induced promoter occupancy in vivo by a dominant negative RXR. Genes Cells 1996;1(2):209–221.
19. Bogan AA, Dallas-Yang Q, Ruse Jr MD, Maeda Y, Jiang G, Nepomuceno L, Scanlan TS, Cohen FE, Sladek FM. Analysis of protein dimerization and ligand binding of orphan receptor HNF4alpha. J Mol Bio 2000;302(4):831–851.
20. Boj SF, Parrizas M, Maestro MA, Ferrer J. A transcription factor regulatory circuit in differentiated pancreatic cells. Proc Natl Acad Sci USA 2001;98(25):14481–14486.
21. Braissant O, Foufelle F, Scotto C, Dauca M, Wahli W. Differential expression of peroxisome proliferator-activated receptors (PPARs): tissue distribution of PPAR-alpha, -beta, and -gamma in the adult rat. Endocrinology 1996;137(1):354–366.
22. Cao G, Beyer TP, Yang XP, Schmidt RJ, Zhang Y, Bensch WR, Kauffman RF, Gao H, Ryan TP, Liang Y, Eacho PI, Jiang XC. Phospholipid transfer protein is regulated by liver X receptors in vivo. J Biol Chem 2002;277(42):39561–39565.
23. Cariou B, van Harmelen K, Duran-Sandoval D, van Dijk TH, Grefhorst A, Abdelkarim M, Caron S, Torpier G, Fruchart JC, Gonzalez FJ, Kuipers F, Staels B. The farnesoid X receptor modulates adiposity and peripheral insulin sensitivity in mice. J Biol Chem 2006;281(16): 11039–11049.
24. Castelli WP, Garrison RJ, Wilson PW, Abbott RD, Kalousdian S, Kannel WB. 1986. Incidence of coronary heart disease and lipoprotein cholesterol levels. The Framingham Study. JAMA 1986;256(20):2835–2838.
25. Chartier FL, Bossu JP, Laudet V, Fruchart JC, Laine B. Cloning and sequencing of cDNAs encoding the human hepatocyte nuclear factor 4 indicate the presence of two isoforms in human liver. Gene 1994;147(2):269–272.

26. Chawla A, Boisvert WA, Lee CH, Laffitte BA, Barak Y, Joseph SB, Liao D, Nagy L, Edwards PA, Curtiss LK, Evans RM, Tontonoz P. A PPAR gamma-LXR-ABCA1 pathway in macrophages is involved in cholesterol efflux and atherogenesis. Mol Cell 2001;7(1): 161–171.

27. Chiang JY, Kimmel R, Stroup D. Regulation of cholesterol 7alpha-hydroxylase gene (CYP7A1) transcription by the liver orphan receptor (LXRalpha). Gene 2001;262(1–2):257–265.

28. Cippitelli M, Santoni A. Vitamin D3: a transcriptional modulator of the interferon-gamma gene. Eur J Immunol 1998;28(10):3017–3030.

29. Costet P, Luo Y, Wang N, Tall AR. Sterol-dependent transactivation of the ABC1 promoter by the liver X receptor/retinoid X receptor. J Biol Chem 2000;275(36):28240–28245.

30. Crestani M, Sadeghpour A, Stroup D, Galli G, Chiang JY. Transcriptional activation of the cholesterol 7alpha-hydroxylase gene (CYP7A) by nuclear hormone receptors. J Lipid Res 1998;39(11):2192–2200.

31. Curtiss LK, Boisvert WA. Apolipoprotein E and atherosclerosis. Curr Opin Lipidol 2000;11(3):243–251.

32. De Fabiani E, Mitro N, Anzulovich AC, Pinelli A, Galli G, Crestani M. The negative effects of bile acids and tumor necrosis factor-alpha on the transcription of cholesterol 7alpha-hydroxylase gene (CYP7A1) converge to hepatic nuclear factor-4: a novel mechanism of feedback regulation of bile acid synthesis mediated by nuclear receptors. J Biol Chem 2001;276(33):30708–30716.

33. Denson LA, Sturm E, Echevarria W, Zimmerman TL, Makishima M, Mangelsdorf DJ, Karpen SJ. The orphan nuclear receptor, shp, mediates bile acid-induced inhibition of the rat bile acid transporter, ntcp. Gastroenterology 2001;121(1):140–147.

34. Desvergne B, Wahli W. Peroxisome proliferator-activated receptors: nuclear control of metabolism. Endocr Rev 1999;20(5):649–688.

35. Dreyer C, Keller H, Mahfoudi A, Laudet V, Krey G, Wahli W. Positive regulation of the peroxisomal beta-oxidation pathway by fatty acids through activation of peroxisome proliferator-activated receptors (PPAR). Biol Cell 1993;77(1):67–76.

36. Dreyer C, Krey G, Keller H, Givel F, Helftenbein G, Wahli W. Control of the peroxisomal beta-oxidation pathway by a novel family of nuclear hormone receptors. Cell 1992;68(5): 879–887.

37. Drocourt L, Ourlin JC, Pascussi JM, Maurel P, Vilarem MJ. Expression of CYP3A4, CYP2B6, and CYP2C9 is regulated by the vitamin D receptor pathway in primary human hepatocytes. J Biol Chem 2002;277(28):25125–25132.

38. Du X, Tabeta K, Mann N, Crozat K, Mudd S, Beutler B. An essential role for Rxr alpha in the development of Th2 responses. Eur J Immunol 2005;35(12):3414–3423.

39. Echchgadda I, Song CS, Roy AK, Chatterjee B. Dehydroepiandrosterone sulfotransferase is a target for transcriptional induction by the vitamin D receptor. Mol Pharmacol 2004;65(3): 720–729.

40. Eeckhoute J, Formstecher P, Laine B. Hepatocyte nuclear factor 4alpha enhances the hepatocyte nuclear factor 1alpha-mediated activation of transcription. Nucleic Acids Res 2004;32(8): 2586–2593.

41. Efanov AM, Barrett DG, Brenner MB, Briggs SL, Delaunois A, Durbin JD, Giese U, Guo H, Radloff M, Gil GS, Sewing S, Wang Y, Weichert A, Zaliani A, Gromada J. A novel glucokinase activator modulates pancreatic islet and hepatocyte function. Endocrinology 2005;146(9): 3696–3701.

42. Escriva H, Delaunay F, Laudet V. Ligand binding and nuclear receptor evolution. Bioessays 2000;22(8):717–727.

43. Escriva H, Safi R, Hanni C, Langlois MC, Saumitou-Laprade P, Stehelin D, Capron A, Pierce R, Laudet V. Ligand binding was acquired during evolution of nuclear receptors. Proc Natl Acad Sci USA 1997;94(13):6803–6808.

44. Foger B, Santamarina-Fojo S, Shamburek RD, Parrot CL, Talley GD, Brewer Jr HB, Plasma phospholipid transfer protein. Adenovirus-mediated overexpression in mice leads

to decreased plasma high density lipoprotein (HDL) and enhanced hepatic uptake of phospholipids and cholesteryl esters from HDL. J Biol Chem 1997;272(43):27393–27400.

45. Forman BM. Are those phospholipids in your pocket? Cell Metab 2005;1(3):153–155.

46. Forman BM, Chen J, Evans RM. Hypolipidemic drugs, polyunsaturated fatty acids, and eicosanoids are ligands for peroxisome proliferator-activated receptors alpha and delta. Proc Natl Acad Sci USA 1997;94(9):4312–4317.

47. Forman BM, Goode E, Chen J, Oro AE, Bradley DJ, Perlmann T, Noonan DJ, Burka LT, McMorris T, Lamph WW, Evans RM, Weinberger C. Identification of a nuclear receptor that is activated by farnesol metabolites. Cell 1995;81(5):687–693.

48. Forman BM, Tontonoz P, Chen J, Brun RP, Spiegelman BM, Evans RM. 15-Deoxy-delta 12, 14-prostaglandin J2 is a ligand for the adipocyte determination factor PPAR gamma. Cell 1995;83(5):803–812.

49. Forman BM, Tzameli I, Choi HS, Chen J, Simha D, Seol W, Evans RM, Moore DD. Androstane metabolites bind to and deactivate the nuclear receptor CAR-beta. Nature 1998;395(6702):612–615.

50. Forman BM, Umesono K, Chen J, Evans RM. Unique response pathways are established by allosteric interactions among nuclear hormone receptors. Cell 1995;81(4):541-550.

51. Goldberg IJ. Lipoprotein lipase and lipolysis: central roles in lipoprotein metabolism and atherogenesis. J Lipid Res 1996;37(4):693–707.

52. Goodwin B, Jones SA, Price RR, Watson MA, McKee DD, Moore LB, Galardi C, Wilson JG, Lewis MC, Roth ME, Maloney PR, Willson TM, Kliewer SA. A regulatory cascade of the nuclear receptors FXR, SHP-1, and LRH-1 represses bile acid biosynthesis. Mol Cell 2000;6(3):517–526.

53. Graham TL, Mookherjee C, Suckling KE, CN AP, Patel L. The PPARdelta agonist GW0742X reduces atherosclerosis in LDLR(–/–) mice. Atherosclerosis 2005;181(1):29–37.

54. Grefhorst A, van Dijk TH, Hammer A, van der Sluijs FH, Havinga R, Havekes LM, Romijn JA, Groot PH, Reijngoud DJ, Kuipers F. Differential effects of pharmacological liver X receptor activation on hepatic and peripheral insulin sensitivity in lean and ob/ob mice. Am J Physiol 2005;289(5):E829–E838.

55. Grimes DS, Hindle E, Dyer T. Sunlight, cholesterol and coronary heart disease. QJM 1996;89(8):579–589.

56. Grober J, Zaghini I, Fujii H, Jones SA, Kliewer SA, Willson TM, Ono T, Besnard P. Identification of a bile acid-responsive element in the human ileal bile acid-binding protein gene. Involvement of the farnesoid X receptor/9-cis-retinoic acid receptor heterodimer. J Biol Chem 1999;274(42):29749–29754.

57. Gulick T, Cresci S, Caira T, Moore DD, Kelly DP. The peroxisome proliferator-activated receptor regulates mitochondrial fatty acid oxidative enzyme gene expression. Proc Natl Acad Sci USA 1994;91(23):11012–11016.

58. Hayhurst GP, Lee YH, Lambert G, Ward JM, Gonzalez FJ. Hepatocyte nuclear factor 4alpha (nuclear receptor 2A1) is essential for maintenance of hepatic gene expression and lipid homeostasis. Mol Cell Biol 2001;21(4):1393–1403.

59. He W, Barak Y, Hevener A, Olson P, Liao D, Le J, Nelson M, Ong E, Olefsky JM, Evans RM. Adipose-specific peroxisome proliferator-activated receptor gamma knockout causes insulin resistance in fat and liver but not in muscle. Proc Natl Acad Sci USA 2003;100(26): 15712–15717.

60. Hebuterne X, Wang XD, Johnson EJ, Krinsky NI, Russell RM. Intestinal absorption and metabolism of 9-cis-beta-carotene in vivo: biosynthesis of 9-cis-retinoic acid. J Lipid Res 1995;36(6):1264–1273.

61. Hertz R, Magenheim J, Berman I, Bar-Tana J. Fatty acyl-CoA thioesters are ligands of hepatic nuclear factor-4alpha. Nature 1998;392(6675):512–516.

62. Hevener AL, He W, Barak Y, Le J, Bandyopadhyay G, Olson P, Wilkes J, Evans RM, Olefsky J. Muscle-specific Pparg deletion causes insulin resistance. Nat Med 2003;9(12): 1491–1497.

63. Heyman RA, Mangelsdorf DJ, Dyck JA, Stein RB, Eichele G, Evans RM, Thaller C. 9-cis
     retinoic acid is a high affinity ligand for the retinoid X receptor. Cell 1992;68(2):397–406.
64. Hirohashi T, Suzuki H, Sugiyama Y. Characterization of the transport properties of cloned rat
     multidrug resistance-associated protein 3 (MRP3). J Biol Chem 1999;274(21):15181–15185.
65. Hollenberg SM, Weinberger C, Ong ES, Cerelli G, Oro A, Lebo R, Thompson EB, Rosenfeld
     MG, Evans RM. Primary structure and expression of a functional human glucocorticoid
     receptor cDNA. Nature 1985;318(6047):635–641.
66. Holt JA, Luo G, Billin AN, Bisi J, McNeill YY, Kozarsky KF, Donahee M, Wang DY,
     Mansfield TA, Kliewer SA, Goodwin B, Jones SA. Definition of a novel growth factor-
     dependent signal cascade for the suppression of bile acid biosynthesis. Genes Dev
     2003;17(13):1581–1591.
67. Honkakoski P, Moore R, Washburn KA, Negishi M. Activation by diverse xenochemicals of
     the 51-base pair phenobarbital-responsive enhancer module in the CYP2B10 gene. Mol
     Pharmacol 1998;53(4):597–601.
68. Honkakoski P, Zelko I, Sueyoshi T, Negishi M. The nuclear orphan receptor CAR-retinoid X
     receptor heterodimer activates the phenobarbital-responsive enhancer module of the CYP2B
     gene. Mol Cell Biol 1998;18(10):5652–5658.
69. Huang W, Zhang J, Chua SS, Qatanani M, Han Y, Granata R, Moore DD. Induction of
     bilirubin clearance by the constitutive androstane receptor (CAR). Proc Natl Acad Sci USA
     2003;100(7):4156–4161.
70. Hunt AN, Clark GT, Attard GS, Postle AD. Highly saturated endonuclear phosphatidylcho-
     line is synthesized in situ and colocated with CDP-choline pathway enzymes. J Biol
     Chem 2001;276(11):8492–8499.
71. Inagaki T, Choi M, Moschetta A, Peng L, Cummins CL, McDonald JG, Luo G, Jones SA,
     Goodwin B, Richardson JA, Gerard RD, Repa JJ, Mangelsdorf DJ, Kliewer SA. Fibroblast
     growth factor 15 functions as an enterohepatic signal to regulate bile acid homeostasis. Cell
     Metab 2005;2(4):217–225.
72. Issemann I, Green S. Activation of a member of the steroid hormone receptor superfamily
     by peroxisome proliferators. Nature 1990;347(6294):645–650.
73. Iwata M, Eshima Y, Kagechika H. Retinoic acids exert direct effects on T cells to suppress
     Th1 development and enhance Th2 development via retinoic acid receptors. Int Immunol
     2003;15(8):1017–1025.
74. Jaari S, van Dijk KW, Olkkonen VM, van der Zee A, Metso J, Havekes L, Jauhiainen M,
     Ehnholm C. Dynamic changes in mouse lipoproteins induced by transiently expressed
     human phospholipid transfer protein (PLTP): importance of PLTP in prebeta-HDL genera-
     tion. Comp Biochem Physiol 2001;128(4): 781–792.
75. Janowski BA, Willy PJ, Devi TR, Falck JR, Mangelsdorf DJ. An oxysterol signalling pathway
     mediated by the nuclear receptor LXR alpha. Nature 1996;383(6602):728–731.
76. Joseph SB, Castrillo A, Laffitte BA, Mangelsdorf DJ, Tontonoz P. Reciprocal regulation of
     inflammation and lipid metabolism by liver X receptors. Nat Med 2003;9(2):213–219.
77. Karin M. New twists in gene regulation by glucocorticoid receptor: is DNA binding dispen-
     sable? Cell 1998;93(4):487–490.
78. Kawamoto T, Sueyoshi T, Zelko I, Moore R, Washburn K, Negishi M. Phenobarbital-responsive
     nuclear translocation of the receptor CAR in induction of the CYP2B gene. Mol Cell Biol
     1999;19(9):6318–6322.
79. Kerr TA, Saeki S, Schneider M, Schaefer K, Berdy S, Redder T, Shan B, Russell DW,
     Schwarz M. Loss of nuclear receptor SHP impairs but does not eliminate negative feedback
     regulation of bile acid synthesis. Dev Cell 2002;2(6):713–720.
80. Kersten S, Seydoux J, Peters JM, Gonzalez FJ, Desvergne B, Wahli W. Peroxisome proliferator-
     activated receptor alpha mediates the adaptive response to fasting. J Clin Invest 1999;103(11):
     1489–1498.
81. Kliewer SA, Lenhard JM, Willson TM, Patel I, Morris DC, Lehmann JM. A prostaglandin
     J2 metabolite binds peroxisome proliferator-activated receptor gamma and promotes adi-
     pocyte differentiation. Cell 1995;83(5):813–819.

82. Kliewer SA, Moore JT, Wade L, Staudinger JL, Watson MA, Jones SA, McKee DD, Oliver BB, Willson TM, Zetterstrom RH, Perlmann T, Lehmann JM. An orphan nuclear receptor activated by pregnanes defines a novel steroid signaling pathway. Cell 1998;92(1):73–82.

83. Kliewer SA, Sundseth SS, Jones SA, Brown PJ, Wisely GB, Koble CS, Devchand P, Wahli W, Willson TM, Lenhard JM, Lehmann JM. Fatty acids and eicosanoids regulate gene expression through direct interactions with peroxisome proliferator-activated receptors alpha and gamma. Proc Natl Acad Sci USA 1997;94(9):4318–4323.

84. Klug A, Schwabe JW. Protein motifs 5. Zinc fingers. Faseb J 1995;9(8):597–604.

85. Koelle MR, Talbot WS, Segraves WA, Bender MT, Cherbas P, Hogness DS. The Drosophila EcR gene encodes an ecdysone receptor, a new member of the steroid receptor superfamily. Cell 1991;67(1):59–77.

86. Krey G, Braissant O, L'Horset F, Kalkhoven E, Perroud M, Parker MG, Wahli W. Fatty acids, eicosanoids, and hypolipidemic agents identified as ligands of peroxisome proliferator-activated receptors by coactivator- dependent receptor ligand assay. Mol Endocrinol 1997;1(6):779–791.

87. Krylova IN, Sablin EP, Moore J, Xu RX, Waitt GM, MacKay JA, Juzumiene D, Bynum JM, Madauss K, Montana V, Lebedeva L, Suzawa M, Williams JD, Williams SP, Guy RK, Thornton JW, Fletterick RJ, Willson TM, Ingraham HA. Structural analyses reveal phosphatidyl inositols as ligands for the NR5 orphan receptors SF-1 and LRH-1. Cell 2005;120(3): 343–355.

88. Kubota N, Terauchi Y, Miki H, Tamemoto H, Yamauchi T, Komeda K, Satoh S, Nakano R, Ishii C, Sugiyama T, Eto K, Tsubamoto Y, Okuno A, Murakami K, Sekihara H, Hasegawa G, Naito M, Toyoshima Y, Tanaka S, Shiota K, Kitamura T, Fujita T, Ezaki O, Aizawa S, Kadowaki T, et al. 1PPAR gamma mediates high-fat diet-induced adipocyte hypertrophy and insulin resistance. Mol Cell 1999;4(4):597–609.

89. Kuo LC, Makinen MW. Hydrolysis of esters by carboxypeptidase A requires a penta-coordinate metal ion. J Biol Chem 1982;257(1):24–27.

90. Ladias JA, Hadzopoulou-Cladaras M, Kardassis D, Cardot P, Cheng J, Zannis V, Cladaras C. Transcriptional regulation of human apolipoprotein genes ApoB, ApoCIII, and ApoAII by members of the steroid hormone receptor superfamily HNF-4, ARP-1, EAR-2, and EAR-3. J Biol Chem 1992;267(22):15849–15860.

91. Laffitte BA, Joseph SB, Chen M, Castrillo A, Repa J, Wilpitz D, Mangelsdorf D, Tontonoz P. The phospholipid transfer protein gene is a liver X receptor target expressed by macrophages in atherosclerotic lesions. Mol Cell Biol 2003;23(6):2182–2191.

92. Laffitte BA, Repa JJ, Joseph SB, Wilpitz DC, Kast HR, Mangelsdorf DJ, Tontonoz P. LXRs control lipid-inducible expression of the apolipoprotein E gene in macrophages and adipocytes. Proc Natl Acad Sci USA 2001;98(2):507–512.

93. Lavrentiadou SN, Hadzopoulou-Cladaras M, Kardassis D, Zannis VI. Binding specificity and modulation of the human ApoCIII promoter activity by heterodimers of ligand-dependent nuclear receptors. Biochemistry 1999;38(3):964–975.

94. Lee CH, Chawla A, Urbiztondo N, Liao D, Boisvert WA, Evans RM, Curtiss LK. Transcriptional repression of atherogenic inflammation: modulation by PPARdelta. Science 2003;302(5644):453–457.

95. Lee CH, Kang K, Mehl IR, Nofsinger R, Alaynick WA, Chong LW, Rosenfeld JM, Evans RM. Peroxisome proliferator-activated receptor delta promotes very low-density lipoprotein-derived fatty acid catabolism in the macrophage. Proc Natl Acad Sci USA 2006;103(7): 2434–2439.

96. Lee CH, Olson P, Hevener A, Mehl I, Chong LW, Olefsky JM, Gonzalez FJ, Ham J, Kang H, Peters JM, Evans RM. PPAR{delta} regulates glucose metabolism and insulin sensitivity. Proc Natl Acad Sci USA 2006;103(9): 3444–3449.

97. Lehmann JM, Kliewer SA, Moore LB, Smith-Oliver TA, Oliver BB, Su JL, Sundseth SS, Winegar DA, Blanchard DE, Spencer TA, Willson TM. Activation of the nuclear receptor LXR by oxysterols defines a new hormone response pathway. J Biol Chem 1997;272(6): 3137–3140.

98. Lehto M, Bitzen PO, Isomaa B, Wipemo C, Wessman Y, Forsblom C, Tuomi T, Taskinen MR, Groop L. Mutation in the HNF-4alpha gene affects insulin secretion and triglyceride metabolism. Diabetes 1999;48(2):423–425.

99. Lemberger T, Saladin R, Vazquez M, Assimacopoulos F, Staels B, Desvergne B, Wahli W, Auwerx J. Expression of the peroxisome proliferator-activated receptor alpha gene is stimulated by stress and follows a diurnal rhythm. J Biol Chem 1996;271(3):1764–1769.

100. Leone TC, Weinheimer CJ, Kelly DP. A critical role for the peroxisome proliferator-activated receptor alpha (PPARalpha) in the cellular fasting response: the PPARalpha-null mouse as a model of fatty acid oxidation disorders. Proc Natl Acad Sci USA 1999;96(13): 7473–7478.

101. Levin AA, Sturzenbecker LJ, Kazmer S, Bosakowski T, Huselton C, Allenby G, Speck J, Kratzeisen C, Rosenberger M, Lovey A, et al. 9-cis retinoic acid stereoisomer binds and activates the nuclear receptor RXR alpha. Nature 1992;355(6358):359–361.

102 Li AC, Brown KK, Silvestre MJ, Willson TM, Palinski W, Glass CK. Peroxisome proliferator-activated receptor gamma ligands inhibit development of atherosclerosis in LDL receptor-deficient mice. J Clin Invest 2000;106(4):523–531.

103. Li Y, Choi M, Cavey G, Daugherty J, Suino K, Kovach A, Bingham NC, Kliewer SA, Xu HE. Crystallographic identification and functional characterization of phospholipids as ligands for the orphan nuclear receptor steroidogenic factor-1. Mol Cell 2005;17(4):491–502.

104. Linton MF, Atkinson JB, Fazio S. Prevention of atherosclerosis in apolipoprotein E-deficient mice by bone marrow transplantation. Science 1995;267(5200):1034–1037.

105. Lu TT, Makishima M, Repa JJ, Schoonjans K, Kerr TA, Auwerx J, Mangelsdorf DJ. Molecular basis for feedback regulation of bile acid synthesis by nuclear receptors. Mol Cell 2000;6(3):507–515.

106. Luo Y, Tall AR. Sterol upregulation of human CETP expression in vitro and in transgenic mice by an LXR element. J Clin Invest 2000;105(4):513–520.

107. Luquet S, Lopez-Soriano J, Holst D, Fredenrich A, Melki J, Rassoulzadegan M, Grimaldi PA. Peroxisome proliferator-activated receptor delta controls muscle development and oxidative capability. Faseb J 2003;17(15):2299–2301.

108. Ma K, Saha PK, Chan L, Moore DD. Farnesoid X receptor is essential for normal glucose homeostasis. J Clin Invest 2006;116(4):1102–1109.

109. Mak PA, Laffitte BA, Desrumaux C, Joseph SB, Curtiss LK, Mangelsdorf DJ, Tontonoz P, Edwards PA. Regulated expression of the apolipoprotein E/C-I/C-IV/C-II gene cluster in murine and human macrophages. A critical role for nuclear liver X receptors alpha and beta. J Biol Chem 2002;277(35):31900–31908.

110. Makishima M, Lu TT, Xie W, Whitfield GK, Domoto H, Evans, RM, Haussler MR, Mangelsdorf DJ. Vitamin D receptor as an intestinal bile acid sensor. Science 2002;296(5571): 1313–1316.

111. Makishima M, Okamoto AY, Repa JJ, Tu H, Learned RM, Luk A, Hull MV, Lustig KD, Mangelsdorf DJ, Shan B. Identification of a nuclear receptor for bile acids. Science 1999: 284(5418):1362–1365.

112. Mangelsdorf DJ, Thummel C, Beato M, Herrlich P, Schutz G, Umesono K, Blumberg B, Kastner P, Mark M, Chambon P, et al. The nuclear receptor superfamily: the second decade. Cell 1995;83(6):835–839.

113. McCarthy TC, Li X, Sinal CJ. Vitamin D receptor-dependent regulation of colon multidrug resistance-associated protein 3 gene expression by bile acids. J Biol Chem 2005;280(24): 23232–23242.

114. Mertz JR, Shang E, Piantedosi R, Wei S, Wolgemuth DJ, Blaner WS. Identification and characterization of a stereospecific human enzyme that catalyzes 9-cis-retinol oxidation. A possible role in 9-cis-retinoic acid formation. J Biol Chem 1997;272(18):11744–11749.

115. Miesfeld R, Okret S, Wikstrom AC, Wrange O, Gustafsson JA, Yamamoto KR. Characterization of a steroid hormone receptor gene and mRNA in wild-type and mutant cells. Nature 1984;312(5996):779–781.

116. Mietus-Snyder M, Sladek FM, Ginsburg GS, Kuo CF, Ladias JA, Darnell JE, Jr, Karathanasis, SK. Antagonism between apolipoprotein AI regulatory protein 1, Ear3/COUP-TF, and

hepatocyte nuclear factor 4 modulates apolipoprotein CIII gene expression in liver and intestinal cells. Mol Cell Biol 1992;12(4):1708–1718.

117. Mitro N, Mak PA, Vargas L, Godio C, Hampton E, Molteni V, Kreusch A, Saez E. The nuclear receptor LXR is a glucose sensor. Nature 2007;445(7124):219–223.

118. Mortimer Jr, EA, Monson RR, MacMahon B. Reduction in mortality from coronary heart disease in men residing at high altitude. N Engl J Med 1977;296(11):581–585.

119. Muerhoff AS, Griffin KJ, Johnson EF. The peroxisome proliferator-activated receptor mediates the induction of CYP4A6, a cytochrome P450 fatty acid omega-hydroxylase, by clofibric acid. J Biol Chem 1992;267(27):19051–19053.

120. Muoio DM, MacLean PS, Lang DB, Li S, Houmard JA, Way JM, Winegar DA, Corton JC, Dohm GL, Kraus WE. Fatty acid homeostasis and induction of lipid regulatory genes in skeletal muscles of peroxisome proliferator-activated receptor (PPAR) alpha knock-out mice. Evidence for compensatory regulation by PPAR delta. J Biol Chem 2002;277(29): 26089–26097.

121. Nagy L, Tontonoz P, Alvarez JG, Chen H, Evans RM. Oxidized LDL regulates macrophage gene expression through ligand activation of PPARgamma. Cell 1998;93(2):229–240.

122. Nakamura K, Kennedy MA, Baldan A, Bojanic DD, Lyons K, Edwards, PA. Expression and regulation of multiple murine ATP-binding cassette transporter G1 mRNAs/isoforms that stimulate cellular cholesterol efflux to high density lipoprotein. J Biol Chem 2004;279(44): 45980–45989.

123. Nishimura T, Utsunomiya Y, Hoshikawa M, Ohuchi H, Itoh N. Structure and expression of a novel human FGF, FGF-19, expressed in the fetal brain. Biochim Biophys Acta 1999; 1444(1):148–151.

124. Nissinen MJ, Gylling H, Jarvinen HJ, Miettinen TA. Ileal pouch-anal anastomosis, conventional ileostomy and ileorectal anastomosis modify cholesterol metabolism. Digest Dis Sci 2004;49(9):1444–1453.

125. Nordestgaard BG, Zilversmit DB. Comparison of arterial intimal clearances of LDL from diabetic and nondiabetic cholesterol-fed rabbits. Differences in intimal clearance explained by size differences. Arteriosclerosis 1989;9(2):176–183.

126. Nuclear Receptors Nomenclature Committee. A unified nomenclature system for the nuclear receptor superfamily. Cell 1999;97(2):161–163.

127. Oliveira HC, Ma L, Milne R, Marcovina SM, Inazu A, Mabuchi H, Tall AR. Cholesteryl ester transfer protein activity enhances plasma cholesteryl ester formation. Studies in CETP transgenic mice and human genetic CETP deficiency. Arterioscler Thromb Vasc Biol 1997; 17(6):1045–1052.

128. Oliver WR, Jr, Shenk JL, Snaith MR, Russell CS, Plunket KD, Bodkin NL, Lewis MC, Winegar DA, Sznaidman ML, Lambert MH, Xu HE, Sternbach DD, Kliewer SA, Hansen BC, Willson TM. A selective peroxisome proliferator-activated receptor delta agonist promotes reverse cholesterol transport. Proc Natl Acad Sci USA 2001;98(9): 5306–5311.

129. Ortlund EA, Lee Y, Solomon IH, Hager JM, Safi R, Choi Y, Guan Z, Tripathy A, Raetz CR, McDonnell DP, Moore DD, Redinbo MR. Modulation of human nuclear receptor LRH-1 activity by phospholipids and SHP. Nat Struct Mol Biol 2005;12(4):357–363.

130. Otte K, Kranz H, Kober I, Thompson P, Hoefer M, Haubold B, Remmel B, Voss H, Kaiser C, Albers M, Cheruvallath Z, Jackson D, Casari G, Koegl M, Paabo S, Mous J, Kremoser C, Deuschle U. Identification of farnesoid X receptor beta as a novel mammalian nuclear receptor sensing lanosterol. Mol Cell Biol 2003;23(3):864–872.

131. Ou J, Tu H, Shan B, Luk A, DeBose-Boyd RA, Bashmakov Y, Goldstein JL, Brown MS. Unsaturated fatty acids inhibit transcription of the sterol regulatory element-binding protein-1c (SREBP-1c) gene by antagonizing ligand-dependent activation of the LXR. Proc Natl Acad Sci USA 2001;98(11):6027–6032.

132. Overbergh L, Decallonne B, Valckx D, Verstuyf A, Depovere J, Laureys J, Rutgeerts O, Saint-Arnaud R, Bouillon R, Mathieu C. Identification and immune regulation of 25-hydroxy-vitamin D-1-alpha-hydroxylase in murine macrophages. Clin Exp Immunol 2000;120(1): 139–146.

133. Owen K, Hattersley AT. Maturity-onset diabetes of the young: from clinical description to molecular genetic characterization. Best Pract Res Clin Endocrinol Metab 2001; 15(3):309–323.

134. Pare JF, Malenfant D, Courtemanche C, Jacob-Wagner M, Roy S, Allard D, Belanger L. The fetoprotein transcription factor (FTF) gene is essential to embryogenesis and cholesterol homeostasis and is regulated by a DR4 element. J Biol Chem 2004;279(20): 21206–21216.

135. Parks DJ, Blanchard SG, Bledsoe RK, Chandra G, Consler TG, Kliewer SA, Stimmel JB, Willson TM, Zavacki AM, Moore DD, Lehmann JM. Bile acids: natural ligands for an orphan nuclear receptor. Science 1999;284(5418):1365–1368.

136. Peet DJ, Turley SD, Ma W, Janowski BA, Lobaccaro JM, Hammer RE, Mangelsdorf DJ. Cholesterol and bile acid metabolism are impaired in mice lacking the nuclear oxysterol receptor LXR alpha. Cell 1998;93(5):693–704.

137. Pei L, Waki H, Vaitheesvaran B, Wilpitz DC, Kurland IJ, Tontonoz P. NR4A orphan nuclear receptors are transcriptional regulators of hepatic glucose metabolism. Nat Med 2006;12(9): 1048–1055.

138. Peters JM, Hennuyer N, Staels B, Fruchart JC, Fievet C, Gonzalez FJ, Auwerx J. Alterations in lipoprotein metabolism in peroxisome proliferator-activated receptor alpha-deficient mice. J Biol Chem 1997;272(43):27307–27312.

139. Peters JM, Lee SS, Li W, Ward JM, Gavrilova O, Everett C, Reitman ML, Hudson LD, Gonzalez FJ. Growth, adipose, brain, and skin alterations resulting from targeted disruption of the mouse peroxisome proliferator-activated receptor beta(delta). Mol Cell Biol 2000; 20(14):5119–5128.

140. Reichardt HM, Tuckermann JP, Gottlicher M, Vujic M, Weih F, Angel P, Herrlich P, Schutz G. Repression of inflammatory responses in the absence of DNA binding by the glucocorticoid receptor. Embo J 2001;20(24):7168–7173.

141. Repa JJ. Mangelsdorf DJ. The role of orphan nuclear receptors in the regulation of cholesterol homeostasis. Annu Rev Cell Dev Biol 2000;16:459–481.

142. Repa JJ, Turley SD, Lobaccaro JA, Medina J, Li L, Lustig K, Shan B, Heyman RA, Dietschy JM, Mangelsdorf DJ. Regulation of absorption and ABC1-mediated efflux of cholesterol by RXR heterodimers. Science 2000;289(5484):1524–1529.

143. Ricote M, Li AC, Willson TM, Kelly CJ, Glass CK. The peroxisome proliferator-activated receptor-gamma is a negative regulator of macrophage activation. Nature 1998;391(6662): 79–82.

144. Romert A, Tuvendal P, Simon A, Dencker L, Eriksson U. The identification of a 9-cis retinol dehydrogenase in the mouse embryo reveals a pathway for synthesis of 9-cis retinoic acid. Proc Natl Acad Sci USA 1998;95(8):4404–4409.

145. Rosen ED, Sarraf P, Troy AE, Bradwin G, Moore K, Milstone DS, Spiegelman BM, Mortensen RM. PPAR gamma is required for the differentiation of adipose tissue in vivo and in vitro. Mol Cell 1999;4(4):611–617.

146. Rowley CW, Staloch LJ, Divine JK, McCaul SP, Simon TC. Mechanisms of mutual functional interactions between HNF-4alpha and HNF-1alpha revealed by mutations that cause maturity onset diabetes of the young. Am J Physiol 2006;290(3):G466–475.

147. Ryffel GU. Mutations in the human genes encoding the transcription factors of the hepatocyte nuclear factor (HNF)1 and HNF4 families: functional and pathological consequences. J Mol Endocrinol 2001;27(1):11–29.

148. Schoonjans K, Watanabe M, Suzuki H, Mahfoudi A, Krey G, Wahli W, Grimaldi P, Staels B, Yamamoto T, Auwerx J. Induction of the acyl-coenzyme A synthetase gene by fibrates and fatty acids is mediated by a peroxisome proliferator response element in the C promoter. J Biol Chem 1995;270(33):19269–19276.

149. Schuler M, Ali F, Chambon C, Duteil D, Bornert JM, Tardivel A, Desvergne B, Wahli W, Chambon P, Metzger D. PGC1alpha expression is controlled in skeletal muscles by PPARbeta, whose ablation results in fiber-type switching, obesity, and type 2 diabetes. Cell Metab 2006; 4(5):407–414.

150. Schwartz K, Lawn RM, Wade DP. ABC1 gene expression and ApoA-I-mediated cholesterol efflux are regulated by LXR. Biochem Biophys Res Commun 2000;274(3):794–802.
151. Seol W, Choi HS, Moore DD. Isolation of proteins that interact specifically with the retinoid X receptor: two novel orphan receptors. Mol Endocrinol 1995;9(1):72–85.
152. Shaish A, Harari A, Hananshvili L, Cohen H, Bitzur R, Luvish T, Ulman E, Golan M, Ben-Amotz A, Gavish D, Rotstein Z, Harats D. 9-cis beta-carotene-rich powder of the alga Dunaliella bardawil increases plasma HDL-cholesterol in fibrate-treated patients. Atherosclerosis 2006;189(1):215–221.
153. Shih SJ, Allan C, Grehan S, Tse E, Moran C, Taylor JM. Duplicated downstream enhancers control expression of the human apolipoprotein E gene in macrophages and adipose tissue. J Biol Chem 2000;275(41):31567–31572.
154. Shin HD, Park BL, Kim LH, Jung HS, Cho YM, Moon MK, Park YJ, Lee HK, Park KS. Genetic polymorphisms in peroxisome proliferator-activated receptor delta associated with obesity. Diabetes 2004;53(3):847–851.
155. Sinal CJ, Tohkin M, Miyata M, Ward JM, Lambert G, Gonzalez FJ. Targeted disruption of the nuclear receptor FXR/BAR impairs bile acid and lipid homeostasis. Cell 2000;102(6): 731–744.
156. Skogsberg J, McMahon AD, Karpe F, Hamsten A, Packard CJ, Ehrenborg E. Peroxisome proliferator activated receptor delta genotype in relation to cardiovascular risk factors and risk of coronary heart disease in hypercholesterolaemic men. J Intern Med 2003;254(6): 597–604.
157. Sladek F. Desperately seeking...something. Mol Cell 2002;10(2):219–221.
158. Sladek FM, Zhong WM, Lai E, Darnell JE, Jr. Liver-enriched transcription factor HNF-4 is a novel member of the steroid hormone receptor superfamily. Genes Dev 1990;4(12B): 2353–2365.
159. Sood V, Colleran K, Burge MR. Thiazolidinediones: a comparative review of approved uses. Diabetes Technol Ther 2000;2(3):429–440.
160. Spilianakis CG, Lee GR, Flavell RA. Twisting the Th1/Th2 immune response via the retinoid X receptor: lessons from a genetic approach. Eur J Immunol 2005;35(12): 3400–3404.
161. Staudinger JL, Goodwin B, Jones SA, Hawkins-Brown D, MacKenzie KI, LaTour A, Liu Y, Klaassen CD, Brown KK, Reinhard J, Willson TM, Koller BH, Kliewer SA. The nuclear receptor PXR is a lithocholic acid sensor that protects against liver toxicity. Proc Natl Acad Sci USA 2001;98(6):3369–3374.
162. Stulnig TM, Steffensen KR, Gao H, Reimers M, Dahlman-Wright K, Schuster GU, Gustafsson JA. Novel roles of liver X receptors exposed by gene expression profiling in liver and adipose tissue. Mol Pharmacol 2002;62(6):1299–1305.
163. Stunnenberg HG. Mechanisms of transactivation by retinoic acid receptors. Bioessays 1993; 15(5):309–315.
164. Sucov HM, Dyson E, Gumeringer CL, Price J, Chien KR, Evans RM. RXR alpha mutant mice establish a genetic basis for vitamin A signaling in heart morphogenesis. Genes Dev 1994;8(9):1007–1018.
165. Sueyoshi T, Negishi M. Phenobarbital response elements of cytochrome P450 genes and nuclear receptors. Annu Rev Pharmacol Toxicol 2001;41:123–143.
166. Takeuchi A, Reddy GS, Kobayashi T, Okano T, Park J, Sharma S. Nuclear factor of activated T cells (NFAT) as a molecular target for 1alpha,25-dihydroxyvitamin D3-mediated effects. J Immunol 1998;160(1):209–218.
167. Tamori Y, Masugi J, Nishino N, Kasuga M. Role of peroxisome proliferator-activated receptor-gamma in maintenance of the characteristics of mature 3T3-L1 adipocytes. Diabetes 2002; 51(7):2045–2055.
168. Tanaka T, Yamamoto J, Iwasaki S, Asaba H, Hamura H, Ikeda Y, Watanabe M, Magoori K, Ioka RX, Tachibana K, Watanabe Y, Uchiyama Y, Sumi K, Iguchi H, Ito S, Doi T, Hamakubo T, Naito M, Auwerx J, Yanagisawa M, Kodama T, Sakai J. Activation of peroxisome proliferator-activated receptor delta induces fatty acid beta-oxidation in

skeletal muscle and attenuates metabolic syndrome. Proc Natl Acad Sci USA 2003;100(26): 15924–15929.

169. Tangirala RK, Bischoff ED, Joseph SB, Wagner BL, Walczak R, Laffitte BA, Daige CL, Thomas D, Heyman RA, Mangelsdorf DJ, Wang X, Lusis AJ, Tontonoz P, Schulman IG. Identification of macrophage liver X receptors as inhibitors of atherosclerosis. Proc Natl Acad Sci USA 2002;99(18):11896–11901.

170. Thompson PD, Remus LS, Hsieh JC, Jurutka PW, Whitfield GK, Galligan MA, Encinas Dominguez C, Haussler CA, Haussler MR. Distinct retinoid X receptor activation function-2 residues mediate transactivation in homodimeric and vitamin D receptor heterodimeric contexts. J Mol Endocrinol 2001;27(2):211–227.

171. Tontonoz P, Hu E, Graves RA, Budavari AI, Spiegelman BM. mPPAR gamma 2: tissue-specific regulator of an adipocyte enhancer. Genes Dev 1994;8(10):1224–1234.

172. Tontonoz P, Mangelsdorf DJ. Liver X receptor signaling pathways in cardiovascular disease. Mol Endocrinol 2003;17(6):985–993.

173. Tontonoz P, Nagy L, Alvarez JG, Thomazy VA, Evans RM. PPARgamma promotes monocyte/macrophage differentiation and uptake of oxidized LDL. Cell 1998;93(2):241–252.

174. Tribble DL, Holl LG, Wood PD, Krauss RM. Variations in oxidative susceptibility among six low density lipoprotein subfractions of differing density and particle size. Atherosclerosis 1992;93(3):189–199.

175. Veldman CM, Cantorna MT, DeLuca HF. Expression of 1,25-dihydroxyvitamin D(3) receptor in the immune system. Arch Biochem Biophys 2000;374(2):334–338.

176. Venkateswaran A, Laffitte BA, Joseph SB, Mak PA, Wilpitz DC, Edwards PA, Tontonoz P. Control of cellular cholesterol efflux by the nuclear oxysterol receptor LXR alpha. Proc Natl Acad Sci USA 2000;97(22):12097–12102.

177. Venkateswaran A, Repa JJ, Lobaccaro JM, Bronson A, Mangelsdorf DJ, Edwards PA. Human white/murine ABC8 mRNA levels are highly induced in lipid-loaded macrophages. A transcriptional role for specific oxysterols. J Biol Chem 2000;275(19):14700–14707.

178. Voors AW, Johnson WD. Altitude and arteriosclerotic heart disease mortality in white residents of 99 of the 100 largest cities in the United States. J Chronic Dis 1979;32(1–2):157–162.

179. Vu-Dac N, Schoonjans K, Laine B, Fruchart JC, Auwerx J, Staels B. Negative regulation of the human apolipoprotein A-I promoter by fibrates can be attenuated by the interaction of the peroxisome proliferator-activated receptor with its response element. J Biol Chem 1994;269(49):31012–31018.

180. Wallace JM, Schwarz M, Coward P, Houze J, Sawyer JK, Kelley KL, Chai A, Rudel LL. Effects of peroxisome proliferator-activated receptor alpha/delta agonists on HDL-cholesterol in vervet monkeys. J Lipid Res 2005;46(5):1009–1016.

181. Walter P, Green S, Greene G, Krust A, Bornert JM, Jeltsch JM, StaubA, Jensen E, Scrace G, Waterfield M, et al. Cloning of the human estrogen receptor cDNA. Proc Natl Acad Sci USA 1985;82(23):7889–7893.

182. Wan YJ, An D, Cai Y, Repa JJ, Hung-Po Chen T, Flores M, Postic C, Magnuson MA, Chen J, Chien KR, French S, Mangelsdorf DJ, Sucov HM. Hepatocyte-specific mutation establishes retinoid X receptor alpha as a heterodimeric integrator of multiple physiological processes in the liver. Mol Cell Biol 2000;20(12):4436–4444.

183. Wang H, Chen J, Hollister K, Sowers LC, Forman BM. Endogenous bile acids are ligands for the nuclear receptor FXR/BAR. Mol Cell 1999;3(5):543–553.

184. Wang L, Lee YK, Bundman D, Han Y, Thevananther S, Kim CS, Chua SS, Wei P, Heyman RA, Karin M, Moore DD. Redundant pathways for negative feedback regulation of bile acid production. Dev Cell 2002;2(6):721–731.

185. Wang XD, Krinsky NI, Benotti PN, Russell RM. Biosynthesis of 9-cis-retinoic acid from 9-cis-beta-carotene in human intestinal mucosa in vitro. Arch Biochem Biophys 1994; 313(1):150–155.

186. Wang YX, Lee CH, Tiep S, Yu RT, Ham J, Kang H, Evans RM. Peroxisome-proliferator-activated receptor delta activates fat metabolism to prevent obesity. Cell 2003;113(2): 159–170.

187. Wang YX, Zhang CL, Yu RT, Cho HK, Nelson MC, Bayuga-Ocampo CR, Ham J, Kang H, Evans RM. Regulation of muscle fiber type and running endurance by PPARdelta. PLoS Biol 2004;2(10):E294.
188. Weinberger C, Hollenberg SM, Ong ES, Harmon JM, Brower ST, Cidlowski J, Thompson EB, Rosenfeld MG, Evans RM. Identification of human glucocorticoid receptor complementary DNA clones by epitope selection. Science 1985;228(4700):740–742.
189. Weinshilboum RM, Otterness DM, Aksoy IA, Wood TC, Her C, Raftogianis RB. Sulfation and sulfotransferases 1: Sulfotransferase molecular biology: cDNAs and genes. Faseb J 1997;11(1):3–14.
190. Wolfrum C, Borrmann CM, Borchers T, Spener F. Fatty acids and hypolipidemic drugs regulate peroxisome proliferator-activated receptors alpha - and gamma-mediated gene expression via liver fatty acid binding protein: a signaling path to the nucleus. Proc Natl Acad Sci USA 2001;98(5):2323–2328.
191. Xie MH, Holcomb I, Deuel B, Dowd P, Huang A, Vagts A, Foster J, Liang J, Brush J, Gu Q, Hillan K, Goddard A, Gurney AL. FGF-19, a novel fibroblast growth factor with unique specificity for FGFR4. Cytokine 1999;11(10):729–735.
192. Xie W, Radominska-Pandya A, Shi Y, Simon CM, Nelson MC, Ong ES, Waxman DJ, Evans RM. An essential role for nuclear receptors SXR/PXR in detoxification of cholestatic bile acids. Proc Natl Acad Sci USA 2001;98(6):3375–3380.
193. Yoshikawa T, Shimano H, Yahagi N, Ide T, Amemiya-Kudo M, Matsuzaka T, Nakakuki M, Tomita S, Okazaki H, Tamura Y, Iizuka Y, Ohashi K, Takahashi A, Sone H, Osuga Ji J, Gotoda T, Ishibashi S, Yamada N. Polyunsaturated fatty acids suppress sterol regulatory element-binding protein 1c promoter activity by inhibition of liver X receptor (LXR) binding to LXR response elements. J Biol Chem 2002;277(3):1705–1711.
194. Yu L, Hammer RE, Li-Hawkins J, Von Bergmann K, Lutjohann D, Cohen JC, Hobbs HH. Disruption of Abcg5 and Abcg8 in mice reveals their crucial role in biliary cholesterol secretion. Proc Natl Acad Sci USA 2002;99(25):16237–16242.
195. Zhang Y, Lee FY, Barrera G, Lee H, Vales C, Gonzalez FJ, Willson TM, Edwards PA. Activation of the nuclear receptor FXR improves hyperglycemia and hyperlipidemia in diabetic mice. Proc Natl Acad Sci USA 2006;103(4):1006–1011.
196. Zhang Y, Repa JJ, Gauthier K, Mangelsdorf DJ. Regulation of lipoprotein lipase by the oxysterol receptors, LXRalpha and LXRbeta. J Biol Chem 2001;276(46):43018–43024.
197. Zollner G, Marschall HU, Wagner M, Trauner M. Role of nuclear receptors in the adaptive response to bile acids and cholestasis: pathogenetic and therapeutic considerations. Mol Pharm 2006;3(3):231–251.

Chapter 7
Diabetes and Oxidant Stress

Alicia J. Jenkins, Michael A. Hill, and Kevin G. Rowley

Abstract Diabetes is associated with chronic micro- and macrovascular complications. Oxidative stress has been defined as 'a "shift in the pro-oxidant – anti-oxidant balance in the pro-oxidant direction'." Oxidant stress may initiate and exacerbate vascular (endothelial) damage through excess production of reactive oxygen species, depletion of nitric oxide, and damage to lipids, proteins, and DNA. Experimental results and theoretical constructs suggest oxidative stress is increased in diabetes, at least in some tissues, though not all studies are supportive. Potential markers of oxidation and glycoxidation are discussed. Pharmacological suppression of intracellular oxidative stress has prevented adverse biochemical and functional changes in cultured cells and animal models, and in some cases surrogate end-points of vascular damage in humans. Definitive clinical studies are awaited.

Keywords: diabetes; complications; atherosclerosis; oxidative stress; glycoxidation

Abbreviations

ACE Angiotensin converting enzyme
AGEs Advanced glycation end-products
ALEs Advanced lipoxidation end-products
AOPPs Advanced oxidation protein products
C Cholesterol
CAD Coronary artery disease
CML Carboxymethyl-lysine
CEL Carboxyethyl-lysine
DCCT Diabetes Control and Complications Trial
EDC (Pittsburgh) Epidemiology of diabetes complications
EDIC Epidemiology of diabetes interventions and complications

J.L. Holtzman (ed.), *Atherosclerosis and Oxidant Stress: A New Perspective*.
© Springer 2008

ELISA Enzyme linked immunosorbent assay
FRAP Ferric reducing anti-oxidant power
ESRD End stage renal disease
Glut-Hb Glutathionyl hemoglobin
GOLD Glyoxal-derived lysine dimer
HDL High density lipoprotein
HMG CoA 3-Hydroxy-3-methylglutaryl coenzyme A
HO-1 Heme-oxygenase-1
HOPE Heart outcomes prevention evaluation
HPLC High pressure liquid chromatography
IC Immune complex
IDL Intermediate density lipoprotein
IMT Intima media thickness
LDL Low density lipoprotein
MetSo Methionine sulfoxide
MOLD Methylglyoxal-derived lysine dimer
MPO Myeloperoxidase
NF-κB Nuclear transcription factor kappa B
NO Nitric oxide
NOS Nitric oxide synthase
Ox-LDL Oxidized LDL
PAFAH Platelet activating factor acetohydrolase
PAI-1 Plasminogen activator inhibitor-1
PKC Protein kinase C
PON Paraoxonase
RAGE Receptor for advanced glycation end-products
RBC Red blood cell
RCEC Retinal capillary endothelial cell
RIA Radio-immunoassay
RENAAL Reduction of end-points in type 2 diabetes with the Angiotensin II antagonist losartan
ROS Reactive oxygen species
SAE Small artery elasticity
4S Scandinavian Simvastatin Survival Study
O_2^- Superoxide anion
SOD Superoxide dismutase
TBARS Thiobarbituric acid reactive substance
TGFβ Transforming growth factor β
TRAP Total reactive antioxidant potential
tPA Tissue plasminogen activator
UKPDS United Kingdom Prospective Diabetes Study
VEGF Vascular endothelium derived growth factor

Definition and Prevalence of Diabetes

Diabetes mellitus, a condition characterized by hyperglycemia, is a chronic disorder of carbohydrate, lipid, and protein metabolism due to the absolute or relative lack of insulin. In 1997, there were an estimated 124 million people with diabetes worldwide, and 221 million affected people are predicted by 2010.[1] While oxidative stress has also been implicated in the pathogenesis of diabetes,[2] this chapter will focus on the relationship between oxidative stress and atherosclerosis in diabetes, with an emphasis on the clinical perspective. The basic mechanisms of oxidative stress are reviewed elsewhere.[3–5] The presentation, diagnosis, and classification of diabetes have been reviewed elsewhere.[6] Approximately 90% of cases have Type 2 diabetes, and the prevalence of both Type 1 and Type 2 diabetes is increasing,[1] including a disturbing increase in Type 2 diabetes in children, usually associated with adiposity and a relatively poor prognosis with respect to the subsequent development of vascular complications.[7] People with both common forms of diabetes are susceptible to long-term complications, which may even be present at the time of formal diagnosis of Type 2 diabetes and can occur five5 to –10 years after Type 1 diabetes onset. Atherosclerosis is also accelerated in hyperinsulinemic non-diabetic subjects.[8]

Chronic Complications of Diabetes and Risk Factors

The chronic complications of diabetes are predominantly vascular, and are usually categorized as macrovascular or microvascular.[9–15] Diabetes is associated with at least a two-fold increased risk of macrovascular disease (coronary artery, cerebrovascular, and peripheral vascular disease), and is the cause of death in 70–80% of people with diabetes.[9–13] The microvascular complications of diabetes are nephropathy, retinopathy, and (peripheral and autonomic) neuropathy.[14,15] Diabetes accounts for over a third of all patients with end stage renal disease (ESRD), and diabetic retinopathy is the most common cause of adult-onset blindness in the Western world.[9,14,15] Subjects with microvascular complications are particularly prone to accelerated atherosclerosis and premature death.[16,17]

Both men and women with diabetes are at heightened risk of atherosclerosis, with loss of female cardioprotection in diabetes, even prior to the menopause.[11] Atheroma develops earlier, progresses at a faster rate than in the non-diabetic population, and extends more distally in the vasculature,[18] often making angioplasty and vascular bypass surgery less feasible in patients with diabetes. In addition to *quantitative* changes in atheroma in diabetes, *qualitative* changes have also been suggested. This area merits further research, as it may suggest additional interventions for people with diabetes. Nevertheless, in recent clinical trials of lipid and blood pressure lowering agents with vascular end-points, the diabetic groups responded at least as well as the non-diabetic groups,[19–21] in keeping with there being common underlying risk factors, pathology, and pathophysiology.

The diagnosis of clinically significant vascular disease may be more problematic in diabetes, as clinical events such as myocardial ischemia may be silent[22,23] or present with atypical pain. The prognosis of vascular events such as a myocardial infarction or of vascular interventions in people with diabetes is worse than that of non-diabetic subjects,[24] perhaps related to more extensive disease and end-organ damage and co-morbidities. There should be a high index of suspicion of vascular disease in people with diabetes, but as yet there are limitations to the routine use of non-invasive measurements of atherosclerosis in clinical practice.

There are pathophysiologic, histologic, and risk factor similarities between atherosclerosis and the related microvascular complications.[25–31] Epidemiologic and family studies suggest that in addition to genetic factors, acquired factors such as poor glycemic control, hypertension, dyslipidemia, oxidative stress, inflammation, and perhaps the propensity to form and break down advanced glycation end-products (AGEs), contribute to vascular damage.[28,31,32] Potential risk factors for diabetic vascular damage are listed in Table 7.1 and major proposed mechanisms underlying accelerated atherosclerosis in diabetes are listed in Table 7.2. Many of the risk factors and mechanisms are inter-related. For example, poor glycemic control causes dyslipidemia, which may exacerbate inflammation. Oxidative stress may

Table 7.1 Potential promoters of atherosclerosis in diabetes

- Increasing age
- Increasing diabetes duration
- Younger age of diabetes onset
- Positive family history of vascular disease
- Race (which may also be a surrogate for socioeconomic and psychosocial factors)
- Increased blood pressure
- Smoking
- Adiposity
- Insulin resistance

Dyslipidemia
  - *Quantitative* changes: ↓ LDL concentration and small dense LDL particles, ↓ triglycerides, ↓ IDL, ↓ Lp(a), ↓ HDL (in particular HDL_2 or large HDL)
  - *Qualitative* changes, e.g., non-enzymatic glycation, oxidation, AGE modification, small Lp(a)
- Poor glycemic control
- Renal damage
- Inflammation

Table 7.2 Mechanisms/pathways of accelerated atherosclerosis in diabetes

- Oxidative stress
- Carbonyl stress
- AGEs/ALEs
- Reductive stress (pseudohypoxia)
- Polyol pathway – Aldose reductase
- PKC activation
- Altered activities of growth factors and cytokines

increase AGE formation and AGEs themselves may induce oxidative stress.[32] A unifying hypothesis based on the overproduction of superoxide by endothelial cell mitochondria, discussed further below, has been suggested by Dr. Michael Brownlee's group.[33,34]

While much progress has been made, the relative importance of the various clinical, genetic, and biochemical factors to atherosclerosis initiation and/or progression in diabetes has not been fully elucidated. This complex and controversial area of research has been hampered by the slow development of atherosclerosis (over decades, commencing in childhood), lack of well-validated surrogate measures of atherosclerosis in diabetes, lack of good animal models for the complications of diabetes, the high cost of long-term clinical research, and the major challenge of quantifying oxidative stress. Even with well-validated, standardized, inexpensive, widely available assays of glycemia (i.e., HbA_{1c}), evidence for the role of glycemia in diabetic vascular disease, and that intensive diabetes management centered around improved glycemia (which also favorably impacts other factors such as dyslipidemia) can attenuate atherosclerosis is only just becoming available.[35–38]

Definition and Mechanisms of Oxidative Stress

Oxidative stress has been defined as the "steady state level of reactive oxygen or oxygen free radicals in a biologic system", or "a shift in the pro-oxidant – anti-oxidant balance in the pro-oxidant direction." It is implicated in diabetes, atherosclerosis, renal failure (which is often associated with diabetes), and many other disease processes, as well as normal aging.[39,40] Exposure to oxidative stress is an unavoidable part of life. Reactive oxygen species (ROS) (such as in Table 7.3), normal byproducts of many enzyme reactions, are always being formed in vivo, and play a vital role in host defense, such as in the phagocytosis of foreign organisms and substances, and in modulation of hormones, growth factors, and cytokine activity.[41–43]

Recently, Brownlee and colleagues proposed a unifying hypothesis based on hyperglycemia hyperglycemia-induced endothelial cell mitochondrial overproduction of superoxide (O_2^-), which links hyperglycemia, oxidative stress, and the vascular complications of diabetes.[33,34] Basically, it is suggested that excess glucose entering (for example) vascular endothelial cells via the insulin independent GLUT-1

Table 7.3 Reactive oxygen species

• Free radicals	• Non-radical species
Alkoxyl radical $RO^{\bullet}$	Hydrogen peroxide H_2O_2
Hydroxyl radical $HO^{\bullet}$	Hypochlorite ClO^-
Hydroperoxyl radical $HOO^{\bullet}$	Peroxynitrite $ONOO^-$
Nitric oxide $NO^{\bullet}$	Singlet oxygen $^1O_2$
Peroxyl radical ROO	
Superoxide anion O_2^-	

transporter, induces mitochondrial overproduction of O_2^-, which then activates other pathways including protein kinase C (PKC), nuclear factor-κB (NF-κB), the polyol pathway, induces NAD(P)H oxidase, and promotes formation of AGEs and advanced lipoxidation end-products (ALEs) and (the highly pro-oxidant and long-lived) peroxynitrite.[33,34,44] There is much evidence relating endothelial dysfunction and vascular damage in general and in diabetes to disturbed nitric oxide (NO) metabolism,[25,44–50] and the Brownlee hypothesis is consistent with this. NO is generated from L-arginine by nitric oxide synthase (NOS), an enzyme with three isoforms; constitutive brain (bNOS), endothelial (eNOS), and inducibile (iNOS). iNOS can be induced by hyperglycemia and O_2^- can inhibit eNOS and quench NO, (by reacting with it to form peroxynitrite), thereby reducing its bioavailability, a feature of diabetic endothelial dysfunction.[44–50] The O_2^- -induced peroxynitrite can induce DNA damage, which activates the nuclear enzyme poly(ADP-ribose) polymerase, which depletes intracellular NAD^+ and induces endothelial dysfunction.[51]

While the hyperglycemia induction of O_2^- hypothesis is theoretically sound, is supported by positive cell culture and animal model data, and is in keeping with observations in human diabetes based on surrogate measures of vascular disease, we await definitive proof - – the amelioration of vascular complications in human diabetic subjects by interventions which disrupt mitochondrial superoxide production. Understanding the mechanisms, their inter-relationships, and relative contributions of oxidative stress and other factors, such as hyperglycemia and dyslipidemia, are important for designing rational interventions. Based on such mechanistic insights from biochemical, cell culture, and animal models, novel antioxidant agents are in development, and laboratory-based studies are promising. Suppression of intracellular oxidative stress by low molecular weight inhibitors, Mn-SOD, lipoic acid, or L-propionyl-carnitine, catalysis of peroxynitrite decomposition, or inhibition of related cell signaling pathways (with PKCβ inhibitors) has prevented adverse changes in cultured cells and animal models ,[44,51–61] and in some cases surrogate end-points of vascular damage in humans.[62,63]

Measurement of Oxidative Stress

Oxidative stress is a dynamic process, and as yet there is no single measurement or panel of tests that adequately reflects oxidative stress or damage in vivo. Oxidative stress and damage is likely to vary between and within individuals, and to be influenced by such factors as prandial status, the type of food eaten, circadian rhythm, exercise, hormonal status, disease status, and medications. Oxidative stress may differ between organs and tissues, and between cells and subcellular compartments. The sites of formation and action of pro-oxidant species and accessibility and efficacy of antioxidants may differ. These factors have important implications for the measurement and modification of oxidative stress and damage.

Due to their very short half-lives, high reactivity, low concentrations, and difficulty in accessing relevant sites of generation in vivo, ROS (Table 7.3) are not readily measured. Because oxidative stress cannot be readily measured directly, its presence is usually inferred by measuring substrates, by assessing antioxidant defenses, by measuring products of free radical damage, and by assessing oxidative stress-induced cell signaling or gene responses (Tables 7.4 and 7.5). Specific assays are described elsewhere.[64–67] Primary products of protein oxidation (Table 7.4) are those generated directly by the interaction of ROS and proteins. Secondary products of oxidation are formed by the interaction of proteins with products of oxidation of lipids, carbohydrates, and amino acids. The intermediates in these reactions are carbonyl and dicarbonyl compounds such as glyoxal, methylglyoxal, and malondialdehyde, the levels of which are usually increased in diabetes. However, not all carbonyl intermediates are oxidatively derived. Carbonyl stress, likely to be increased in diabetes and also relevant to its vascular complications, is well reviewed elsewhere.[31,40,68–70]

Table 7.4 Measures of " 'oxidative stress' "

• Specific measures of ROS
  See Table 7.3
• Specific anti-oxidant levels
  Aqueous phase
    Albumin; ascorbate; bilirubin; flavanoids; glutathione
  Metal sequestration related
    Transferrin, ceruloplasmin; ubiquinone; urate
  Lipid soluble
    Carotenes (α, β); lutein; lycopene; tocopherols (α,γ)
• Measures of oxidative damage
  DNA
    Urothymi(di)ne glycol; 8-hydroxyguanine and 8-hydroxydeoxyguanosine;
  Protein-related primary oxidation products
    Amino acid hydroperoxides, e.g., valine, leucine, isoleucine; aromatic, e.g., *o*-tyrosine, dityrosine, chlorotyrosine, nitrotyrosine; protein carbonyls, e.g., adipic semialdehyde; sulphydryl, e.g., methionine sulphoxide;
  Protein-related secondary oxidation products
    Some AGEs, e.g., CML, CEL, pentosidine, MOLD (methylglyoxal-derived lysine dimer), GOLD (glyoxal-derived lysine dimer), crosslines; glutathionyl hemoglobin
  Lipid related
    Lipid peroxides; 4-hydroxynonenal; isoprostanes; malondialdehyde
• Activity of oxidative stress stress-related enzymes
  Antioxidant enzymes
    PON; PAFAH (platelet activating factor acetohydrolase); SOD; catalase; xanthine oxidase; glutathione peroxidase
  Pro-oxidant enzymes
    MPO; NADH/NADPH oxidase; Nitric oxide synthase
  • Activation of cell signaling
    PKC; Activated Protein-1; NF-κB
  • Expression of oxidative stress related genes or gene products
    HO-1; TGF-ß; VEGF; RAGE (receptor for advanced glycation end-products)

Table 7.5 Other "oxidative stress/damage" assays

- TRAP/FRAP (Total reactive antioxidant potential/Ferric reducing antioxidant power) assays (contributed to by albumin, bilirubin, urate, transferrintransferring, and ascorbate)
- Antioxidant capacity assays
- LDL oxidizibility (influenced by lipid soluble antioxidant content, lipid composition)
- Ox-LDL by ELISA (and anti-bodies to Ox-LDL and immune-complexes)
- TBARS (thiobarbituric acid reactive substance)
- AGE assays by ELISA, RIA or AGE-peptide assays by HPLC
- Protein carbonyls (by ELISA)
- Advanced Oxidation Protein Products (AOPPs)

There are several important considerations in the interpretation of experiments suggested as demonstrating increased oxidative stress in diabetes and its related vascular damage. Increased levels of oxidative damage may reflect increased oxidative stress per se, increased substrate or reduced detoxification pathways, or a combination thereof. Therefore, increased levels of secondary oxidation products, e.g., carboxymethy-lysine (CML) or of lipid oxidation products such as circulating oxidized LDL (Ox-LDL) may reflect increased substrate availability rather than increased oxidative stress per se. In keeping with these observations, Baynes and colleagues have demonstrated increased levels of some secondary protein oxidation products such as CML in skin collagen in diabetes,[71,72] but levels of the skin collagen primary oxidation product methionine sulfoxide (MetSo) were not increased in diabetes.[73]

Induction of hemoxygenase-1, an intracellular anti-oxidant, in cell or tissues is often regarded as evidence of increased oxidative stress.[74] However, other factors such as osmotic stress (such as induced by hyperglycemia), reductive stress, heat, and endotoxin contamination of stressors such as in vitro generated oxidized LDL and AGEs may also activate such pathways. Reduction in antioxidant defences (such as lipid soluble antioxidants) could be interpreted as either evidence of increased oxidative stress or a reflection of lower oxidative stress.

Is Oxidative Stress per se Increased in Diabetes and Vascular Damage?

There are many theoretical reasons why oxidative stress should be increased in diabetes, including hyperglycemia hyperglycemia-related glucose autoxidation, increased glucose flux through the polyol pathway, and activation of reduced forms of NADPH oxidase, therefore Brownlee's unifying hypothesis[33,34] is appealing. There are several excellent review articles.[3,39,40,45,47,49,75–77] However there are other areas of research, such as with vitamin E, in which the theory, biochemistry, cell culture and animal model data, and even human surrogate end-point data has been positive, yet human trials with hard clinical end-points of the successful interventions have not proven beneficial.[78] While biochemical studies, cell culture, and animal models contribute valuable knowledge regarding mechanisms of damage, and facilitate development and preclinical testing of interventions, they may not adequately reflect the whole human condition – that most relevant to clinical practice. Yet as evidenced by numerous publications and ongoing studies (including in our laboratories), it is still controversial as to whether or not "'oxidative stress'" is increased in human diabetes per se, or as a result of its association with its macro- and microvascular complications.

In view of the difficulty in obtaining vascular tissue from living subjects, (especially that from healthy non-diabetic control subjects) and the current lack of a clinically applicable assay (such as a HbA_{1c} equivalent for oxidative stress), the majority of human studies relate to indirect measures of oxidative stress in plasma, serum, blood cells, or urine. These sites may not be ideal for reflecting oxidative damage to tissues given the antioxidant-rich nature of plasma. Examples of oxidative stress-related measures in readily accessible tissues, suitable for clinical practice, are discussed below. Some of the more promising measures in clinical research (discussed) are oxidized LDL, isoprostanes, some AGE measures, paraoxonase, and myeloperoxidase.

Lipoprotein Oxidation

Post-synthetic lipoprotein modifications such as glycation and oxidation may adversely alter lipoprotein composition and function and promote atherosclerosis, even in the setting of favorable lipid levels. Oxidation of LDL, as first suggested by Chisholm and Sgteinberg over 20 years ago (reviewed in [79–81]), is still central to current theories of atherosclerosis, and has also been implicated in renal damage[82,83] and diabetic retinopathy.[84,85] We have previously reviewed the area of the relationship between modified lipoproteins (including oxidized lipoproteins) and the vascular complications of diabetes.[86–88]

Studies of Ox-LDL exposure in cultured vascular cells and isolated vessels have demonstrated many responses pertinent to atherosclerosis and diabetic vascular complications: increased cell adhesion molecule expression, impaired vasorelaxation, enhanced arteriolar vasoconstriction due to increased Ca^{2+} sensitivity, prothrombotic effects (enhanced platelet adhesion and increased PAI-1 production), transformation of smooth muscle cells into foam cells, induction of growth factors, cell proliferation, and apoptosis.[27,79–85,87–91] Lopes-Virella et al. demonstrated enhanced macrophage uptake of in vivo modified LDL from diabetic subjects,[92] and of in vitro glycated LDL.[93] We have demonstrated adverse effects of oxidized LDL on cultured cells relevant to macrovascular and microvascular complications of diabetes, including heme-oxygenase-1 (HO-1) induction, reduced cell viability, pro-thrombotic changes in retinal capillary endothelial cell (RCEC) tissue plasminogen activator (tPA) and plasminogen activator inhibitor-1 (PAI-1) production and vasoconstrictory changes in RCEC enothelin-1 and nitrite.[28,85,94–96] In these cell cell-based assays we have found that toxicity of modified LDL can be inhibited by LDL vitamin E enrichment,[85] the antioxidant enzyme SOD, dicarbonyl scavengers (aminoguanidine,[96] metformin), and non-specific and specific inhibitors of Protein Kinase C (PKC) (unpublished observations). However, while these and other data implicate modified lipoproteins and cell signaling in vascular toxicity, as stated earlier, antioxidants have not yet proven effective in preventing vascular complications in humans[78] with diabetes or atherosclerosis in diabetic or non-diabetic subjects. Similarly PKC inhibitors have shown vasoprotective effects in vitro and in animal studies,[60,61] but favorable outcomes of studies in human diabetes are awaited.

Glycation of LDL[27,86,87] correlates with other measures of glycemia and increases matrix binding in vitro[97,98] such that it may be more likely to be retained in the arterial subendothelial space in vivo, where it is susceptible to further modification, such as oxidation. It is controversial as to whether LDL glycation increases susceptibility to oxidation. Relative to healthy controls, Tsai et al. demonstrated increased susceptibility of LDL from Type 1 diabetic patients with poor glycemic control to in vitro (copper-induced) oxidation.[99] However, we did not find any difference in susceptibility to copper oxidation of LDL from healthy controls and complication-free Type 1 diabetic subjects in moderate glycemic control.[100] Nor did we find greater susceptibility to copper oxidation of in vivo glycated LDL fractions from Type 1 diabetic subjects than their relatively non-glycated LDL fractions, nor were there significant differences in the lipid soluble antioxidant content, CML, carboxyethyl-lysine (CEL), or pentosidine of these in vivo modified lipoproteins.[101] Further, in cross-sectional analyses of the DCCT/EDIC (Diabetes Control and Complications Trial/Epidemiology of diabetes interventions and complications) cohort we did not observe any relationship between LDL susceptibility to oxidation and HbA1c[102] and severity of nephropathy[103] or retinopathy[104] or carotid intima media thickness (IMT) (personal communication, Timothy J. Lyons, MD), a surrogate measure of atherosclerosis. A prospective component of the study is in progress.

Oxidized LDL and Lp(a) have been demonstrated in human atheroma,[105,106] but to our knowledge, there are as yet no studies specifically in vascular tissues from Type 1 and Type 2 diabetic subjects. Plaque Ox-LDL levels are increased almost 70-fold to that in the circulation,[105] in keeping with its formation and preferential retention in the extravascular space. Levels of circulating Ox-LDL measured by commercially available enzyme linked immunosorbent assays (ELISAs) have been shown to be positively associated with coronary artery disease (CAD) severity, predictive of clinical vascular events in the general population[106-109] and to be associated with diabetic nephropathy.[110] In a cross-sectional study we have observed similar circulating concentrations of Ox-LDL and Ox-LDL/LDL in healthy non-diabetic subjects and complication-free Type 1 diabetic subjects, but higher levels in those with vascular complications (unpublished observations). Diabetes specific cross-sectional and prospective studies which adjust for substrate stress of LDL levels are merited.

Antibodies and Immune Complex Formation with Modified LDL

Antibodies to, and immune complexes (IC) with modified lipoproteins such as Ox-LDL, glycated, and AGE-modified LDL are also implicated in human vascular damage.[111–115] Such immune complexes (IC) can increase foam cell formation and have pro-inflammatory effects, both of which are features of atherosclerosis. Lopes-Virella and colleagues have demonstrated increased Ox-LDL-anti-Ox-LDL IC levels in a cross-sectional study of Type 1 diabetic subjects with vs. without proteinuria[116] and in a prospective study within the Pittsburgh Epidemiology of diabetes complications (EDC) (of Type 1 diabetic subjects) the apoB and cholesterol content of circulating IC were significantly higher in subjects who developed CAD and nephropathy compared to matched subjects who did not.[117] Recently Lopes-Virella et al. evaluated antibodies to modified LDL and circulating IC in a cross-sectional study of the DCCT/EDIC cohort. There were no statistically significant relationships between evaluated complications and levels of circulating antibodies to Ox-LDL, glycated-LDL and AGE-modified LDL, however the IC apoB and cholesterol content was significantly elevated in subjects with increased urinary albumin loss and with moderate to severe retinopathy (personal communication, Maria Lopes-Virella, MD). These observations suggest that interaction of the immune system with modified lipids and proteins may potentiate vascular damage in diabetes.

Thus, there are contrasting results regarding oxidized LDL and vascular damage in diabetes. It may be that Ox-LDL and other measures of oxidative damage and related factors are increased only as a result of diabetic vascular complications and may be relevant to only certain stages of atherosclerosis (such as initiation, propagation, or complication such as plaque rupture).

Isoprostanes

A promising measure of lipid oxidation (which occurs in lipoproteins, and cell membranes), and one which can be measured in plasma and urine by gas chromatography or by ELISA is that of isoprostanes (reviewed in [118–121]). As they are cell permeable, isoprostanes measured in plasma or urine may also include cellular-derived isoprostanes. Increasing age, cigarette smoking, coronary artery disease, renal disease, and diabetes have been associated with high levels of F2-isoprostanes.[118–122] Isoprostanes are vasoconstrictory and may modulate tissue ischemia.[123–125] Relative to healthy controls and long-term Type 1 diabetic subjects with no clinical evidence of complications, we have found plasma isoprostane levels to be significantly ($p < 0.05$) higher in Type 1 diabetic subjects with vascular complications (2,480 ± 269 pmol/IL, $n = 20$), but there was no statistically significant difference between healthy controls (1,723 ± 225, $n = 20$) and complication-free diabetic subjects with at least 15 years of diabetes (1,775 ± 202, $n = 20$) (unpublished data). In cross-sectional studies we also noted statistically significant inverse relationships between plasma isoprostanes and small artery elasticity (SAE) as measured non-invasively by pulse-wave analysis in diabetic subjects and in healthy subjects (unpublished observations). Lower SAE, which we have demonstrated correlates with flow mediated dilatation,[126] and is NO-related,[127] has been reported in Type 1[128] and Type 2 diabetes,[129] and it has been suggested to be associated with and predictive of macrovascular events in the general population.[130]

Isoprostane concentrations in humans can be lowered by antioxidants[131,132] and by HMG CoA reductase inhibitors,[133] but evidence as to whether this reduces atherosclerosis in diabetes is awaited.

Dietary Antioxidants

Lower circulating levels of dietary dietary-derived antioxidants, which may be secondary to low anti-oxidant intake or because of increased degradation in vivo, are suggested to reflect increased oxidative stress. In cross-sectional case case–control studies in diabetes, there are reports of normal, increased, and decreased levels of aqueous phase and lipid soluble antioxidants (summarized[134]). The weight of evidence is in favor of normal levels, at least in non-disadvantaged communities, and supplementation is not recommended in diabetes unless a specific deficiency is documented. We have demonstrated very low plasma antioxidant levels in Australian Aboriginal and Torres Strait Islander communities including many diabetic subjects, arising from low intakes of fruit and vegetables (in association with poor food supply in remote areas). In these populations, plasma carotenoid concentrations were inversely related to markers of inflammation and vascular dysfunction (C-reactive protein, cell adhesion molecules, and microalbuminuria), and were positively related to activity of paraoxonase (PON), a putative anti-oxidant enzyme,[135] implicated in atherosclerosis (discussed later). As mentioned earlier, lower antioxidants may be interpreted as reflecting increased oxidative stress or a lack thereof. Furthermore, even if the former applies, a weakened defense, may still be adequate to protect against oxidative damage and vascular complications, and its supplementation (at least in non-deficient subjects) may not be protective against oxidative damage and atherosclerosis. Thus studies of antioxidant vitamin levels in diabetes do not provide strong evidence for increased oxidative stress in diabetes in general.

Markers of Oxidative Damage in Proteins

Advanced Glycation End-Products

Advanced glycation end-products (AGEs), which have been implicated in the macro- and microvascular complications of diabetes, form in vivo in diabetic and non-diabetic subjects, in a range of tissues, including long-lived connective tissue (skin collagen, vascular matrix, and lens), shorter shorter-lived circulating proteins (albumin, immunoglobulins, and lipoproteins), in cell membranes, and intracellularly (e.g., on hemoglobin). There are many excellent review papers on AGEs and their related receptors.[27,32,39,40,65,68,70,136–142] The majority of human studies addressing the role of AGEs in vascular disease are cross-sectional. In most, but not all studies, AGEs are higher in people with diabetes as opposed to those without, and are higher in diabetic subjects with complications compared to those without complications. In a cross-sectional study of non-diabetic controls and Type 1 diabetic subjects, McCance et al. demonstrated elevated levels of total fluorescence and specific (secondary protein oxidation products) CML and pentosidine measured by gas chromatography/mass spectroscopy in skin collagen from subjects with evidence of diabetic microvascular damage.[71] In a similar cross-sectional study of immunoreactive AGEs in skin collagen, Beisswenger et al. found a significant increase in tissue AGEs in Type 1 diabetic subjects with high normal urinary ("pre-microalbuminuric") albumin excretion, and as expected, further increases in AGEs with microalbuminuria and macroalbuminuria.[143] However as suggested by Baynes et al., these increases in skin collagen AGEs could be accounted for by increased substrate rather than increased oxidative stress per se. In the Baynes laboratory, levels of a primary oxidation product MetSo in skin collagen did not differ between diabetic subjects and healthy controls. Thus, at least in the extracellular milieu, the evidence favors a lack of increase in oxidative stress in diabetes per se.

In collaboration with the Baynes and Thorpe group we quantified specific markers of glycation and glycoxidation in (more readily available) red blood cell (RBC) membranes, plasma, and lipoproteins (LDL and HDL) of Type 1 diabetic subjects with and without nephropathy using gas chromatography/mass spectroscopy and reverse phase high pressure liquid chromatography (HPLC). In spite of higher levels of glycation (fructoselysine) in diabetes, we found similar levels of the AGEs (carboxymethyl-lysine [CML], carboxyethyl-lysine [CEL], and pentosidine) in RBC membrane and plasma proteins of non-diabetic controls, microalbuminuria-prone and resistant subjects (with normal serum creatinine).[144–146] This is further evidence of a lack of increase in oxidation -related products at the interface of the extracellular and intracellular milieu in diabetes. In another series of patients, we found significantly elevated plasma protein CML, CEL, and pentosidine only in diabetic and non-diabetic subjects with elevated serum creatinine (unpublished data). This is likely to represent an elevating effect of impaired renal clearance on circulating AGE levels.

However, using immunoreactive measures, which may detect non-oxidatively derived products, and cross-react with other epitopes, there are positive data showing increased AGEs in diabetes and in relationship to complications. Using a polyclonal AGE antibody and a monoclonal CML antibody Hanssen's Oslo Oslo-based group has demonstrated: (a) increased serum CML and AGEs in Type 1 diabetics vs. non-diabetic subjects; (b) predictive value of baseline serum AGE, but not CML, for renal disease progression assessed by kidney biopsy in young Type 1 diabetic patients with microalbuminuria; (c) association of AGE but not CML with left ventricular dysfunction in Type 1 diabetes; (d) increased serum AGE and CML in Type 2 diabetes vs. non-diabetic controls, and association of serum AGE, but not CML, with coronary artery disease in a cross-sectional study of Type 2 diabetes; (e) increased serum methylglyoxal -derived hydroimidazolone in Type 2 diabetes, with higher levels in the presence of CAD.[147–151] However, also using an AGE ELISA with anti-sera from Bucala, Tan et al. found that serum AGEs did not differ between Type 2 diabetic subjects and controls, but noted negative correlations between serum AGEs and brachial artery endothelium-dependent and –independent vasodilatation.[152]

In studies in progress in our laboratory we have found that non-specific AGE-peptide levels are about 50% higher in Type 1 diabetic patients ($n = 148$) and 150% higher in Type 2 ($n = 23$) diabetic patients versus. non-diabetic control subjects

($n = 71$). The higher levels in the Type 1 diabetic group were driven by high AGE-peptide levels in those with early renal damage. AGE-peptide levels correlated significantly with measures of renal dysfunction, but not with concurrent HbA1c levels, nor other measures of oxidative stress (serum oxidized LDL, isoprostanes, and paraoxonase-1 activity). We are also comparing serum AGE levels using two types of anti-sera generated by Dr. George Jerums' group. In preliminary studies, serum AGE levels (using an anti-serum to aerobically modified protein) were about 2-twofold higher in Type 1 diabetic subjects ($n = 25$) versus. healthy controls ($n = 13$), but did not differ between diabetic subjects with versus. without vascular complications. In contrast, relative to healthy control subjects, serum AGEs (measured by an antibody to an anaerobically generated antigen) were higher in 25 Type 1 diabetes subjects per se and 2–3 two- to threefold higher in complication-prone versus. complication-free diabetics (unpublished observations). Thus, data relating to AGEs in diabetes and its vascular complications are contrasting, though this may reflect differences in epitopes and populations studied. While there is supportive evidence of increases in at least some types of AGEs in diabetes, not all are oxidatively derived, and elevations may reflect increased substrate stress or impaired catabolism, rather than increased oxidative stress per se.

Protein Carbonyls

Protein carbonyl assays have been proposed as stable measures of tissue injury by oxidative stress and a general measure of oxidative stress.[153] The identity of products measured is not fully elucidated, but they may be derived from fragmentation and amine oxidation mediated by metal cations or hypochlorous acid. Plasma protein carbonyl levels increase with age, are higher in intensive care patients vs. healthy controls.[153,154] Relative to healthy subjects, circulating protein carbonyl levels have been found to be increased in Type 1 diabetes, and higher in subjects with vs. without microvascular complications,[155] but not in Type 2 diabetes.[156] In our laboratory we found no difference in protein carbonyl levels between complication-free Type 1 diabetic subjects and healthy controls, but high levels in ESRD subjects.[157] While there may be differences between assays and populations evaluated, these conflicting results do not support a general diabetes-related increase in oxidative damage, as measured by protein carbonyls. To our knowledge, there are no studies relating protein carbonyl levels to macrovascular disease or events, particularly in diabetes.

Glutathionyl Hemoglobin (Glut-Hb)

Oxidative stress may differ between the extra- and intracellular environments, and between subcellular compartments. Intracellular oxidative stress is less readily measured, but is appealing, particularly in light of Brownlee's findings,[33,34] and the value of HbA$_{1c}$, an intracellular measure of glycation, to clinical practice. Glut-Hb, formed by the reaction of hemoglobin with oxidized thiol groups has been suggested as a measure of intracellular oxidative stress.[158,159] Glut-Hb has a higher affinity for oxygen than does native Hb, hence may contribute to tissue hypoxia[158] as well as being a marker of oxidative stress. Niwa et al. demonstrated that Glut-Hb levels are increased in Type 2 diabetes, hyperlipidemia,[160] and in renal failure,[161] relative to a (poorly defined) control group, and can be lowered in Type 2 diabetes by vitamin E supplementation.[162] We recently measured Glut-Hb levels in Type 1 diabetic subjects with and without microvascular complications and in relationship to non-invasively determined vascular elasticity, in Type 2 diabetic subjects with and without coronary artery disease, and in a non-diabetic group of subjects of similar age and gender distribution. Measures of hemoglobin glycation were increased in diabetes and related to complications and vascular elasticity as expected. However, we found no difference in Glut-Hb between subjects with diabetes compared to those without diabetes, and between diabetic subjects with vascular damage compared to those without vascular damage. Nor were there any significant relationships between this putative oxidative stress measure and smoking status (a pro-oxidant stress), lipids, or plasma isoprostanes (manuscript in preparation). There are no prospective studies of Glut-Hb and vascular events, particularly in diabetes.

Antioxidant Enzymes, Their Related Genes and Vascular Damage in Diabetes

Various extracellular and intracellular enzymes act as pro-oxidants and antioxidants. Altered levels or activity of such enzymes may contribute to increased oxidative stress and damage in diabetes, and represent therapeutic targets. Furthermore, genetic polymorphisms of some of these enzymes may contribute to the heritability of atherosclerosis susceptibility in the general and diabetic populations and to that of the related microvascular complications in diabetes. Enzymes currently of interest in the field of diabetes research are superoxide dismutase, paraoxonase (an HDL-associated enzyme which can inhibit lipoprotein oxidation) and myeloperoxidase, a pro-oxidant enzyme.

Superoxide Dismutase

Superoxide dismutase (SOD), an enzyme that exists in several forms in both the extracellular and intracellular milieu, catalyzes the breakdown of O_2^-, and is implicated in hypertension and vascular damage.[163,164] Impaired endothelium-dependent vasodilatation, a feature of diabetes, occurs in the SOD knockout mice.[165] High glucose and methylglyoxal, features of the diabetic milieu, can induce O_2^- and lower SOD activity[166–167] in model systems. High glucose[168] and Ox-LDL[169] can increase SOD activity, perhaps as an adaptive protective response. Increasing SOD activity can reverse adverse effects of the diabetic milieu in animal models,[170,171] short-term human studies,[172] and cultured cells, including blockade of three pathways implicated in vascular damage in diabetes.[173]

In human studies, SOD concentration does not seem to be altered in diabetes, but the majority of studies find lower *activity* of intracellular (erythrocyte and leukocyte) and extracellular SOD, usually inversely related to HbA_{1c} and associated with higher levels of oxidative damage (as reflected by markers of DNA damage and lipid oxidation).[174–180] However, there are also similar cross-sectional studies in which SOD activity is unchanged[180–185] or even higher[186–188] in diabetic subjects compared with control subjects. In most, but not all studies, the presence of diabetic microvascular complications was associated with even lower SOD activity in diabetes. In the general population, including some diabetic subjects, SOD activity was lower in subjects with vs. without coronary artery disease.[189,190] However, in another study there was no significant difference in SOD activity of diabetic subjects with vs. without peripheral vascular disease.[191] Furthermore, in a prospective study in the general population, including people with diabetes, SOD activity was not predictive of future vascular events.[192] There are few SOD genotype genotype-related studies in diabetes. Polymorphisms of SOD genes have been associated with neuropathy in Type 1 diabetes[193] and with nephropathy in Type 2 diabetes,[194] but not with macrovascular disease in Type 2 diabetes.[195] Further prospective and interventional studies of SOD activity and genotypes and vascular events in human diabetes are required. As yet, to our knowledge, there are no reported SOD SOD-related intervention studies with vascular event end-points in human diabetes.

Paraoxonase (PON)

There are at least three paraoxonase (PON) genes (PON 1,2, and 3), but the most well well-studied gene product is PON-1, located on HDL. PON is also present in tissues. PON protects against exogenous organophosphate poisons and is thought to hydrolyze phospholipid oxidation products. It may therefore protect against damaging modifications of lipoproteins and cell membranes, and high PON activity should be protective.[196–199] Acute-phase HDL, which has greatly reduced PON activity is less protective against LDL oxidation.[200] Enyzme activity is usually assessed in vitro by hydrolysis of artificial substrates such as paraoxon and phenylacetate, but more (patho)physiologically relevant substrates would be preferable.[201] Nevertheless, there are numerous cross-sectional and longitudinal studies evaluating vascular disease risk in relationship to hydrolysis of the artificial substrates. In most, but not all studies, low serum PON activity has been associated with or predictive of vascular disease.[196–199,202]

Major determinants of PON activity (at least against paraoxon) are PON genotypes, which have also been associated with cardiovascular disease in some, but not all, studies.[198,199,203] Data with regard to the relationship of PON activity, related genotypes, and diabetes complications are contrasting. Cross-sectional studies report lower serum PON activity in diabetic subjects with vs. without vascular complications.[204–206]. However others find no difference [207] (our unpublished results) or higher (supposedly protective) activity.[208] PON genotypes differ in their ability to protect lipoproteins against in vitro oxidation,[209] but in the DCCT/EDIC cohort of Type 1 diabetic subjects we did not find any difference between LDL oxidizibility and PON genotypes. Polymorphisms in genes for PON-1, a PON-1 promotor region, and PON-2 have been studied in relation to atherosclerosis and to diabetic macro- and microvascular complications. In the general population, including diabetic subjects, PON-1 55 L/L phenotype was an independent risk factor for atheroma verified at autopsy.[210] Case–control studies in Type 2 diabetes have found associations between PON genotypes and macrovascular disease[211–215] and nephropathy,[216] and a relationship between PON-1 55 polymorphisms and markers of oxidative DNA damage[217] and isoprostanes.[218] However, in Type 1 diabetes Araki et al. did not find any difference in three PON genotypes in subjects prone or resistant to diabetic nephropathy.[219] As yet there are no publications relating PON genotypes or activities to atherosclerotic events in Type 1 diabetes. These inconsistent studies may reflect relatively small numbers, different ethnic backgrounds, ages and diabetes duration, differences in glycemia, smoking, medications, the definition of complications, and unevaluated gene—gene interactions. There is also a paradox in PON research in that vascular disease, including diabetic complications, has been associated with PON genotypes coding for (allegedly protective) high serum PON activity.[203,220] Thus, the association of PON with vascular damage, including in diabetes, is complex, and may differ at different stages of disease.

While genotypes cannot be changed, they may increase our understanding of mechanisms of vascular damage and aid in the identification of high-risk patients. In contrast, lifestyle and pharmaceutical interventions can modulate PON activity.[201,221–226] Healthy diets,[135,221,222] including dietary-modification induced increases in antioxidant levels,[135] smoking cessation,[223] lipid modulating drugs (simvastatin[224] and gemfibrozil[225]), and hormone replacement in postmenopausal diabetic women[226] can increase PON activity, but as yet this change has not been shown to be associated with reduced vascular events in any population.

Myeloperoxidase

Myeloperoxidase (MPO) is a leukocyte enzyme which generates ROS and reactive nitrogen species as part of its vital role in normal host defense. However, these MPO-generated oxidants have also been implicated in lipid oxidation, endothelial dysfunction, inflammation, plaque instability, and poor ventricular remodeling after myocardial infarction (reviewed in [227]). MPO activity is increased in the leukocytes from (Type 2) diabetic subjects.[228,229] MPO is present and active in human atherosclerotic lesions, and MPO MPO-generated oxidation products including the MPO specific oxidation product chlorotyrosine, and of nitrotyrosine, dityrosine, and isoprostanes have been identified in human atherosclerotic lesions.[227,230] The relative abundance of enzyme and related oxidation products in diabetic vs. non-diabetic atherosclerotic lesions is as yet unknown.

In keeping with a major role of MPO in atherosclerosis, inherited MPO deficiency is associated with lower rate of cardiovascular disease,[231] and MPO gene polymorphisms (−463G/A and −129G/A), in studies including diabetic subjects, have been associated with altered MPO activity, angiographically proven coronary artery disease,[232] autopsy autopsy-verified aortic atheroma,[233] reduced coronary flow reserve in healthy young men,[234] size and functional outcome of cerebral infarction,[235] and higher pentosidine levels and cardiovascular disease in end-stage renal disease.[236]

MPO levels have also been associated with and predictive of coronary artery disease in studies including diabetic and non-diabetic subjects. In a case—control coronary angiographic study Zhang et al. recently demonstrated that blood and leukocyte myeloperoxidase levels were independent predictors of cardiovascular disease presence and burden.[237] In a prospective study, Brennan et al. demonstrated that plasma myeloperoxidase levels were predictive of acute, 30 -day and 6six-month outcome in patients presenting with chest pain (with or without evidence of troponin T rise).[238] Further supportive evidence is the predictive power of (NO - derived oxidants, catalyzed by MPO) such as nitrotyrosine, for atherosclerosis risk and burden[239] in a mixed population of diabetic and non-diabetic subjects.

While vitamin E does not inhibit MPO-induced oxidation in vitro, HMG CoA Reductase inhibitors can lower MPO/NO -generated oxidation products, as suggested by cross-sectional and intervention studies.[239,240] Further Type 1 and Type 2 diabetes specific studies are warranted.

Therefore, there are several oxidative stress enzymes and related products that are strong candidates for potentiating atherosclerosis in diabetes. Antioxidant enzyme levels or activities are abnormal in many, but not all, published studies in diabetes, and related genotypes have been associated with atherosclerosis in some studies. These enzymes (or their products) have been located at the site of vascular damage. There is associative and predictive power for atherosclerosis atherosclerosis-related events, and related interventions in the laboratory ameliorate vascular damage or surrogate end-points. Thus, evidence to date is supportive, but not conclusive, of a role for these oxidative stress -related factors in vascular damage. Measurement of such factors merits inclusion in human cross-sectional, longitudinal, and intervention studies of vascular disease in Type 1 and Type 2 diabetic subjects, and further exploration in diabetes relevant biochemical, cell culture, and animal model systems.

The Link Between Oxidative Stress and Vascular Damage in Diabetes

We currently lack good measures of oxidative stress and oxidative damage in human Type 1 and Type 2 diabetes specific studies to make a definitive decision as to whether oxidative stress is increased in diabetes per se, or in relationship to its vascular complications. Once an appropriate measure, or more likely panel of

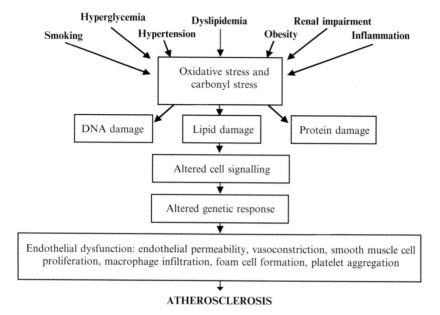

Fig. 7.1 Schema of risk factors and mechanisms for accelerated atherosclerosis in diabetes

measures, are validated and standardized, a reference range in healthy non-diabetic subjects over a wide age range must be determined. Oxidative stress and damage damage-related levels can then be compared in well well-characterized Type 1 and Type 2 diabetic subjects with and without micro- and macrovascular complications, over a range of glycemic control, and with known lifestyle (e.g., smoking) and medications (which may have antioxidant activity). Based on current knowledge, oxidative stress is likely to be increased in some parts of some cells in some tissues, for at least some of the time. Even if oxidative stress, an inevitable part of living, is not increased in diabetes per se, then it may still contribute to the progression of vascular complications of diabetes. A simple schema is suggested (Figure 7.1) .

Thus, it remains conceivable that, even if not increased in diabetes, lowering oxidative stress and oxidative damage may reduce vascular complications in diabetes, in the same way that lowering supposedly 'normal' levels of cholesterol has resulted in further reduction of vascular events in at-risk groups. Much further (long-term human based) research is required to prove this.

Treatment of Oxidative Stress

Potential mechanisms of macrovascular damage by oxidative stress are shown in Table 7.6. Antioxidant supplementation can reduce some measures of oxidative damage in people with diabetes, and high high-dose vitamin E (at doses also likely to have

Table 7.6 Potential mechanisms of macrovascular damage by oxidative stress or related products

- Altered cell viability
- Cell proliferation – ↓ smooth muscle cells, ↓ in endothelial scells
- Apoptosis and necrosis, e.g., smooth muscle cells
- Increased foam cell formation
- Uptake of modified LDL, e.g., Ox-LDL and immune complexes with LDL
- Cell activation and altered cell function
  e.g., PKC, NF-κB, MAPK, and TGF-β activation
  e.g., ↑ Matrix production and ↓ degradation
- Abnormal vascular tone and blood flow
  e.g., ↑; Endothelin-1, ↓ nitric oxide bioavailability
- Increased endothelial barrier permeability
- Pro-inflammatory effects
  ↑ Cell adhesion molecules
  ↑ Monocyte chemoattractant activity and vascular ingress
- Proclotting effects
  ↑ PAI-1
  ↓ tPA
  ↓ Tissue factor pathway inhibitor
  ↑ Platelet aggregation
- AGEs
- Vascular stiffening
- Modulation of above effects

↓ Increased, ↓ decreased, PKC protein kinase C, TGF-β transforming growth factor-beta, PAI-1 plasminogen activator inhibitor-1, tPA tissue plasminogen activator, NF-κB nuclear factor-kappa B, MAPK mitogen activated kinase pathway, Ox-LDL oxidized low density lipoprotein.

PKC inhibitory activity)[241] can also improve surrogate measures of retinal[242] and macrovascular endothelial dysfunction[243] in young people with relatively short duration Type 1 diabetes. However, the recent negative trials of antioxidant supplementation for clinical vascular disease end-points in the general and Type 2 diabetic populations[78,244] have reduced enthusiasm for antioxidant supplementation in diabetes. Mitigating factors in these negative antioxidant trials may be the type, site of action, dose, and duration of antioxidant supplementation and stage of pre-existing vascular damage (influenced by patient age and diabetes duration). Therefore, the American Diabetes Association does not currently recommend vitamin supplementation in diabetes unless a deficiency state is evident.[245]

As knowledge is gained regarding the mechanisms and sites of oxidative stress, our understanding of the negative outcome in the vitamin E intervention studies improves. As well as anti-oxidant actions, vitamin E can have both pro-oxidant effects, at least in model systems,[246,247] and does not reduce some systemic markers of oxidative stress. Unfortunately a broad panel of oxidative stress measures (e.g., including Ox-LDL, isoprostanes, and MPO) was not included in the negative vitamin E intervention studies. Vitamin E is located predominantly in lipophilic/hydrophobic environments (such as lipoproteins and cell membranes), yet many

ROS are generated in the cytosol or extracellular compartments. Furthermore, antioxidants may only act on a limited number of pro-oxidant pathways. For example, vitamin E scavenges already formed oxidation products, predominantly from lipid peroxidation and does not reduce peroxynitrite.

Another lipid -soluble free radical scavenger of interest is lipoic acid. This antioxidant acts in the mitochondria and can reduce lipid oxidation measures and improve neural blood flow in animal models of diabetes. In humans, lipoic acid has improved some measures of peripheral and cardiac autonomic neuropathy and endothelial dysfunction,[248] but studies regarding macrovascular end-points are not available.

While prospective vitamin E supplementation intervention studies have not reduced vascular events, intensive diabetes management and lipid and blood pressure lowering have proven effective.[35–37,249,250] Intensive diabetes management reduced vascular events in the United Kingdom Prospective Diabetes Study (UKPDS) of Type 2 diabetes,[37,249] and in the younger Type 1 diabetic DCCT/EDIC cohort reduced microvascular complications[35,250] and the surrogate atherosclerosis end-point of carotid intima media thickness.[36] Benefit may partly relate to a reduction in hyperglycemia -induced oxidative stress. As yet, to our knowledge, there are no published measures of oxidative stress or damage-related markers in these studies.

Clinical trials of lipid lowering and blood pressure lowering agents have shown beneficial effects on macrovascular events and survival in diabetes, and these may be partly mediated by the antioxidant effects of these drugs. HMG CoA Reductase inhibitors ("'statins'") proved successful in the Scandinavian Simvastatin Survival Study (4S) study[21,251] and the Heart Protection Study.[19] In addition to favorable effects on the lipid profile, lowering total- and LDL-C, triglycerides and increasing HDL-C, statins have pleiotropic effects which include anti–inflammatory and anti-oxidant effects. Statins increase PON activity and NO bioavailability, decrease O_2^- production, and decrease MPO- and NO-derived oxidants (e.g., chlorotyrosine and dityrosine).[252–255] They can rapidly improve endothelial dysfunction in diabetic patients.[256] Similarly, the blood pressure and microalbuminuria lowering angiotensin converting enzyme (ACE) inhibitors and angiotensin-1 receptor antagonists, which reduced diabetic vascular events in the Heart Outcomes Prevention Evaluation (HOPE)[78] and reduction of end-points in type 2 diabetes with the angiotensin II antagonist losartan (RENAAL)[258,257] studies are also strong intracellular antioxidants. Other agents already in clinical practice may have antioxidant effects that partly mediate their benefit. For example, thiazolidinediones have intracellular antioxidant effects, inhibit iNOS, and reduce peroxynitrite production.[2598–2643]

A better understanding of the mechanisms of oxidative stress and the vascular complications of diabetes, facilitated by biochemical, cell culture, and animal studies has resulted in the design of novel antioxidant drugs. Such drugs (discussed earlier) include low molecular weight agents that mimic the antioxidant enzymes catalase and SOD, an intracellular O_2^- scavenger L-propionyl-carnitine, polya(ADP-ribose) polymerase inhibitors (e.g., PJ34), and peroxynitrite decomposition catalysts (e.g., FP15). These agents are based on sound theory and have proven effective in model diabetic systems, but clinical trials in humans are awaited.

Conclusion and Future Directions

The onset and progression of diabetes-related atherosclerosis is likely to involve a wide range of pathogenic mechanisms, including oxidative stress, which as suggested by Brownlee, may have a central role stemming from hyperglycemia hyperglycemia-induced O_2^- production by mitochondria. Research has increased our understanding of oxidative stress in general and in diabetes, and its contribution to atherosclerosis and diabetic vascular complications. Well-validated and standardized assays of oxidative stress and damage are urgently needed. Samples for analysis must be collected and stored appropriately to avoid ex vivo oxidation, an obvious point, but one that can be difficult to achieve in large multicenter clinical trials. Knowledge of oxidative stress-related gene polymorphisms may facilitate identification and treatment of high complication risk diabetic patients and drug choice. Well-tolerated and effective drugs targeting appropriate oxidative stress pathways in appropriate compartments are required.

The relationship of oxidative stress stress-related markers to macrovascular events in both Type 1 and in Type 2 diabetes, levels defining high risk and treatment goals, and response to appropriate interventions requires much further study. Further biochemical, cell culture, animal, and human studies are required to elucidate underlying mechanisms of oxidative damage and to design and test effective treatments. Longer -term observational and intervention studies in well-characterized Type 1 and in Type 2 diabetic patients, focusing on macrovascular end-points and including measures of oxidative stress and damage are required. Surrogate measures of macrovascular damage will facilitate such studies, but knowledge of their relationship to clinical events and survival is vital.

Until such data and more specific guidelines and antioxidant drugs are available, aggressive management of diabetes according to currently accepted guidelines for lifestyle, glycemia, blood pressure, and dyslipidemia[265] dyslipidemia[264] should be continued for the prevention of macrovascular disease. These have proven successful, although atherosclerosis and the related microvascular complications still remain major causes of morbidity and premature mortality in this increasingly common condition. As diabetes complications are multi-factorial in origin, it is appropriate that a multi-faceted approach to prevention and treatment should be taken, and in the future, this may include new antioxidant therapies guided by measures of oxidative stress.

Acknowledgements The authors thank our colleagues for input into discussed research from the authors' laboratories, including: Professors James Best, George Jerums, Bruce Kemp, Timothy Lyons, John Baynes, Suzanne Thorpe, Maria Lopes-Virella, and W. Tim Garvey, and Drs Rick Klein, Deanna Cheek, Peter Hoffman, Christine Winterbourn, George Kalogerakis, Arthur Baker, Craig Nelson, Andrew Wilson, Kevin Croft, Trevor Mori, Andrzej Januszewski, Jasmine Chung, SQ Chan, and also Ms. Connie Karschimkus and Jade Woon, and Mr. George Dragicevic. Grant support for the research was provided by the Australian National Heart Foundation, VicHealth, the Juvenile Diabetes Research Foundation, Diabetes Australia Research Trust, the American Diabetes Association Lions SightFirst Diabetic Retinopathy Research Program, National Health and Medical Research Council, and the Ophthalmic Research Institute of Australia.

References

1. Amos AF, McCarty DJ, Zimmet P. The rising global burden of diabetes and its complications: estimates and projections to the year 2010. Diabetic Med 1997;14(Suppl 5): S1–S85.
2. Mandrup-Poulsen T. Beta cell death and protection. Ann N Y Acad Sci 2003;1005:32–42.
3. Kuroki T, Isshiki K, King GL. Oxidative stress: the lead or supporting actor in the pathogenesis of diabetic complications. J Am Soc Nephrol 2003;14(8 Suppl 3):S216–S220.
4. Rosen P, Nawroth PP, King G, Moller W, Tritschler HJ, Packer L. The role of oxidative stress in the onset and progression of diabetes and its complications: a summary of a Congress Series sponsored by UNESCO-MCBN, the American Diabetes Association and the German Diabetes Society. Diabetes Metab Res Rev 2001;17(3):189–212.
5. Ceriello A. New insights on oxidative stress and diabetic complications may lead to a "causal" antioxidant therapy. Diabetes Care 2003;26(5):1589–1596.
6. American Diabetes Association. Diagnosis and classification of diabetes mellitus. Diabetes Care 2004;(Suppl 1):S5–S10.
7. American Diabetes Association Consensus Statement. Type 2 Diabetes in Children and Adolescents. Diabetes Care 2000;23:381–389.
8. Despres JP, Lamarche B, Mauriege P, Cantin B, Dagenais GR, Moorjani S, Lupien PJ. Hyperinsulinemia as an independent risk factor for ischemic heart disease. N Engl J Med 1996;334(15):952–957.
9. Uwaifo GI, Ratner RE. Diabetes 1996 Vital Statistics. American Diabetes Association.
10. Pickup JC, Williams G (Eds). Chronic complications of diabetes. Melbourne: Blackwell Press, 1994.
11. Pyorala K. Diabetes and heart disease. In: Mogensen CE, Standl E (Eds). Prevention and Treatment of the Diabetic Late Complications. New York: Walter de Gruyter 1989, pp. 151–168.
12. American Diabetes Association Position Statement. Diabetic nephropathy. Diabetes Care 2003;(Suppl 1):S94–S98.
13. Bloomgarden ZT. The epidemiology of complications. Diabetes Care 2002;25(5):924–932.
14. Scott AR. Diabetic nephropathy. In: Donnelly R, Jonas J (Eds). Vascular Complications of Diabetes. Oxford: Blackwell Publishers, 2002, pp. 21–31.
15. American Diabetes Association Position Statement. Diabetic retinopathy. Diabetes Care 2003;(Suppl 1):S99–S102.
16. Borch-Johnsen K, Kreiner S. Proteinuria: value as a predictor of cardiovascular mortality in insulin dependent diabetes mellitus. Br Med J 1987;294:1651–1654.
17. Bakis GL. Microalbuminuria: prognostic implications. Curr Opin Nephrol Hypertens 1996;5:219–223.
18. Donahue RP, Orchard TJ. Diabetes mellitus and macrovascular complications. An epidemiological perspective. Diabetes Care 1992;15(9):1141–1155.
19. Collins R, Armitage J, Parish S, Sleigh P, Peto R, Heart Protection Study Collaborative Group. MRC/BHF Heart Protection Study of cholesterol-lowering with simvastatin in 5963 people with diabetes: a randomised placebo-controlled trial. Lancet 2003;361(9374):2005–2016.
20. Yusuf S, Sleight P, Pogue J, Bosch J, Davies R, Dagenais G. Effects of an angiotensin-converting-enzyme inhibitor, ramipril, on cardiovascular events in high-risk patients. The Heart Outcomes Prevention Evaluation Study Investigators. N Engl J Med 2000;342(3): 145–153.
21. Herman WH, Alexander CM, Cook JR, Boccuzzi SJ, Musliner TA, Pedersen TR, Kjekshus J, Pyorala K. Effect of simvastatin treatment on cardiovascular resource utilization in impaired fasting glucose and diabetes. Findings from the Scandinavian Simvastatin Survival Study. Diabetes Care 1999;22(11):1771–1778.
22. Larsen J, Brekke M, Sandvik L, Arnesen H, Hanssen KF, Dahl-Jorgensen K. Silent coronary atheromatosis in type 1 diabetic patients and its relation to long-term glycemic control. Diabetes 2002;51(8):2637–2641.

23. Penfornis A, Zimmermann C, Boumal D, Sabbah A, Meneveau N, Gaultier-Bourgeois S, Bassand JP, Bernard Y. Use of dobutamine stress echocardiography in detecting silent myocardial ischaemia in asymptomatic diabetic patients: a comparison with thallium scintigraphy and exercise testing. Diabet Med 2001;18(11):900–905.

24. Arcavi L, Behar S, Caspi A, Reshef N, Boyko V, Knobler H. High fasting glucose levels as a predictor of worse clinical outcome in patients with coronary artery disease: results from the Bezafibrate Infarction Prevention (BIP) study. Am Heart J 2004;147(2):239–245.

25. Tooke JE. Possible pathophysiological mechanisms for diabetic angiopathy in type 2 diabetes. J Diabetes Complicat 2000;14(4):197–200.

26. Giardino I, Brownlee M. The biochemical basis of microvascular disease. In: Pickup JC, Williams G, (Eds). Textbook of Diabetes. Melbourne: Blackwell Press, 1997.

27. Klein R, Sharrett AR, Klein BE, Moss SE, Folsom AR, Wong TY, et al. The association of atherosclerosis, vascular risk factors, and retinopathy in adults with diabetes: the Atherosclerosis Risk in Communities study. Ophthalmology 2002;109(7):1225–1234.

28. Jenkins AJ, Best JD, Klein RL, Lyons TJ. Lipoproteins, glycoxidation and diabetic angiopathy. Diabetes Metab Res Rev 2004;20(5):349–368.

29. Shore AC, Tooke JE. Microvascular function and haemodynamic disturbances in diabetes mellitus and its complications. In: Pickup JC, Williams G (Eds). Textbook of Diabetes. Melbourne: Blackwell Press, 1997.

30. Diamond JR. Analogous pathobiologic mechanisms in glomerulosclerosis and atherosclerosis. Kidney Int 1991;31(Suppl):S29–S34.

31. Lyons TJ, Jenkins AJ. Glycation, oxidation, and lipoxidation in the development of the complications of diabetes: a carbonyl stress hypothesis. Diabetes Rev 1997;5:365–391.

32. Stitt AW, Jenkins AJ, Cooper ME. Advanced glycation end products and diabetic complications. Expert Opin Investig Drugs 2002;11(9):1205–1223.

33. Brownlee M. Biochemistry and molecular cell biology of diabetic complications. Nature 2001;414(6865):813–820.

34. Nishikawa T, Edelstein D, Du XL, Yamagishi S, Matsumura T, Kaneda Y, Yorek MA, Beebe D, Oates PJ, Hammes HP, Giardino I, Brownlee M. Normalizing mitochondrial superoxide production blocks three pathways of hyperglycaemic damage. Nature 2000;404(6779): 787–790.

35. The Diabetes Control and Complications Trial Research Group. The effect of intensive treatment of diabetes on the development and progression of long-term complications in insulin dependent diabetes mellitus. New Engl J Med 1993;329:977–986.

36. Nathan DM, Lachin J, Cleary P, Orchard T, Brillon DJ, Backlund JY, O'Leary DH, Genuth S, Diabetes Control and Complications Trial, Epidemiology of Diabetes Interventions and Complications Research Group. Intensive diabetes therapy and carotid intima-media thickness in type 1 diabetes mellitus. N Engl J Med 2003;348(23):2294–2303.

37. UKPDS Group. Intensive blood-glucose control with sulphonylureas or insulin compared with conventional treatment and risk of complications in patients with type 2 diabetes UKPDS 33. Lancet 1998;352:837–853.

38. Herman WH, Crofford OB. The relationship between metabolic control and complications. In: Pickup JC, Williams G, (Eds). Textbook of Diabetes. Melbourne: Blackwell Press, 1997.

39. Baynes JW, Thorpe SR. Oxidative stress in diabetes. In: Packer L, Rosen P, Tritschler HJ, King GL (Eds). Antioxidants in Diabetes Management. New York: Marcel Decker, 2000, pp. 77–91.

40. Baynes JW, Thorpe SR. Role of oxidative stress in diabetic complications: a new perspective on an old paradigm. Diabetes 1999;48(1):1–9.

41. Droge W. Free radicals in the physiological control of cell function. Physiol Rev 2002;82(1):47–95.

42. Rice Evans CA, Diplock AT, Symons MCR. Introduction to free radicals. Techniques in Free Radical Research. In: Burdon RH and, van Knippenberg PH (Eds). Laboratory Techniques in Biochemistry and Molecular Biology. Amsterdam: Elsevier, 1991, pp. 1–18.

43. Taniyama Y, Griendling KK. Reactive oxygen species in the vasculature: molecular and cellular mechanisms. Hypertension 2003;42(6):1075–1081.
44. Ceriello A. New insights on oxidative stress and diabetic complications may lead to a "causal" antioxidant therapy. Diabetes Care 2003;26(5):1589–1596.
45. Giugliano D, Ceriello A, Paolisso G. Oxidative stress and diabetic vascular complications. Diabetes Care 1996;19(3):257–267.
46. Farkas K, Sarman B, Jermendy G, Somogyi A. Endothelial nitric oxide in diabetes mellitus: too much or not enough? Diabetes Nutr Metab 2000;13(5):287–297.
47. Bonnefont-Rousselot D. Glucose and reactive oxygen species. Curr Opin Clin Nutr Metab Care 2002;5(5):561–568.
48. Rosen P, Du X, Sui GZ. Molecular mechanisms of endothelial dysfunction in the diabetic heart. Adv Exp Med Biol 2001;498:75–86.
49. Piconi L, Quagliaro L, Ceriello A. Oxidative stress in diabetes. Clin Chem Lab Med 2003;41(9):1144–1149.
50. Cai H, Harrison DG. Endothelial dysfunction in cardiovascular diseases: the role of oxidant stress. Circ Res 2000;87(10):840–844.
51. Garcia Soriano F, Virag L, Jagtap P, Szabo E, Mabley JG, Liaudet L, Marton A, Hoyt DG, Murthy KG, Salzman AL, Southan GJ, Szabo C. Diabetic endothelial dysfunction: the role of poly(ADP-ribose) polymerase activation. Nat Med 2001;7(1):108–113.
52. Szabo C, Mabley JG, Moeller SM, Shimanovich R, Pacher P, Virag L, Soriano FG, Van Duzer JH, Williams W, Salzman AL, Groves JT. Part I: Pathogenetic role of peroxynitrite in the development of diabetes and diabetic vascular complications: studies with FP15, a novel potent peroxynitrite decomposition catalyst. Mol Med 2002;8(10):571–580.
53. Pacher P, Liaudet L, Soriano FG, Mabley JG, Szabo E, Szabo C. The role of poly(ADP-ribose) polymerase activation in the development of myocardial and endothelial dysfunction in diabetes. Diabetes 2002;51(2):514–521.
54. Haj-Yehia AI, Nassar T, Assaf P, Nassar H, Anggard EE. Effects of the superoxide dismutase-mimic compound TEMPOL on oxidant stress-mediated endothelial dysfunction. Antioxid Redox Signal 1999;1(2):221–232.
55. Nassar T, Kadery B, Lotan C, Da'as N, Kleinman Y, Haj-Yehia A. Effects of the superoxide dismutase-mimetic compound tempol on endothelial dysfunction in streptozotocin-induced diabetic rats. Eur J Pharmacol 2002;436(1–2):111–118.
56. Packer L, Kraemer K, Rimbach G. Molecular aspects of lipoic acid in the prevention of diabetes complications. Nutrition 2001;17(10):888–895.
57. Vanella A, Russo A, Acquaviva R, Campisi A, Di Giacomo C, Sorrenti V, Barcellona ML. L-propionyl-carnitine as superoxide scavenger, antioxidant, and DNA cleavage protector. Cell Biol Toxicol 2000;16(2):99–104.
58. Cotter MA, Jack AM, Cameron NE. Effects of the protein kinase C beta inhibitor LY333531 on neural and vascular function in rats with streptozotocin-induced diabetes. Clin Sci (Lond) 2002;103(3):311–321.
59. Cameron NE, Jack AM, Cotter MA. Effect of alpha-lipoic acid on vascular responses and nociception in diabetic rats. Free Radic Biol Med 2001;31(1):125–135.
60. Tuttle KR, Anderson PW. A novel potential therapy for diabetic nephropathy and vascular complications: protein kinase C beta inhibition. Am J Kidney Dis 2003;42(3):456–465.
61. Way KJ, Katai N, King GL. Protein kinase C and the development of diabetic vascular complications. Diabet Med 2001;18(12):945–959.
62. Beckman JA, Goldfine AB, Gordon MB, Garrett LA, Creager MA. Inhibition of protein kinase C beta prevents impaired endothelium-dependent vasodilation caused by hyperglycemia in humans. Circ Res 2002;90(1):107–111.
63. Heitzer T, Finckh B, Albers S, Krohn K, Kohlschutter A, Meinertz T. Beneficial effects of alpha-lipoic acid and ascorbic acid on endothelium-dependent, nitric oxide-mediated vasodilation in diabetic patients: relation to parameters of oxidative stress. Free Radic Biol Med 2001;31(1):53–61.

64. Abuja PM, Albertini R. Methods for monitoring oxidative stress, lipid peroxidation and oxidation resistance of lipoproteins. Clin Chim Acta 2001;306(1–2):1–17.
65. Onorato JM, Thorpe SR, Baynes JW. Immunohistochemical and ELISA assays for biomarkers of oxidative stress in aging and disease. Ann N Y Acad Sci 1998;854:277–290.
66. Wu LL, Chiou CC, Chang PY, Wu JT. Urinary 8-OHdG: a marker of oxidative stress to DNA and a risk factor for cancer, atherosclerosis and diabetics. Clin Chim Acta 2004;339(1–2):1–9.
67. Oxidative stress biomarkers and antioxidant protocols. In: Armstrong D (Ed.)., Methods in Molecular Biology Volume 186. Totowa: Humana Press, 2002.
68. Miyata T, van Yprsele de Strihou C, Kurokawa K, Baynes JW. Alterations in nonenzymatic biochemistry in uremia: origin and significance of "carbonyl stress" in long-term uremic complications. Kidney Int 1999;55(2):389–399.
69. Suzuki D, Miyata T, Kurokawa K. Carbonyl stress. Contrib Nephrol 2001;134:36–45.
70. Baynes JW, Thorpe SR. Glycoxidation and lipoxidation in atherogenesis. Free Radic Biol Med 2000;28(12):1708–1716.
71. McCance DR, Dyer DG, Dunn JA, Bailie KE, Thorpe SR, Baynes JW, Lyons TJ. Maillard reaction products and their relation to complications in insulin-dependent diabetes mellitus. J Clin Invest 1993;91(6):2470–2478.
72. Dyer DG, Dunn JA, Thorpe SR, Bailie KE, Lyons TJ, McCance DR, Baynes JW. Accumulation of Maillard reaction products in skin collagen in diabetes and aging. J Clin Invest 1993;91(6):2463–2469.
73. Wells-Knecht MC, Lyons TJ, McCance DR, Thorpe SR, Baynes JW. Age-dependent increase in ortho-tyrosine and methionine sulfoxide in human skin collagen is not accelerated in diabetes. Evidence against a generalized increase in oxidative stress in diabetes. J Clin Invest 1997;100(4):839–846.
74. Wang LJ, Lee TS, Lee FY, Pai RC, Chau LY. Expression of heme oxygenase-1 in atherosclerotic lesions. Am J Pathol 1998;152:711–720.
75. Chung SS, Ho EC, Lam KS, Chung SK. Contribution of polyol pathway to diabetes-induced oxidative stress. J Am Soc Nephrol 2003;14(8 Suppl 3):S233–S236.
76. Li JM, Shah AM. ROS generation by nonphagocytic NADPH oxidase: potential relevance in diabetic nephropathy. J Am Soc Nephrol 2003;14(8 Suppl 3):S221–S226.
77. Maritim AC, Sanders RA, Watkins JB. Diabetes, oxidative stress, and antioxidants: a review. J Biochem Mol Toxicol 2003;17(1):24–38.
78. Lonn E, Yusuf S, Hoogwerf B, Pogue J, Yi Q, Zinman B, Bosch J, Dagenais G, Mann JF, Gerstein HC, HOPE Study, MICRO-HOPE Study. Effects of vitamin E on cardiovascular and microvascular outcomes in high-risk patients with diabetes: results of the HOPE study and MICRO-HOPE substudy. Diabetes Care 2002;25(11):1919–1927.
79. Chisolm GM, Steinberg D. The oxidative modification hypothesis of atherogenesis: an overview. Free Radic Biol Med 2000;28(12):1815–1826.
80. Penn MS, Chisolm GM. Oxidized lipoproteins, altered cell function and atherosclerosis. Atherosclerosis 1994;108(Suppl):S21–S29.
81. Albertini R, Moratti R, De Luca G. Oxidation of low-density lipoprotein in atherosclerosis from basic biochemistry to clinical studies. Curr Mol Med 2002;2(6):579–592.
82. Schlondorff D. Cellular mechanisms of lipid injury in the glomerulus. Am J Kidney Dis 1993;22(1):72–82.
83. Heeringa P, Tervaert JW. Role of oxidized low-density lipoprotein in renal disease. Curr Opin Nephrol Hypertens 2002;11(3):287–293.
84. Lyons TJ, Li W, Wells-Knecht MC, Jokl R. Toxicity of mildly modified low-density lipoproteins to cultured retinal capillary endothelial cells and pericytes. Diabetes 1994;43(9):1090–1095.
85. Jenkins AJ, Li W, Moller K, Klein RL, Fu MX, Baynes JW, Thorpe SR, Lyons TJ. Pre-enrichment of modified low density lipoproteins with alpha-tocopherol mitigates adverse effects on cultured retinal capillary cells. Curr Eye Res 1999;19(2):137–145.
86. Lyons TJ, Jenkins AJ. Lipoprotein glycation and its metabolic consequences. Curr Opin Lipidol 1997;8(3):174–180

87. Jenkins AJ, Rowley KG, Lyons TJ, Best JD, Hill MA, Klein RL. Lipoproteins and diabetic microvascular complications. Curr Pharm Des 2004;10(27):3395–3418.
88. Lyons TJ. Oxidized low density lipoproteins – a role in the pathogenesis of atherosclerosis in diabetes? Diabet Med 1991;8:411–419.
89. Relou IA, Hackeng CM, Akkerman JW, Malle E. Low-density lipoprotein and its effect on human blood platelets. Cell Mol Life Sci 2003;60(5):961–971.
90. Kuo Hein TW, Liao JC, Kuo L. oxLDL specifically impairs endothelium-dependent, NO-mediated dilation of coronary arterioles. Am J Physiol Heart Circ Physiol 2000;278(1): H175–H183.
91. Bolz SS, Galle J, Derwand R, de Wit C, Pohl U. Oxidized LDL increases the sensitivity of the contractile apparatus in isolated resistance arteries for Ca(2+) via a rho- and rho kinase-dependent mechanism. Circulation 2000;102(19):2402–2410.
92. Lyons TJ, Klein RL, Baynes JW, Stevenson HC, Lopes-Virella MF. Stimulation of choles-teryl ester synthesis in human monocyte-derived macrophages by lipoproteins from Type 1 diabetic subjects: the influence of non-enzymatic glycosylation of low-density lipoproteins. Diabetologia 1987;30:916–923.
93. Lopes-Virella MF, Klein RL, Lyons TJ, Stevenson HC, Witztum JL. Glycosylated low den-sity lipoprotein enhances cholesteryl ester synthesis in human monocyte-derived macro-phages. Diabetes 1988;37:550–557.
94. Jenkins AJ, Velarde V, Klein RL, Joyce KC, Phillips KD, Mayfield RK, Lyons TJ, Jaffa AA. Native and modified LDL activate extracellular signal-regulated kinases in mesangial cells. Diabetes 2000;49(12):2160–2169.
95. Velarde V, Jenkins AJ, Christopher J, Lyons TJ, Jaffa AA. Activation of MAPK by modified low-density lipoproteins in vascular smooth muscle cells. J Appl Physiol 2001;91(3): 1412–1420.
96. Lyons TJ, Li W, Wojciechowski B, Wells-Knecht MC, Wells-Knecht KJ, Jenkins AJ. Aminoguanidine and the effects of modified LDL on cultured retinal capillary cells. Invest Ophthalmol Vis Sci 2000;41:1176–1180.
97. Edwards IJ, Wagner JD, Litwak KN, Rudel LL, Cefalu WT. Glycation of plasma low density lipoproteins increases interaction with arterial proteoglycans. Diabetes Res Clin Pract 1999;46(1):9–18.
98. Edwards IJ, Terry JG, Bell-Farrow AD, Cefalu WT. Improved glucose control decreases the interaction of plasma low-density lipoproteins with arterial proteoglycans. Metabolism 2002;51(10):1223–1229.
99. Tsai EC, Hirsch IB, Brunzell JD, Chait A. Reduced plasma peroxyl radical trapping capacity and increased susceptibility of LDL to oxidation in poorly controlled IDDM. Diabetes 1994;43(8):1010–1014.
100. Jenkins AJ, Klein RL, Chassereau CN, Hermayer KL, Lopes-Virella MF. LDL from patients with well-controlled IDDM is not more susceptible to in vitro oxidation. Diabetes 1996;45(6):762–767.
101. Jenkins AJ, Thorpe SR, Alderson NL, Hermayer KL, Lyons TJ, King LP, et al. In vivo gly-cated LDL is not more susceptible to oxidation than non-glycated LDL in type 1 diabetes. Metabolism 2004;53(8):969–976.
102. Jenkins AJ, Lyons TJ, Zheng D, Otvos JD, Lackland DT, McGee D, et al. Serum lipoproteins in the diabetes control and complications trial/epidemiology of diabetes intervention and complications cohort: associations with gender and glycemia. Diabetes Care 2003;26(3): 810–818.
103. Jenkins AJ, Lyons TJ, Zheng D, Otvos JD, Lackland DT, McGee D, Garvey WT, Klein RL, DCCT/EDIC Research Group. Lipoproteins in the DCCT/EDIC cohort: associations with diabetic nephropathy. Kidney Int 2003;64(3):817–828.
104. Jenkins AJ, Lyons TJ, Zheng D, Lackland DT, McGee D, Garvey WT, Klein RL. Diabetic retinopathy and serum lipoprotein subclasses in the DCCT/EDIC Cohort. Invest Ophthalmol Vis Sci 2004;45(3):910–918.

105. Nishi K, Itabe H, Uno M, Kitazato KT, Horiguchi H, Shinno K, Nagahiro S. Oxidized LDL in carotid plaques and plasma associates with plaque instability. Arterioscler Thromb Vasc Biol 2002;22(10):1649–1654.

106. Ehara S, Ueda M, Naruko T, Haze K, Itoh A, Otsuka M, et al. Elevated levels of oxidized low density lipoprotein show a positive relationship with the severity of acute coronary syndromes. Circulation 2001;103(15):1955–1960.

107. Nordin Fredrikson G, Hedblad B, Berglund G, Nilsson J. Plasma oxidized LDL: a predictor for acute myocardial infarction? J Intern Med 2003;253(4):425–429.

108. Tsutsui T, Tsutamoto T, Wada A, Maeda K, Mabuchi N, Hayashi M, et al. Plasma oxidized low-density lipoprotein as a prognostic predictor in patients with chronic congestive heart failure. J Am Coll Cardiol 2002;39(6):957–962.

109. Holvoet P, Mertens A, Verhamme P, Bogaerts K, Beyens G, Verhaeghe R, et al. Circulating oxidized LDL is a useful marker for identifying patients with coronary artery disease. Arterioscler Thromb Vasc Biol 2001;21(5):844–848.

110. Ujihara N, Sakka Y, Takeda M, Hirayama M, Ishii A, Tomonaga O, et al. Association between plasma oxidized low-density lipoprotein and diabetic nephropathy. Diabetes Res Clin Pract 2002;58(2):109–114.

111. Virella G, Thorpe SR, Alderson NL, Stephan EM, Atchley D, Wagner F, et al. Autoimmune response to advanced glycosylation end-products of human LDL. J Lipid Res 2003;44(3):487–493.

112. Virella G, Atchley D, Koskinen S, Zheng D, Lopes-Virella MF, DCCT/EDIC Research Group. Proatherogenic and proinflammatory properties of immune complexes prepared with purified human oxLDL antibodies and human oxLDL. Clin Immunol 2002;105(1): 81–92.

113. Turk Z, Sesto M, Skodlar J, Ferencak G, Turk N, Stavljenic-Rukavina A. Soluble LDL-immune complexes in type 2 diabetes and vascular disease. Horm Metab Res 2002;34(4):196–201.

114. Lopes-Virella MF, Virella G, Orchard TJ, Koskinen S, Evans RW, Becker DJ, et al. Antibodies to oxidized LDL and LDL-containing immune complexes as risk factors for coronary artery disease in diabetes mellitus. Clin Immunol 1999;90(2):165–172.

115. Lopes-Virella MF, Virella G. The role of immune and inflammatory processes in the development of macrovascular disease in diabetes. Front Biosci 2003;8:s750–s768.

116. Atchley DH, Lopes-Virella MF, Zheng D, Kenny D, Virella G. Oxidized LDL-anti-oxidized LDL immune complexes and diabetic nephropathy. Diabetologia 2002;45(11):1562–1571.

117. Orchard TJ, Virella G, Forrest KY, Evans RW, Becker DJ, Lopes-Virella MF. Antibodies to oxidized LDL predict coronary artery disease in type 1 diabetes: a nested case-control study from the Pittsburgh Epidemiology of Diabetes Complications Study. Diabetes 1999;48(7):1454–1458.

118. Fam SS, Morrow JD. The isoprostanes: unique products of arachidonic acid oxidation–a review. Curr Med Chem 2003;10(17):1723–1740.

119. Schwedhelm E, Boger RH. Application of gas chromatography-mass spectrometry for analysis of isoprostanes: their role in cardiovascular disease. Clin Chem Lab Med 2003;41(12):1552–1561.

120. Cracowski JL, Durand T, Bessard G. Isoprostanes as a biomarker of lipid peroxidation in humans: physiology, pharmacology and clinical implications. Trends Pharmacol Sci 2002;23(8):360–366.

121. Mezzetti A, Cipollone F, Cuccurullo F. Oxidative stress and cardiovascular complications in diabetes: isoprostanes as new markers on an old paradigm. Cardiovasc Res 2000;47(3): 475–488.

122. Ikizler TA, Morrow JD, Roberts LJ, Evanson JA, Becker B, Hakim RM, Shyr Y, Himmelfarb J. Plasma F2-isoprostane levels are elevated in chronic hemodialysis patients. Clin Nephrol 2002;58(3):190–197.

123. Michoud E, Lecomte M, Lagarde M, Wiernsperger N. In vivo effect of 8-epi-PGF2alpha on retinal circulation in diabetic and non-diabetic rats. Prostaglandins Leukot Essent Fatty Acids 1998;59(6):349–355.

124. Gardan B, Cracowski JL, Sessa C, Hunt M, Stanke-Labesque F, Devillier P, Bessard G. Vasoconstrictor effects of iso-prostaglandin F2alpha type-III (8-iso-prostaglandin F2alpha) on human saphenous veins. J Cardiovasc Pharmacol 2000;35(5):729–734.
125. Hou X, Roberts LJ, Gobeil F, Taber D, Kanai K, Abran D, Brault S, Checchin D, Sennlaub F, Lachapelle P, Varma D, Chemtob S. Isomer-specific contractile effects of a series of synthetic F(2)-isoprostanes on retinal and cerebral microvasculature. Free Radic Biol Med 2004;36(2):163–172.
126. Wilson AM, O'Neal D, Nelson CL, Prior DL, Best JD, Jenkins AJ. Comparison of arterial assessments in low and high vascular disease risk groups. Am J Hypertens 2004;17(4): 285–291.
127. McVeigh GE, Allen PB, Morgan DR, Hanratty CG, Silke B. Nitric oxide modulation of blood vessel tone identified by arterial waveform analysis. Clin Sci (Lond) 2001;100(4): 387–393.
128. Romney JS, Lewanczuk RZ. Vascular compliance is reduced in the early stages of type 1 diabetes. Diabetes Care 2001;24(12):2102–2106.
129. McVeigh G, Brennan G, Hayes R, Cohn J, Finkelstein S, Johnston D. Vascular abnormalities in non-insulin-dependent diabetes mellitus identified by arterial waveform analysis. Am J Med 1993;95(4):424–430.
130. Grey E, Bratteli C, Glasser SP, Alinder C, Finkelstein SM, Lindgren BR, Cohn JN. Reduced small artery but not large artery elasticity is an independent risk marker for cardiovascular events. Am J Hypertens 2003;16(4):265–269.
131. Jialal I, Devaraj S, Venugopal SK. Oxidative stress, inflammation, and diabetic vasculopathies: the role of alpha tocopherol therapy. Free Radic Res 2002;36(12):1331–1336.
132. Upritchard JE, Schuurman CR, Wiersma A, Tijburg LB, Coolen SA, Rijken PJ, Wiseman SA. Spread supplemented with moderate doses of vitamin E and carotenoids reduces lipid peroxidation in healthy, nonsmoking adults. Am J Clin Nutr 2003;78(5):985–992.
133. Desideri G, Croce G, Tucci M, Passacquale G, Broccoletti S, Valeri L, Santucci A, Ferri C. Effects of bezafibrate and simvastatin on endothelial activation and lipid peroxidation in hypercholesterolemia: evidence of different vascular protection by different lipid-lowering treatments. J Clin Endocrinol Metab 2003;88(11):5341–5347.
134. Leonhardt W. Concentrations of antioxidative vitamins in plasma and low-density lipoprotein of diabetic patients. In: Packer L, Rosen P, Tritschler HJ, King GL (Eds). Antioxidants in Diabetes Management. New York: Marcel Decker, 2000, pp. 65–76.
135. Cohen J, Jenkins AJ, Karschimkus C, Qing S, Lee CT, O'Dea K, Best JD, Rowley KG. Paraoxonase and other coronary risk factors in a community-based cohort. Redox Rep 2002;7(5):304–307.
136. Jerums G, Panagiotopoulos S, Forbes J, Osicka T, Cooper M. Evolving concepts in advanced glycation, diabetic nephropathy, and diabetic vascular disease. Arch Biochem Biophys 2003;419(1):55–62.
137. Forbes JM, Cooper ME, Oldfield MD, Thomas MC. Role of advanced glycation end products in diabetic nephropathy. J Am Soc Nephrol 2003;14(8 Suppl 3):S254–S258.
138. Silacci P. Advanced glycation end-products as a potential target for treatment of cardiovascular disease. J Hypertens 2002;20(8):1483–1485.
139. Stern DM, Yan SD, Yan SF, Schmidt AM. Receptor for advanced glycation endproducts (RAGE) and the complications of diabetes. Ageing Res Rev 2002;1(1):1–15.
140. Wendt T, Bucciarelli L, Qu W, Lu Y, Yan SF, Stern DM, Schmidt AM. Receptor for advanced glycation endproducts (RAGE) and vascular inflammation:insights into the pathogenesis of macrovascular complications in diabetes. Curr Atheroscler Rep 2002;4(3):228–237.
141. Vlassara H, Palace MR. Diabetes and advanced glycation endproducts. J Intern Med 2002;251(2):87–101.
142. Wautier JL, Guillausseau PJ. Advanced glycation end products, their receptors and diabetic angiopathy. Diabetes Metab 2001;27(5 Pt 1):535–542.
143. Beisswenger PJ, Makita Z, Curphey TJ, Moore LL, Jean S, Brinck-Johnsen T, Bucala R, Vlassara H. Formation of immunochemical advanced glycosylation end products precedes

and correlates with early manifestations of renal and retinal disease in diabetes. Diabetes 1995;44:824–829.

144. Requena JR, Ahmed MU, Reddy SR, Fountain CW, Degenhardt TP, Jenkins AJ, Smyth B, Lyons TJ, Thorpe SR. Detection of AGE-lipids in vivo: glycation and carboxymethylation of aminophosholipids in red-cell membranes. Proceedings of the 1997 International Malliard Meeting.

145. Lyons TJ, Requena JR, Fountain CW, Jenkins AJ, Perez CP, Gates D, Hermayer KL, King LP, Baynes JW, Thorpe SR. Glycoxidation and lipoxidation products in red blood cell membranes in poorly controlled diabetes. Diabetologia 1997;40(Suppl 1):A589.

146. Jenkins AJ, Lyons TJ, Smyth B, Requena JR, Fountain CW, Dagenhart T, Hermayer KL, Phillips KD, King LP, Baynes JW, Thorpe SR. Glycoxidation and lipoxidation products in red blood cell membranes in IDDM – relationship to glycemic control and microvascular complications. Diabetes 1998;47(Suppl 1):A127.

147. Berg TJ, Bangstad HJ, Torjesen PA, Osterby R, Bucala R, Hanssen KF. Advanced glycation end products in serum predict changes in the kidney morphology of patients with insulin-dependent diabetes mellitus. Metabolism 1997;46:661–665.

148. Berg TJ, Torjesen PA, Dahl-Jørgensen K, Hanssen KF. Increased serum levels of AGEs in serum from children and adolescents with Type 1 diabetes. Diabetes Care 1997;21: 1006–1008.

149. Kilhovd BK, Berg TJ, Birkeland KI, Thorsby P, Hanssen KF. Serum levels of advanced glycation end products are increased in patients with Type 2 diabetes and coronary heart disease. Diabetes Care 1999;22:1543–1548.

150. Berg TJ, Snorgaard O, Faber J, Torjesen PA, Hildebrandt P, Mehlsen JK, Hanssen KF. Serum levels of AGEs are associated with left ventricular diastolic function in patients with Type 1 diabetes. Diabetes Care 1999;22:1186–1190.

151. Kilhovd BK, Giardino I, Torjesen PA, Birkeland KI, Berg TJ, Thornalley PJ, Brownlee M, Hanssen KF. Increased serum levels of the specific AGE-compound methylglyoxal-derived hydroimidazolone in patients with type 2 diabetes. Metabolism 2003;52(2):163–167.

152. Tan KC, Chow WS, Ai VH, Metz C, Bucala R, Lam KS. Advanced glycation end products and endothelial dysfunction in type 2 diabetes. Diabetes Care 2002;25(6):1055–1059.

153. Buss H, Chan TP, Sluis KB, Domigan NM, Winterbourn CC. Protein carbonyl measurement by a sensitive ELISA method. Free Rad Res 1997;23:361–366.

154. Winterbourn CC, Buss IH, Chan TP, Plank LD, Clark MA, Windsor JA. Protein carbonyl measurements show evidence of early oxidative stress in critically ill patients. Crit Care Med 2000;28(1):143–149.

155. Martin-Gallan P, Carrascosa A, Gussinye M, Dominguez C. Biomarkers of diabetes-associated oxidative stress and antioxidant status in young diabetic patients with or without subclinical complications. Free Radic Biol Med 2003;34(12):1563–1574.

156. Odetti P, Garibaldi S, Noberasco G, Aragno I, Valentini S, Traverso N, Marinari UM. Levels of carbonyl groups in plasma proteins of type 2 diabetes mellitus subjects. Acta Diabetol 1999;36(4):179–183.

157. Kalogerakis G, Baker AM, Christov S, Dwyer K, Lee P, Buss H, Winterbourn C, Best JD, Jenkins AJ. Oxidative stress and high density lipoprotein (HDL) function in end stage renal disease (ESRD) and type 1 diabetes mellitus. Annual Scientific Meeting of the Australian Atherosclerosis Society, Sydney, Australia, November 2000.

158. Naito C, Kajita M, Niwa T. Determination of glutathionyl hemoglobin in hemodialysis patients using electrospray ionization liquid chromatography-mass spectrometry. J Chromatogr B–Biomed Sci Appl 1999;731(1):121–124.

159. Bursell SE, King GL. The potential use of glutathionyl hemoglobin as a clinical marker of oxidative stress. Clin Chem 2000;46(2):145–146.

160. Niwa T, Naito C, Mawjood AHM, Imai K. Increased glutathionyl hemoglobin in diabetes mellitus and hyperlipidemia demonstrated by liquid chromatography/electronspray ionization-mass spectroscopy. Clin Chem 2000;46:82–88.

161. Takayama F, Tsutsui S, Horie M, Shimokata K, Niwa T. Glutathionyl hemoglobin in uremic patients undergoing hemodialysis and continuous ambulatory peritoneal dialysis. Kidney Int Suppl 2001;78:S155–S158.

162. Naito C, Niwa T. Analysis of glutathionyl hemoglobin levels in diabetic patients by electrospray ionization liquid chromatography–mass spectrometry: effect of vitamin E administration. J Chromatogr B - Biomed Sci Appl 2000;746(1):91–94.

163. Maytin M, Leopold J, Loscalzo J. Oxidant stress in the vasculature. Curr Atheroscler Rep 1999;1(2):156–164.

164. Fukai T, Folz RJ, Landmesser U, Harrison DG. Extracellular superoxide dismutase and cardiovascular disease. Cardiovasc Res 2002;55(2):239–249.

165. Cooke CL, Davidge ST. Endothelial-dependent vasodilation is reduced in mesenteric arteries from superoxide dismutase knockout mice. Cardiovasc Res 2003;60(3):635–642.

166. Du Y, Miller CM, Kern TS. Hyperglycemia increases mitochondrial superoxide in retina and retinal cells. Free Radic Biol Med 2003;35(11):1491–1499.

167. Kang JH. Modification and inactivation of human Cu, Zn-superoxide dismutase by methylglyoxal. Mol Cells 2003;15(2):194–199.

168. Gupta S, Chough E, Daley J, Oates P, Tornheim K, Ruderman NB, Keaney JF Jr. Hyperglycemia increases endothelial superoxide that impairs smooth muscle cell Na+- K+-ATPase activity. Am J Physiol Cell Physiol 2002;282(3):C560–C566.

169. Kinscherf R, Deigner HP, Usinger C, Pill J, Wagner M, Kamencic H, Hou D, Chen M, Schmiedt W, Schrader M, Kovacs G, Kato K, Metz J. Induction of mitochondrial manganese superoxide dismutase in macrophages by oxidized LDL: its relevance in atherosclerosis of humans and heritable hyperlipidemic rabbits. FASEB J 1997;11(14): 1317–1328.

170. Voinea M, Georgescu A, Manea A, Dragomir E, Manduteanu I, Popov D, Simionescu M. Superoxide dismutase entrapped-liposomes restore the impaired endothelium-dependent relaxation of resistance arteries in experimental diabetes. Eur J Pharmacol 2004;484(1): 111–118.

171. Zanetti M, Sato J, Katusic ZS, O'Brien T. Gene transfer of superoxide dismutase isoforms reverses endothelial dysfunction in diabetic rabbit aorta. Am J Physiol Heart Circ Physiol 2001;280(6):H2516–H2523.

172. Rodriguez-Manas L, Lopez-Doriga P, Petidier R, Neira M, Solis J, Pavon I, Peiro C, Sanchez-Ferrer CF. Effect of glycaemic control on the vascular nitric oxide system in patients with type 1 diabetes. J Hypertens 2003;21(6):1137–1143.

173. Nishikawa T, Edelstein D, Du XL, Yamagishi S, Matsumura T, Kaneda Y, Yorek MA, Beebe D, Oates PJ, Hammes HP, Giardino I, Brownlee M. Normalizing mitochondrial superoxide production blocks three pathways of hyperglycaemic damage. Nature 2000;404(6779): 787–790.

174. Kotake M, Shinohara R, Kato K, Hayakawa N, Hayashi R, Uchimura K, Makino M, Nagata M, Kakizawa H, Nakagawa H, Nagasaka A, Itoh M. Reduction of activity, but no decrease in concentration, of erythrocyte Cu,Zn-superoxide dismutase by hyperglycaemia in diabetic patients. Diabet Med 1998;15(8):668–671.

175. Bhatia S, Shukla R, Venkata Madhu S, Kaur Gambhir J, Madhava Prabhu K. Antioxidant status, lipid peroxidation and nitric oxide end products in patients of type 2 diabetes mellitus with nephropathy. Clin Biochem 2003;36(7):557–562.

176. Dincer Y, Akcay T, Ilkova H, Alademir Z, Ozbay G. DNA damage and antioxidant defense in peripheral leukocytes of patients with Type 1 diabetes mellitus. Mutat Res 2003;527(1–2): 49–55.

177. Muchova J, Liptakova A, Orszaghova Z, Garaiova I, Tison P, Carsky J, Durackova Z. Antioxidant systems in polymorphonuclear leucocytes of Type 2 diabetes mellitus. Diabet Med 1999;16(1):74–78.

178. Skrha J, Hodinar A, Kvasnicka J, Hilgertova J. Relationship of oxidative stress and fibrinolysis in diabetes mellitus. Diabet Med 1996;13(9):800–805.

179. Kedziora-Kornatowska KZ, Luciak M, Blaszczyk J, Pawlak W. Lipid peroxidation and activities of antioxidant enzymes in erythrocytes of patients with non-insulin dependent diabetes with or without diabetic nephropathy. Nephrol Dial Transplant 1998;13(11):2829–2832.

180. Merzouk S, Hichami A, Madani S, Merzouk H, Berrouiguet AY, Prost J, Moutairou K, Chabane-Sari N, Khan NA. Antioxidant status and levels of different vitamins determined by high performance liquid chromatography in diabetic subjects with multiple complications. Gen Physiol Biophys 2003;22(1):15–27.

181. Memisogullari R, Taysi S, Bakan E, Capoglu I. Antioxidant status and lipid peroxidation in Type II diabetes mellitus. Cell Biochem Funct 2003;21(3):291–296.

182. Roussel AM, Kerkeni A, Zouari N, Mahjoub S, Matheau JM, Anderson RA. Antioxidant effects of zinc supplementation in Tunisians with type 2 diabetes mellitus. J Am Coll Nutr 2003;22(4):316–321.

183. Ruiz C, Alegria A, Barbera R, Farre R, Lagarda MJ. Lipid peroxidation and antioxidant enzyme activities in patients with type 1 diabetes mellitus. Scand J Clin Lab Invest 1999;59(2):99–105.

184. Akkus I, Kalak S, Vural H, Caglayan O, Menekse E, Can G, Durmus B. Leukocyte lipid peroxidation, superoxide dismutase, glutathione peroxidase and serum and leukocyte vitamin C levels of patients with Type II diabetes mellitus. Clin Chim Acta 1996;244(2):221–227.

185. Leonard MB, Lawton K, Watson ID, Patrick A, Walker A, MacFarlane I. Cigarette smoking and free radical activity in young adults with insulin-dependent diabetes. Diabet Med 1995;12(1):46–50.

186. Kimura F, Hasegawa G, Obayashi H, Adachi T, Hara H, Ohta M, Fukui M, Kitagawa Y, Park H, Nakamura N, Nakano K, Yoshikawa T. Serum extracellular superoxide dismutase in patients with type 2 diabetes: relationship to the development of micro- and macrovascular complications. Diabetes Care 2003;26(4):1246–1250.

187. Palanduz S, Ademoglu E, Gokkusu C, Tamer S. Plasma antioxidants and type 2 diabetes mellitus. Res Commun Mol Pathol Pharmacol 2001;109(5–6):309–318.

188. Martin-Gallan P, Carrascosa A, Gussinye M, Dominguez C. Biomarkers of diabetes-associated oxidative stress and antioxidant status in young diabetic patients with or without subclinical complications. Free Radic Biol Med 2003;34(12):1563–1574.

189. Landmesser U, Merten R, Spiekermann S, Buttner K, Drexler H, Hornig B. Vascular extracellular superoxide dismutase activity in patients with coronary artery disease: relation to endothelium-dependent vasodilation. Circulation 2000;101(19):2264–2270.

190. Wang XL, Adachi T, Sim AS, Wilcken DE. Plasma extracellular superoxide dismutase levels in an Australian population with coronary artery disease. Arterioscler Thromb Vasc Biol 1998;18(12):1915–1921.

191. Jandric-Balen M, Bozikov V, Bistrovic D, Jandric I, Bozikov J, Romic Z, Balen I. Antioxidant enzymes activity in patients with peripheral vascular disease, with and without presence of diabetes mellitus. Coll Anthropol 2003;27(2):735–743.

192. Blankenberg S, Rupprecht HJ, Bickel C, Torzewski M, Hafner G, Tiret L, Smieja M, Cambien F, Meyer J, Lackner KJ, AtheroGene Investigators. Glutathione peroxidase 1 activity and cardiovascular events in patients with coronary artery disease. N Engl J Med 2003;23;349(17):1605–1613.

193. Strokov IA, Bursa TR, Drepa OI, Zotova EV, Nosikov VV, Ametov AS. Predisposing genetic factors for diabetic polyneuropathy in patients with type 1 diabetes: a population-based case-control study. Acta Diabetol 2003;40(Suppl 2):S375–S379.

194. Nomiyama T, Tanaka Y, Piao L, Nagasaka K, Sakai K, Ogihara T, Nakajima K, Watada H, Kawamori R. The polymorphism of manganese superoxide dismutase is associated with diabetic nephropathy in Japanese type 2 diabetic patients. J Hum Genet 2003;48(3):138–141.

195. Ukkola O, Erkkila PH, Savolainen MJ, Kesaniemi YA. Lack of association between polymorphisms of catalase, copper–zinc superoxide dismutase (SOD), extracellular SOD and endothelial nitric oxide synthase genes and macroangiopathy in patients with type 2 diabetes mellitus. J Intern Med 2001;249(5):451–459.

196. Mackness MI, Durrington PN. HDL, its enzymes and its potential to influence lipid peroxidation. Atherosclerosis 1995;115:243–253.
197. Mackness MI, Mackness B, Durrington PN, Connelly PW, Hegele RA. Paraoxonase: biochemistry, genetics and relationship to plasma lipoproteins. Genetics Mol Biol 1996:69–76.
198. Mackness MI, Mackness B, Durrington PN. Paraoxonase and coronary heart disease. Atheroscler Suppl 2002;3(4):49–55.
199. Durrington PN, Mackness B, Mackness MI. Paraoxonase and atherosclerosis. Arterioscler Thromb Vasc Biol 2001;21(4):473–480.
200. Van Lenten BJ, Wagner AC, Nayak DP, Hama S, Navab M, Fogelman AM. High-density lipoprotein loses its anti-inflammatory properties during acute influenza A infection. Circulation 2001;103(18):2283–2288.
201. Durrington PN, Mackness B, Mackness MI. The hunt for nutritional and pharmacological modulators of paraoxonase. Arterioscler Thromb Vasc Biol 2002;22(8):1248–1250.
202. Mackness B, Durrington P, McElduff P, Yarnell J, Azam N, Watt M, Mackness M. Low paraoxonase activity predicts coronary events in the Caerphilly Prospective Study. Circulation 2003;107(22):2775–2779.
203. Mackness B, Durrington PN, Mackness MI. The paraoxonase gene family and coronary heart disease. Curr Opin Lipidol 2002;13(4):357–362.
204. Inoue M, Suehiro T, Nakamura T, Ikeda Y, Kumon Y, Hashimoto K. Serum arylesterase/diazoxonase activity and genetic polymorphisms in patients with type 2 diabetes. Metabolism 2000;49(11):1400–1405.
205. Mackness B, Durrington P, Abuashia B, Boulton A, Mackness M. Low PON activity in Type 2 diabetes mellitus complicated by retinopathy. Clin Sci 2000;98:355–363.
206. Ikeda Y, Suehiro T, Inoue M, Nakauchi Y, Morita T, Arii K, et al. Serum paraoxonase activity and its relationship to diabetic complications in patients with non-insulin-dependent diabetes mellitus. Metabolism 1998;47(5):598–602.
207. Mackness MI, Harty D, Bhatnagar D, Winocour PH, Arrol S, Ishola M, et al. Serum paraoxonase activity in familial hypercholesterolaemia and insulin-dependent diabetes mellitus. Atherosclerosis 1990;86:193–199.
208. Kordonouri O, James RW, Bennetts B, Chan A, Kao YL, Danne T, et al. Modulation by blood glucose levels of activity and concentration of paraoxonase in young patients with type 1 diabetes mellitus. Metabolism 2001;50(6):657–660.
209. Kuremoto K, Watanabe Y, Ohmura H, Shimada K, Mokuno H, Daida H. R/R genotype of human paraoxonase (PON1) is more protective against lipoprotein oxidation and coronary artery disease in Japanese subjects. J Atheroscler Thromb 2003;10(2):85–92.
210. Malin R, Jarvinen O, Sisto T, Koivula T, Lehtimaki T. Paraoxonase producing PON1 gene M/L55 polymorphism is related to autopsy-verified artery-wall atherosclerosis. Atherosclerosis 2001;157(2):301–307.
211. Hu Y, Tian H, Liu R. Gln-Arg192 polymorphism of paraoxonase 1 is associated with carotid intima-media thickness in patients of type 2 diabetes mellitus of Chinese. Diabetes Res Clin Pract 2003;61(1):21–27.
212. Koch M, Hering S, Barth C, Ehren M, Enderle MD, Pfohl M. Paraoxonase 1 192 Gln/Arg gene polymorphism and cerebrovascular disease: interaction with type 2 diabetes. Exp Clin Endocrinol Diabetes 2001;109(3):141–145.
213. Pfohl M, Koch M, Enderle MD, Kuhn R, Fullhase J, Karsch KR, et al. Paraoxonase 192 Gln/Arg gene polymorphism, coronary artery disease, and myocardial infarction in type 2 diabetes. Diabetes 1999;483:623–627.
214. James RW, Leviev I, Ruiz J, Passa P, Froguel P, Garin MC. Promoter polymorphism T(-107)C of the paraoxonase PON1 gene is a risk factor for coronary heart disease in type 2 diabetic patients. Diabetes 2000;49(8):1390–1393.
215. Osei-Hyiaman D, Hou L, Mengbai F, Zhiyin R, Zhiming Z, Kano K. Coronary artery disease risk in Chinese type 2 diabetics: is there a role for paraoxonase 1 gene (Q192R) polymorphism? Eur J Endocrinol 2001;144(6):639–644.

216. Pinizzotto M, Castillo E, Fiaux M, Temler E, Gaillard RC, Ruiz J. Paraoxonase2 polymorphisms are associated with nephropathy in Type II diabetes. Diabetologia 2001;44(1): 104–107.

217. Malin R, Laine S, Rantalaiho V, Wirta O, Pasternack A, Jokela H, Alho H, Koivula T, Lehtimaki T. Lipid peroxidation is increased in paraoxonase L55 homozygotes compared with M-allele carriers. Free Radic Res 2001;34(5):477–484.

218. Malin R, Rantalaiho V, Huang XH, Wirta O, Pasternack A, Leinonen JS, Alho H, Jokela H, Koivula T, Tanaka T, Okada K, Ochi H, Toyokuni S, Lehtimaki T. Association between M/L55-polymorphism of paraoxonase enzyme and oxidative DNA damage in patients with type 2 diabetes mellitus and in control subjects. Hum Genet 1999;105(1–2):179–180.

219. Araki S, Makita Y, Canani L, Ng D, Warram JH, Krolewski AS. Polymorphisms of human paraoxonase 1 gene (PON1) and susceptibility to diabetic nephropathy in Type 1 diabetes mellitus. Diabetologia 2000;43(12):1540–1543.

220. Garin MCB, James RW, Dussoix P, Blanche H, Passa P, Froguel P, et al. Paraoxonase polymorphism Met-Leu54 is associated with modified serum concentrations of the enzyme: a possible link between the paraoxonase gene and increased risk of cardiovascular disease in diabetes. J Clin Invest 1997;99:62–66.

221. Kleemola P, Freese R, Jauhiainen M, Pahlman R, Alfthan G, Mutanen M. Dietary determinants of serum paraoxonase activity in healthy humans. Atherosclerosis 2002;160(2):425–432.

222. Aviram M, Dornfeld L, Rosenblat M, Volkova N, Kaplan M, Coleman R, Hayek T, Presser D, Fuhrman B. Pomegranate juice consumption reduces oxidative stress, atherogenic modifications to LDL, and platelet aggregation: studies in humans and in atherosclerotic apolipoprotein E-deficient mice. Am J Clin Nutr 2000;71(5):1062–1076.

223. Nishio E, Watanabe Y. Cigarette smoke extract inhibits plasma paraoxonase activity by modification of the enzyme's free thiols. Biochem Biophys Res Comm 1997;236(2):289–293.

224. Tomas M, Senti M, Garcia-Faria F, Vila J, Torrents A, Covas M, et al. Effect of simvastatin therapy on PON activity and related lipoproteins in familial hypercholesterolemic patients. Arterioscler Thromb Vasc Biol 2000;20:2113–2119.

225. Balogh Z, Seres I, Harangi M, Kovacs P, Kakuk G, Paragh G. Gemfibrozil increases paraoxonase activity in type 2 diabetic patients. A new hypothesis of the beneficial action of fibrates? Diabetes Metab 2001;27(5 Pt 1):604–610.

226. Sutherland WH, Manning PJ, de Jong SA, Allum AR, Jones SD, Williams SM. Hormone-replacement therapy increases serum paraoxonase arylesterase activity in diabetic postmenopausal women. Metabolism 2001;50(3):319–324.

227. Brennan ML, Hazen SL. Emerging role of myeloperoxidase and oxidant stress markers in cardiovascular risk assessment. Curr Opin Lipidol 2003;14(4):353–359.

228. Uchimura K, Nagasaka A, Hayashi R, Makino M, Nagata M, Kakizawa H, Kobayashi T, Fujiwara K, Kato T, Iwase K, Shinohara R, Kato K, Itoh M. Changes in superoxide dismutase activities and concentrations and myeloperoxidase activities in leukocytes from patients with diabetes mellitus. J Diab Compl 1999;13(5–6):264–270.

229. Sato N, Shimizu H, Suwa K, Shimomura Y, Kobayashi I, Mori M. MPO activity and generation of active O_2 species in leukocytes from poorly controlled diabetic patients. Diabetes Care 1992;15(8):1050–1052.

230. Thukkani AK, McHowat J, Hsu FF, Brennan ML, Hazen SL, Ford DA. Identification of alpha-chloro fatty aldehydes and unsaturated lysophosphatidylcholine molecular species in human atherosclerotic lesions. Circulation 2003;108(25):3128–3133.

231. Kutter D, Devaquet P, Vanderstocken G, Paulus JM, Marchal V, Gothot A. Consequences of total and subtotal myeloperoxidase deficiency: risk or benefit? Acta Haematol 2000;104(1):10–15.

232. Nikpoor B, Turecki G, Fournier C, Theroux P, Rouleau GA. A functional myeloperoxidase polymorphic variant is associated with coronary artery disease in French-Canadians. Am Heart J 2001;142(2):336–339.

233. Makela R, Karhunen PJ, Kunnas TA, Ilveskoski E, Kajander OA, Mikkelsson J, Perola M, Penttila A, Lehtimaki T. Myeloperoxidase gene variation as a determinant of atherosclerosis

progression in the abdominal and thoracic aorta: an autopsy study. Lab Invest 2003;83(7):919–925.

234. Makela R, Laaksonen R, Janatuinen T, Vesalainen R, Nuutila P, Jaakkola O, Knuuti J, Lehtimaki T. Myeloperoxidase gene variation and coronary flow reserve in young healthy men. J Biomed Sci 2004;11(1):59–64.

235. Hoy A, Leininger-Muller B, Poirier O, Siest G, Gautier M, Elbaz A, Amarenco P, Visvikis S. Myeloperoxidase polymorphisms in brain infarction. Association with infarct size and functional outcome. Atherosclerosis 2003;167(2):223–230.

236. Pecoits-Filho R, Stenvinkel P, Marchlewska A, Heimburger O, Barany P, Hoff CM, Holmes CJ, Suliman M, Lindholm B, Schalling M, Nordfors L. A functional variant of the myeloperoxidase gene is associated with cardiovascular disease in end-stage renal disease patients. Kidney Int 2003;84(Suppl):S172–S176.

237. Zhang R, Brennan ML, Fu X, Aviles RJ, Pearce GL, Penn MS, Topol EJ, Sprecher DL, Hazen SL. Association between myeloperoxidase levels and risk of coronary artery disease. JAMA 2001;286(17):2136–2142.

238. Brennan ML, Penn MS, Van Lente F, Nambi V, Shishehbor MH, Aviles RJ, Goormastic M, Pepoy ML, McErlean ES, Topol EJ, Nissen SE, Hazen SL. Prognostic value of myeloperoxidase in patients with chest pain. N Engl J Med 2003;349(17):1595–1604.

239. Shishehbor MH, Aviles RJ, Brennan ML, Fu X, Goormastic M, Pearce GL, Gokce N, Keaney JF Jr, Penn MS, Sprecher DL, Vita JA, Hazen SL. Association of nitrotyrosine levels with cardiovascular disease and modulation by statin therapy. JAMA 2003;289(13):1675–1680.

240. Shishehbor MH, Brennan ML, Aviles RJ, Fu X, Penn MS, Sprecher DL, Hazen SL. Statins promote potent systemic antioxidant effects through specific inflammatory pathways. Circulation 2003;108(4):426–431.

241. Bursell SE, King G. Protein kinase C, development of diabetic vascular complications, and role of Vitamin E in preventing these abnormalities. In: Packer L, Rosen P, Tritschler HJ, King GL (Eds). Antioxidants in Diabetes Management. New York: Marcel Decker, 2000, pp. 241–264.

242. Bursell SE, Clermont AC, Aiello LP, Aiello LM, Schlossman DK, Feener EP, Laffel L, King GL. High-dose vitamin E supplementation normalizes retinal blood flow and creatinine clearance in patients with type 1 diabetes. Diabetes Care 1999;22(8):1245–1251.

243. Skyrme-Jones RA, O'Brien RC, Berry KL, Meredith IT. Vitamin E supplementation improves endothelial function in Type 1 diabetes mellitus: a randomized, placebo-controlled study. J Am Coll Cardiol 2000;36(1):94–102.

244. MRC/BHF Heart Protection Study of antioxidant vitamin supplementation in 20,536 high-risk individuals: a randomised placebo-controlled trial. Lancet 2002;360(9326):23–33.

245. Nutrition recommendations and principles for people with diabetes mellitus. Diabetes Care 2000;23(Suppl 1):S43–S46.

246. Bowry VW, Ingold KU, Stocker R. Vitamin E in human low-density lipoprotein. When and how this antioxidant becomes a pro-oxidant. Biochem J 1992;288(Pt 2):341–344.

247. Thomas SR, Stocker R. Molecular action of vitamin E in lipoprotein oxidation: implications for atherosclerosis. Free Radic Biol Med 2000;28(12):1795–1805.

248. Ziegler D. Clinical trials of α-lipoic acid in diabetic polyneuropathy and cardiac autonomic neuropathy. In: Packer L, Rosen P, Tritschler HJ, King GL (Eds). Antioxidants in Diabetes Management. New York: Marcel Decker, 2000, pp. 173–184.

249. UKPDS Group. Tight blood pressure control and risk of macrovascular and microvascular complications in type 2 diabetes: UKPDS 38. UK Prospective Diabetes Study Group. Br Med J 1998;317(7160):703–713.

250. Writing Team For DCCT/EDIC Research Group. Sustained effect of intensive treatment of type 1 diabetes mellitus on development and progression of diabetic nephropathy: the Epidemiology of Diabetes Interventions and Complications (EDIC) study. JAMA 2003;290(16):2159–2167.

251. Pedersen TR. Coronary artery disease: the Scandinavian Simvastatin Survival Study experience. Am J Cardiol 1998;82(10B):53T–56T.

252. Tomas M, Senti M, Garcia-Faria F, Vila J, Torrents A, Covas M, Marrugat J. Effect of simvastatin therapy on PON activity and related lipoproteins in familial hypercholesterolemic patients. Arterioscler Thromb Vasc Biol 2000;20:2113–2119.

253. De Caterina R, Cipollone F, Filardo FP, Zimarino M, Bernini W, Lazzerini G, Bucciarelli T, Falco A, Marchesani P, Muraro R, Mezzetti A, Ciabattoni G. Low-density lipoprotein level reduction by the 3-hydroxy-3-methylglutaryl coenzyme-A inhibitor simvastatin is accompanied by a related reduction of F2-isoprostane formation in hypercholesterolemic subjects: no further effect of vitamin E. Circulation 2002;106(20):2543–2549.

254. Albert MA, Danielson E, Rifai N, Ridker PM. Effect of statin therapy on C-reactive protein levels: the pravastatin inflammation/CRP evaluation (PRINCE): a randomized trial and cohort study. JAMA 2001;286(1):64–70.

255. Wassmann S, Nickenig G. Interrelationship of free oxygen radicals and endothelial dysfunction – modulation by statins. Endothelium 2003;10(1):23–33.

256. Bocan TM. Pleiotropic effects of HMG-CoA reductase inhibitors. Curr Opin Investig Drugs 2002;3(9):1312–1317.

257. Tsunekawa T, Hayashi T, Kano H, Sumi D, Matsui-Hirai H, Thakur NK, Egashira K, Iguchi A. Cerivastatin, a hydroxymethylglutaryl coenzyme a reductase inhibitor, improves endothelial function in elderly diabetic patients within 3 days. Circulation 2001;104(4):376–379.

258. Brenner BM, Cooper ME, de Zeeuw D, Keane WF, Mitch WE, Parving HH, Remuzzi G, Snapinn SM, Zhang Z, Shahinfar S, RENAAL Study Investigators. Effects of losartan on renal and cardiovascular outcomes in patients with type 2 diabetes and nephropathy. N Engl J Med 2001;345(12):861–869.

259. Gumieniczek A. Effect of the new thiazolidinedione-pioglitazone on the development of oxidative stress in liver and kidney of diabetic rabbits. Life Sci 2003;74(5):553–562.

260. Mizushige K, Tsuji T, Noma T. Pioglitazone: cardiovascular effects in prediabetic patients. Cardiovasc Drug Rev 2002;20(4):329–340.

261. May JM, Qu ZC. Troglitazone protects human erythrocytes from oxidant damage. Antioxid Redox Signal 2000;2(2):243–250.

262. Garg R, Kumbkarni Y, Aljada A, Mohanty P, Ghanim H, Hamouda W, Dandona P. Troglitazone reduces reactive oxygen species generation by leukocytes and lipid peroxidation and improves flow-mediated vasodilatation in obese subjects. Hypertension 2000;36(3): 430–435.

263. Cominacini L, Garbin U, Pasini AF, Davoli A, Campagnola M, Rigoni A, Tosetti L, Lo Cascio V. The expression of adhesion molecules on endothelial cells is inhibited by troglitazone through its antioxidant activity. Cell Adhes Comm 1999;7(3):223–231.

264. Cominacini L, Young MM, Capriati A, Garbin U, Fratta Pasini A, Campagnola M, Davoli A, Rigoni A, Contessi GB, Lo Cascio V. Troglitazone increases the resistance of low density lipoprotein to oxidation in healthy volunteers. Diabetologia 1997;40(10):1211–1218.

265. American Diabetes Association. Position Statement. Standards of medical care in diabetes. Diabetes Care 2004;27(Supp 1):S15–S35.

Chapter 8
Molecular Mechanisms of Environmental Atherogenesis

Kimberly P. Miller and Kenneth S. Ramos

Epidemiology of Cardiovascular Disease

Cardiovascular diseases (CVD) are the leading cause of death in both males and females in the United States, and are classified into four major forms: coronary heart disease (CHD), cerebrovascular disease (stroke), hypertensive disease (high blood pressure), and rheumatic fever/rheumatic heart disease.[5] Over 70 million Americans (1 in 4) have one or more types of cardiovascular disease, and in 2002, 38% of all deaths in the U.S. were attributed to cardiovascular diseases, equal to 1 of every 2.6 deaths. In fact, fatalities due to cardiovascular diseases each year are about equal to the next five leading causes of death combined: cancer, chronic lower respiratory diseases, accidents, diabetes mellitus, and pneumonia/influenza.[5] Based on age-adjusted statistics, cardiovascular disease targets 34.3% of male and 32.4% of female non-Hispanic whites; 41.1% of male and 44.7% of female non-Hispanic blacks; and 29.2% of male and 29.3% of female Mexican Americans.[5] According to the Centers for Disease Control and National Center for Health Statistics (CDC/NCHS), if all forms of major cardiovascular diseases were eliminated, life expectancy of the U.S. population would rise by almost 7 years.

A number of risk factors contribute to the onset of cardiovascular diseases, including smoking, high blood pressure, elevated cholesterol, physical inactivity, excess weight and obesity, and diabetes.[5] Exposure to tobacco smoke represents a significant environmental risk factor for cardiovascular diseases. Between 1995 and 1999, an average of 442,398 Americans died each year of smoking-related illnesses, with the largest portion of these deaths related to cardiovascular disease.[5] However, quitting smoking has a significant impact in decreasing cardiovascular disease risk. One year after quitting, there is a 50% decrease in CHD risk, and within 15 years after quitting, the risk of death from CHD approaches that of a long-time nonsmoker.[5]

It should be recognized though that nonsmokers are just as likely to develop cardiovascular diseases as smokers due to general exposure to environmental tobacco smoke. Nearly 35,000 nonsmokers die each year from cardiovascular diseases as a result of exposure to environmental tobacco smoke.[5]

J.L. Holtzman (ed.), *Atherosclerosis and Oxidant Stress: A New Perspective.*
© Springer 2008

Atherosclerosis

Atherosclerosis is a leading cause of deaths due to heart attack (CHD) and stroke.[5] This disease is a form of thickening and/or hardening of the arteries, and is characterized by plaque build-up in both large and medium size vessels such as the aorta or carotid arteries. Atherosclerosis actually accounts for 75% of all deaths from cardiovascular diseases.[5]

The vascular wall is the site of injury where the process of atherosclerosis begins. Both large and medium-sized vessels contain three distinct cellular layers. The innermost layer, the tunica intima, consists of a single layer of endothelial cells (ECs) resting on a thin basal lamina. This layer lines the lumen of the vessel where blood flows. ECs lie parallel to the direction of blood flow and act as a barrier between the blood and sub-endothelial components of the vascular wall. The middle layer, or tunica media, comprises multiple layers of smooth muscle cells interwoven with collagen and elastin. These muscle cells are important in the regulation of vascular tone and the contractile response of the artery. Receptors on the plasma membrane of vascular smooth muscle cells (vSMCs) regulate calcium conductance responsible for activation of the contractile apparatus of these cells. In vSMCs, extracellular calcium stores that permeate the cell via receptor- and/or voltage-operated channels mediate contraction. In addition to contractile functions, vSMCs also regulate extracellular matrix protein synthesis necessary for arterial repair, the metabolism and secretion of bioactive substances, and the regulation of monocyte function. Finally, the outermost layer of the vessel wall, the tunica adventitia, consists of a loose layer of fibroblasts, collagen, elastin, and glycosaminoglycans. The adventitial layer gives structural support to the vessel through fibroblast secretion of collagen and glycosaminoglycans (for a review see [195]).

The formation of atherosclerotic lesions involves migration of smooth muscle cells (SMCs) from the tunica media into the tunica intima coupled to uncontrolled cell proliferation and altered production of extracellular matrix proteins. Other critical elements in atherosclerotic lesions include inflammatory cells, lipids, blood products, and calcium, which are recruited through the injury process and contribute to the progression and complication of the lesion (for a review see [251]) Two major hypotheses, "the response to injury" and "clonal expansion" hypotheses, have guided mechanistic studies of atherosclerosis over the past 30 years.

Response to Injury Hypothesis

In the "response to injury" hypothesis, damage to ECs lining the tunica intima triggers an inflammatory response resulting in the recruitment of platelets and inflammatory cells, along with SMC migration and proliferation from the media to the intima.[213,215,216] These factors ultimately form a vascular lesion that extends into the vessel lumen (Fig. 8.1).

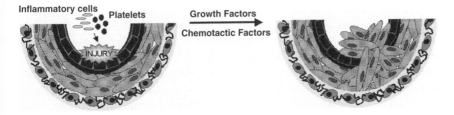

Fig. 8.1 Illustrated representation of the "Response to Injury" hypothesis

The process often begins when lipoproteins carried in the circulation become trapped beneath the endothelium, either due to increased lipid transport or dysfunction of the endothelial cell layer.[237] Glycoproteins then begin to adhere to the surface of the endothelium,[215] followed by recruitment of monocytes and T lymphocytes that attach to these glycoproteins. Migration into the subendothelial space then proceeds. As injury and migration continue, monocytes become macrophages, and lipid accumulation gives rise to foam cells, ultimately resulting in formation of a fatty streak (reviewed in [216, 251]). In humans, the fatty streak mainly consists of lipid-filled macrophages, T lymphocytes, and lipid-containing SMCs.[216,250] As the lesion progresses due to increased injury and migration of SMCs from the media to the intima, these fatty streaks can be converted to SMC-rich lesions. This migration can be induced by macrophages that continue to accumulate lipid, and begin to express genes for chemotactic factors that induce SMC proliferation and replication. Such factors include platelet-derived growth factor (PDGF), transforming growth factor beta (TGFβ), heparin-binding epidermal growth factor (HB-EGF), fibroblast growth factor (FGF), eicosanoids, cytokines, interleukin-1 (IL-1), and tumor necrosis factor alpha (TNFα).[214]

Lesions resulting from the replication of macrophages and SMCs are termed intermediate lesions. Layers of macrophages, T cells, and SMCs within intermediate lesions then begin to form connective tissue. With continued injury, a fibro-proliferative response takes place and a fibrous plaque, or advanced complicated lesion results. A lesion of this type consists of a fibrous cap of connective tissue containing embedded SMCs, monocyte-derived macrophages, and T lymphocytes, which covers a lesion consisting of macrophages, lipid necrotic debris, SMCs, and loose connective tissue.[213] As a result, three different types of lesions can exist in the progression of atherosclerosis: the fatty streak, the intermediate lesion, and the advanced complicated lesion.[213,251] Overall, what begins as a protective inflammatory response mechanism progresses into an injurious fibro-proliferative response.

In this model, the progression of the atherosclerotic lesion and ultimate stage of growth is dependent on gene expression in macrophages at the fatty streak stage. At this point, the lesion can either continue to grow, if genes producing growth stimulatory molecules are activated (PDGF, FGF, HB-EGF), or remain static if genes that produce growth-inhibitory molecules are activated (TGFβ, IL-1, TNFα). In addition, secondary gene expression in SMCs induced by cytokines can result in autocrine growth stimulation.[214]

As shown in Fig. 8.1, toxicants that promote the response to injury model travel through the bloodstream and target vascular cells, both smooth muscle and endothelial cells. Some toxicants bypass the endothelial layer and target the medial smooth muscle cell layer specifically. Smooth muscle cell toxicants that induce this type of injury include a number of environmental agents, such as polycyclic aromatic hydrocarbons, and industrial chemicals such as dinitrotoluenes, allylamine and hydrazine.[199] Endothelial cell injury, if not repaired, can influence injury of the medial layer as well. Endothelial cell toxicants that contribute to this model and potentiate the atherogenic process include acrolein, homocysteine, heavy metals, and cyclophosphamide.[199]

Clonal Expansion Hypothesis

Benditt and Benditt[12] proposed a monoclonal origin of atherosclerotic plaque development, an alternative hypothesis to explain initiation of the atherosclerotic process. The experimental basis in support of this hypothesis was derived from the concept of X-chromosome inactivation first proposed by Lyon.[134] In early embryonic development of females, there is a random inactivation of one or the other of two X chromosomes, and subsequently, each cell population reproduces "true to type" through somatic growth. With a cellular marker to distinguish the two populations, one is able to delineate whether a pathologically new formation is derived from one, or from many cells. The cellular marker used by Benditt and Benditt was glucose-6-phosphate dehydrogenase (G-6-PD), an enzyme found to be heterozygous in one-third of the black female population who exhibit mixtures of the A and B forms of this enzyme.[15] The presence of one or the other of these two enzyme types (A or B) in a tissue would indicate that the cells originated from a single cell population. The presence of both enzyme types (A and B) would indicate that the cells originated from multiple cells. Many investigators have utilized this assay to assess the origin of cell populations in several tumor types.[63,130]

Atherosclerotic plaques are comprised mainly of SMCs, macrophages, lipid deposits, foam cells, and fibrous connective tissue.[251] Examination of 30 atherosclerotic-type plaques and 59 "normal" artery walls using the method described above, found that 80% of the plaques were comprised of a monotypic cell population characterized by the presence of one G-6-PD enzyme type (A or B).[12] Samples of the "normal" artery wall predominantly consisted of multiple cellular types as evidenced by the presence of both A and B G-6-PD isoenzymes (97%). Subsequent studies by Pearson et al.[180] confirmed these results, showing that 89.7% of the fibrous plaques they examined contained only one isoenzyme, while 98% of uninvolved aorta contained both isoenzymes. On the basis of these results, it was considered that three stages of atherosclerotic plaque development exist: (1) initiation – SMCs become mutated, but exist unexpressed in a subthreshold neoplastic state; (2) promotion/progression – a promoting factor induces proliferation of these

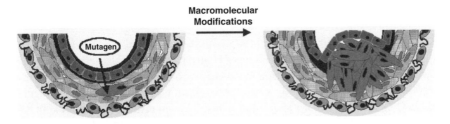

Fig. 8.2 Illustrated representation of the "Monoclonal Expansion" hypothesis

mutated cells; and (3) complication – this mutagenic change is modulated by expression of some of the disadvantages of the conditional neoplastic state.[13]

Overall, this model suggests that injury to the arterial wall transforms SMCs to a genetically altered state. These mutated cell populations, originating from one injured SMC, can proliferate either through exposure to growth promoting factors, or by mutation-induced constitutive production of growth factors within the SMC itself (Fig. 8.2).

The resulting atherosclerotic plaque consisting of highly-proliferative SMCs resembles a benign neoplastic tumor, such as the uterine leiomyoma.[130] Thus, this hypothesis provides a possible link between atherogenesis and carcinogenesis. In both processes, initiation of target cells occur (toxic injury to one cell, for example), followed by promotion of injury (mutated cells proliferate), and finally plaque/tumor formation. On this basis, it has been hypothesized that environmental agents implicated in cell transformation and tumorigenesis may contribute directly to plaque development.[196,198]

The monoclonal hypothesis has been highly debated among the vascular biology community. The controversy is primarily rooted on the often polyclonal nature of atherosclerotic plaques (reviewed by Ramos and Partridge[200]). As a result, the monoclonal hypothesis has been revised to embrace the principles put forth by Benditt and emerging evidence of the complex genetic basis of atherosclerotic vascular disease.

Pathogenesis of Atherosclerosis

Atherosclerotic lesions mainly form within large to medium-sized arteries, such as the coronary, carotid, basilar, vertebral, superficial femoral, iliac, and aorta.[213] Major points of lesion formation within these arteries are found in the entrance regions of arteries, such as the ascending aorta, and in the lateral leading edges of the flow divider at principal branches of the aorta.[38] As noted previously, three processes contribute to formation of the atherosclerotic lesion: proliferation of SMCs, macrophages, and lymphocytes; formation of a connective tissue matrix by SMCs, consisting of elastic fiber proteins, collagen, and proteoglycans; and the accumulation of lipid and cholesterol in surrounding matrix and associated cells.[54,55,142,143,208,209]

Growth factors and cytokines play a significant role in the proliferation and migration processes of multiple cell types contributing to vascular lesion formation. Growth-related signal transduction mechanisms contribute significantly to the progression of vSMCs to a highly proliferative phenotype as a result of atherogenic insult.[198] Growth regulatory molecules involved in cell proliferation include PDGF, bFGF, IGF-1, TNFα, IL-1, and TGFβ (for a review see [215, 216]). PDGF and IGF-1 are also involved in smooth muscle chemotaxis, inducing migration of medial SMCs into the intima of the artery.[215] Both oxidized low density lipoproteins and TGFβ induce monocyte chemotaxis through the endothelium.[215] Cytokines involved in the inflammatory response after the endothelium has been injured include IL-1 and IL-2, TNFα, interferon γ (IFNγ), and colony stimulating factors.[215,216]

The pathogenesis of atherosclerosis has similarities to other disease processes, such as glomerulosclerosis.[45] Functional and morphological similarities between lesion cell types such as the glomerular mesangial cells in glomerulosclerosis and vSMCs in atherosclerosis exist, while activated macrophages are also found in both types of lesions. In addition, calcium-dependent contractile responses characterize both cell types, and both lesions contain the growth regulatory molecule, PDGF.[212] The similarities between these two disease processes may also hold for other inflammatory fibro-proliferative responses such as pulmonary fibrosis, rheumatoid arthritis, and wound repair.[213]

Environmental Risk Factors

Risk factors for cardiovascular disease are numerous and include aspects of the human lifestyle that can and cannot be controlled.[5] Factors that cannot be controlled include age, gender, and heredity. Older people are more at risk for CVD, especially those over 65 years of age. Males aged 35–44 are also at a greater risk for CVD than females, and tend to have heart attacks earlier in life. The risk for females increases after menopause due to hormonal changes. Finally, heredity and race play a large role in risk for CVD. Children who have parents that have experienced heart attack or stroke are likely to develop CVD themselves. In regards to race, African-Americans have a greater risk than Caucasians for CVD due to higher blood pressure levels. Mexican-Americans, American-Indians, native Hawaiians and Asian-Americans are also at a greater risk due to higher rates of obesity and diabetes.

There are risk factors for CVD that can be controlled. Exposure to tobacco smoke, whether through first-hand or second-hand smoke, carries a significant risk. The risk of death from CVD for smokers is 2–3 times that of nonsmokers. A number of the toxicants present in cigarette smoke are damaging to blood vessel walls, and trigger the formation of vascular lesions. High blood cholesterol can also contribute to an increased risk of heart disease, and is a factor that can be controlled through the diet. This factor will be discussed in more detail later.

Other physical factors contributing to increased risk of CVD include high blood pressure, physical inactivity, and obesity. Usually these three are present simultaneously, and this further enhances the morbidity risk. High blood pressure increases the burden on the heart, and subsequently causes both the heart and blood vessels to be more prone to injury. Physical inactivity contributes to CVD by its likely combination with overeating, obesity, high cholesterol levels, and often the development of diabetes. Regular exercise helps to condition the heart, lower blood pressure, and control obesity. Obese or overweight males and females who carry most of their weight around their waist increase their risk of CVD. Added weight places more of a burden on the heart. Many overweight individuals are also more likely to develop diabetes, a disease marked by unstable glucose levels. Heart and blood vessel diseases are significant causes of death for nearly two-thirds of individuals with diabetes.

Factors that are not major risk factors, but can contribute to the onset of CVD, exist as well, including increased levels of stress. Relationships have been found between the risk for CVD and personal stress, health behaviors, and socioeconomic status. Sex hormones, while not entirely controllable, contribute to risk as well, predominantly in women. After menopause, women develop a greater risk for heart attacks due to loss of estrogen than women who continue to cycle. Interestingly, surgical menopause due to hysterectomy causes the risk of heart attack to rise more sharply than the natural loss of hormone through menopause. Finally, the level of alcohol use contributes to the onset of CVD. Large amounts of alcohol consumed on a regular basis increases blood pressure, and can contribute to developing other risk factors such as tobacco use and obesity. However, moderate amounts of alcohol (average of 1 or 2 drinks per day for females and males, respectively) can actually lower the risk of CVD from that of nondrinkers.

Hypercholesterolemia and oxidized low density lipoprotein (OxLDL) are among the most significant risk factors associated with the initiation and progression of atherosclerosis. Three different cholesterol lipoproteins, very low density lipoprotein (VLDL), low density lipoprotein (LDL), and high density lipoprotein (HDL), transport cholesterol and proteins through the blood to peripheral tissues requiring cholesterol for cellular membrane synthesis. VLDLs contain the highest ratio of lipids as compared to LDL and HDL. HDLs contain more protein than lipid, and individuals with high levels of HDL in the blood are less prone to develop CHD than individuals with high VLDL or LDL levels. Elevated levels of LDL in the blood are often due to defects in the apo B, or apo E (LDL) receptors responsible for the normal uptake and catabolism of LDL within cells.[252] LDL is considered to be the major source of cholesterol accumulation in foam cells, cells that contribute to the formation of pre-atherosclerotic fatty streaks.[255] However, LDL requires oxidative modification before it can contribute to the atherosclerotic process.[255] The effects and characteristics of oxidized LDL have largely been studied in vitro, however the mechanisms by which LDL is oxidized in vivo continue to be debated.

Evidence for OxLDL in vivo was firmly established by Steinberg[254]: (1) OxLDL is found in both rabbit and human atherosclerotic lesions; (2) antibodies against OxLDL react with materials in both rabbit and human lesions; (3) autoantibodies against OxLDL are evident in both rabbit and human plasma; and (4) treatment with compounds to prevent oxidation of LDL slow the progression of induced atherosclerosis in rabbits, hamsters, mice, and nonhuman primates. Oxidation of LDL is believed to occur within the artery wall after it has been taken up by intimal ECs by transcytosis, whereby LDL is surrounded by proteoglycans and extracellular matrix components.[78,210,253] The process of LDL oxidation is a free-radical driven lipid peroxidation event where polyunsaturated fatty acids of LDL lipids are converted to lipid hydroperoxides.[192] These lipid hydroperoxide products can be further degraded through free radical reactions to reactive products including malondialdehyde and 4-hydroxynonenal.[53] It is believed that these reactive products are the culprits in overall OxLDL toxicity.[161] In this manner, the toxicity of OxLDL in the vasculature can be compared to oxidative damage caused by chemical atherogens, a concept that mechanistically links seemingly unrelated biochemical processes. As will be addressed later in this review, many polycyclic aromatic hydrocarbon and aliphatic amine atherogens are metabolized by cytochrome P450 enzymes to reactive byproducts, including hydrogen peroxide, superoxide radicals, and hydroxyl radicals. These free radical species can cause significant cellular injury in the vessel wall, including lipid peroxidation, altered redox status/signaling, and damage to both DNA and proteins. As a result, free radical production mechanisms through both pathways indicate the similarity between cholesterol-induced injury and chemically induced injury.

OxLDL was first implicated in vascular lesion formation by Carew et al.[28] and Kita et al.,[113] who showed that WHHL rabbits with a gene defect causing LDL receptor deficiency, and thereby considered hypercholesterolemic, had smaller atherosclerotic lesions upon treatment with the antioxidant probucol. OxLDL is also present in macrophages of human lesions,[213] and is capable of promoting monocyte and T-lymphocyte transmigration through the endothelium and into the arterial wall.[213] In addition, OxLDL stimulates proliferation of SMCs through activation of PDGF.[297]

A recent finding by McMillan and Bradfield[147] has shown that LDL can contribute to vascular disease via an Ah receptor (AHR)-mediated pathway. LDL that was modified by either fluid shear stress or NaOCl activation (to model oxidation) produced activation of AHR signaling in multiple cell lines and species. Since shear stress is such an important factor in vascular biology, this offers another mechanism of LDL involvement in potential lesion formation. These results are also intriguing since AHR has been implicated in activating *c-Ha-ras* gene expression in vSMCs that could lead to a proliferative response.[108] This mechanism will be further considered later in this chapter.

Low HDL is also a risk factor in coronary heart disease, especially in women, and exceeds the risk of high levels of LDL in the blood.[137] HDL provides a protective effect against CHD, and is capable of inhibiting LDL oxidation caused by redox metals in cultured arterial cells.[136] HDL also acts to prevent the formation of lipid peroxides in LDL when they are both incubated under oxidizing conditions.[135] Therefore, low levels of HDL could contribute to the prevalence of potentially oxidizable LDL simply by not providing effective protection against its accumulation.

Atherogens vs. Carcinogens

Mechanisms characteristic of the progression of atherogenesis are analogous to mechanisms representative of carcinogenesis. As mentioned previously, the clonal expansion theory of the progression of atherosclerosis correlates closely with the course of tumor progression in carcinogenesis. The cellular and molecular mechanisms of both atherosclerotic lesion and neoplastic tumor formation are similar in the course of initiation, promotion, and progression of the disease. Of relevance in this context is that a number of toxic environmental chemicals can contribute to both processes.

The first set of compounds classified as both atherogens and carcinogens are the polycyclic aromatic hydrocarbons (PAHs). PAHs such as BaP, 7,12-dimethylbenzanthracene (DMBA), and 3-methylcholanthrene (3-MC) were initially identified for their potent carcinogenic potential. Nearly all PAHs are oxidized by cytochrome P450 enzymes to toxic metabolic intermediates which can be involved in DNA adduct formation or mutation of DNA. Factors such as solubility, distribution to target tissues, and intracellular localization relative to enzymes involved in biotransformation figure prominently in the expression of PAH carcinogenicity.[1] DMBA can be hydroxylated to a benzylic alcohol[152] or oxidized by cytochrome P450s to a radical cation (benzylic carbocation), which is its most highly toxic form.[29] Metabolism of BaP to the secondary metabolite BaP 7,8-diol-9,10-epoxide is considered the ultimate carcinogenic product of metabolism of this compound in that it adducts strongly to DNA. As atherogens, BaP and DMBA are biotransformed through P450 enzymes primarily in the smooth muscle layer of the aorta, and also in the aortic endothelium.[199] DMBA, in combination with methoxamine, induces focal proliferation of SMCs by an initiation–promotion sequence.[199] Others have indicated that several PAHs act as promoters of the atherosclerotic response by increasing the size, and not the frequency of atherosclerotic lesions.[2,185] 3-MC however increases both the number and size of lipid-staining aortic lesions found in animals that have been fed an atherogenic diet for 8 weeks, indicating the action of this PAH as an initiator of the atherosclerotic process.[199]

Occupational exposure to inorganic metals is also a risk factor for the initiation of both carcinogenesis and atherosclerosis. Arsenic, cadmium, chromium, and nickel are all considered carcinogens with a predominant malignancy of pulmonary carcinoma from working in metal refineries.[239] The inorganic metal cadmium is also considered to be a potent atherogen as well. Long-term exposure to cadmium is linked to the development of atherosclerosis and hypertension through its high localization in the elastic lamina of large arteries, especially at arterial branching points.[188]

While atherogenesis and carcinogenesis have similar etiologic mechanisms, some toxicants are primarily atherogens, and possess little carcinogenic potential. Two industrial agents are examples of this: allylamine, used in the synthesis of pharmaceutical and commercial products, and dinitrotoluene, a precursor in the synthesis of polyurethane foams, coatings, elastomers, and explosives. Allylamine is an aliphatic amine that is bioactivated by amine oxidases to acrolein and hydrogen peroxide to induce arterial smooth muscle cell injury and proliferation.[195] Repeated injury of the vasculature by allylamine generates smooth muscle cell hyperplasia and coronary artery and aortic lesions similar to those found in atherosclerotic vessels.[199] Dinitrotoluene exposure in humans can lead to circulatory disorders of atherosclerotic etiology, while repeated in vivo exposure leads to dysplasia and rearrangement of aortic smooth muscle cells.[194,199] Carcinogenic toxicity has been identified with dinitrotoluene exposure in lab animals, however in humans, the toxicity is primarily of cardiovascular etiology.

Natural products also play a role in the onset of atherosclerosis. One such atherogen is homocysteine, a sulfur-containing amino acid that is a byproduct of the biosynthesis of cysteine from methionine. Individuals with genetic defects in enzymes necessary for homocysteine metabolism have high plasma homocysteine concentrations, and often develop atherosclerosis during childhood.[139,174] Homocysteine is responsible for inducing endothelial cell injury that precedes the formation of atherosclerotic plaques, and also increases vascular fragility and the proliferation of vSMCs.[199] The reactive sulfhydryl group of homocysteine may be responsible for its atherogenic properties.

Reactive Oxygen Species and Oxidative Stress

Reactive oxygen species (ROS) are products of the numerous reduction–oxidation (redox) reactions occurring constantly within the cell, and are predominant mediators of a number of signal transduction processes that regulate normal cellular function. These redox mechanisms occur through electron transport in the mitochondria, or through metabolic conversion of chemicals or proteins within the cytosol. ROS are found in the form of superoxide anions ($O_2^{-\bullet}$), hydroxyl radicals ($^\bullet OH$), hydrogen peroxide (H_2O_2), and nitric oxide (NO). When atypical quantities of these species are generated through redox reactions within the cell, cellular redox balance is altered, and a number of different cellular processes can be affected. Alteration in the redox balance of the cell shifting toward the pro-oxidant is termed oxidative stress. Of importance is the fact that oxidative stress is not exclusively attributed to increased levels of ROS in the cell – decreases in redox status also constitute oxidative stress, and can have profound effects on cellular processes as well. Altered conditions in the cell that can lead to oxidative stress include:

(1) increased levels of transition metals or their reactive forms, (2) depletion of nonenzymatic antioxidant defenses, (3) increased generation of ROS, (4) ionizing radiation, and (5) redox cycling.

Cellular Redox Reactions

Free radicals and ROS are produced constantly during the life of the cell, and are a major product of electron transport in the mitochondria. In addition to ROS, other reactive compounds can be generated in the body by normal processes. This is especially true in regards to detoxification and metabolism of xenobiotics by various enzymatic systems. While xenobiotics may not be as directly toxic as parent compounds, their metabolic byproducts may be reactive species and thereby induce toxicity. These reactive metabolic byproducts can include free radicals and electrophiles (for a review see [76]).

Redox Cycling

Free radicals, chemical species characterized by one or more unpaired electrons in the outer shell, can contribute to toxicity in two ways – as an electron donor or an electron acceptor. Reductase enzymes add electrons to parent compounds to increase their hydrophilicity and facilitate excretion from the body. With a lone pair electron, the reactive parent compound can easily donate its free electron to molecular oxygen, regenerating the parent compound, but producing a superoxide radical ($O_2^{-\bullet}$). This continual process is termed "redox cycling." Superoxide radicals continue to be produced and significantly alter the redox balance of the cell, resulting in oxidative stress (Fig. 8.3).

Conversely, peroxidase enzymes remove electrons from nucleophilic parent compounds, such as those containing hydroxyl or amine functional groups, resulting in a free radical species. Hydroquinones, such as that shown in Fig. 8.3, are such compounds that lose one electron to form a semiquinone, and a second electron to form a quinone. Redox cycling also occurs here with reduction back to the hydroquinone species catalyzed by reductase enzymes (e.g., NADPH-cytochrome P450 reductase or NADPH-quinone oxidoreductase). The generation of radical cation forms of the parent compound, as well as ROS through redox cycling, contributes to the toxicity and elevation of oxidative stress within the cell. Quinones generated through the redox cycling event above represent another class of reactive metabolic byproducts – electrophiles. Electrophilic compounds contain reactive functional groups with a partial or full positive charge that are electron acceptors. Such compounds extract electrons from other chemicals containing nucleophilic functional groups, and contribute to their toxication, thereby initiating free radical

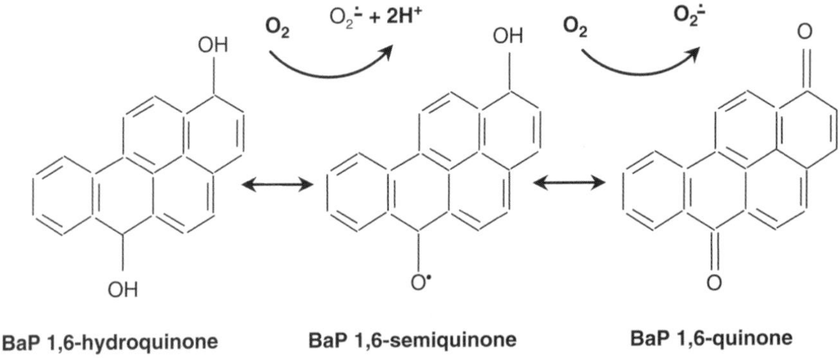

BaP 1,6-hydroquinone   BaP 1,6-semiquinone   BaP 1,6-quinone

Fig. 8.3 Redox cycling of the BaP metabolites, BaP 1,6-hydroquinone and BaP 1,6-quinone

forming redox reactions as mentioned above. Nucleophiles in themselves are not necessarily reactive species, but become so through loss of an electron by electrophilic compounds (for reviews see [76,178]).

Reactive Oxygen Species and Atherosclerosis

Increased levels of ROS that contribute to oxidative stress play a key role in vascular biology and the onset of atherosclerosis. A major source of ROS in blood vessels is the NADH/NADPH oxidase enzyme, which is expressed in endothelial cells, SMCs, and fibroblasts of the vessel wall.[289] Physiologically, ROS regulate vascular tone and structure,[265] induce vascular contraction,[39] and promote SMC growth.[201,264,288] Acute exposures to oxygen radicals can cause loss of contractile function and structural abnormalities of the vessel.[26,77,285] In addition, ROS are proinflammatory molecules and contribute to the metabolism of LDL to OxLDL.[36]

Oxygen free radicals and free radical species are significantly involved in cases of heart failure due to myocardial infarction.[230] In this type of injury, apoptotic events that occur are believed to be the result of oxidative stress.[74,102] Clinical studies of patients undergoing coronary artery bypass graft surgery have also suggested that increased free radical production and decreased antioxidant reserves play a role in the pathogenesis of heart failure.[30,75,230,236]

Oxygen-derived free radicals also play a significant role in ischemic reperfusion injury.[17,62,191] While reperfusion involves introduction of molecular oxygen-containing solutions to the ischemic myocardium, the breakdown of molecular oxygen to ROS and free radicals can actually enhance myocardial injury.[117,296] Of the ROS detected in the pathogenesis of reperfusion injury, superoxide anion ($O_2^{-\bullet}$), hydrogen peroxide (H_2O_2), and hydroxyl radicals ($^\bullet OH$) were most prevalent.[117,296] While the antioxidant enzymes superoxide dismutase, catalase, and glutathione peroxidase are present within the myocardium, the overload of ROS during reperfusion injury may overwhelm their antioxidant capabilities.[61]

Vascular cells are stimulated to generate ROS by a number of factors including cytokines, OxLDL, angiotensin II, high glucose, advanced glycosylation endproducts of proteins, and shear stress. Generated ROS (including $(O_2^{-\bullet})$ and H_2O_2) can thereby increase inflammatory gene transcription through activation of transcription factors such as NFκB and AP-1. Inflammatory genes known to be responsive in the vasculature to ROS are VCAM-1, TNFα, IL-1β, and MCP-1, among others. ROS scavengers and antioxidants can inhibit this inflammatory gene expression and decrease the pathogenesis of atherosclerosis.[32,119] Oxidative stress influences blood flow, inhibits platelet aggregation, inhibits leukocyte adhesion, and moderates cellular growth, thereby affecting vessel diameter, vessel wall remodeling and lesion formation, during the atherogenic process.[4,80]

Reactive Oxygen Species as Second Messengers

ROS can also act as "second messengers" in the body, influencing the regulation of transcription, signal transduction pathways, and the modification of proteins involved in these processes. As mentioned previously, there are many risk factors that contribute to the onset of atherosclerosis, including hypertension, diabetes, hyperlipidemia, and tobacco smoking. A possible link between all of these factors and atherosclerosis may be explained by the second messenger actions of ROS. As reviewed by Kunsch and Medford,[120] one hypothesis suggests that oxidative signals may regulate the expression of vascular inflammatory genes, thus providing a molecular mechanism that links these risk factors. Pro-inflammatory or pro-oxidant stimuli may induce vascular cells to produce ROS, which in turn transmit these signals to elevate the expression of genes involved in the atherosclerotic process, including those responsible for the generation of adhesion molecules and other inflammatory gene products. Nitric oxide (NO) regulates vascular inflammatory gene expression, including the activity of NFκB in ECs, which could implicate a mechanism for suppression of vascular gene expression.[183] H_2O_2 can also regulate NFκB activation by influencing IκB phosphorylation, releasing NFκB to translocate into the nucleus and bind to promoter regions of target genes. Oxidative stress can also activate AP-1 transcription factors to bind target genes within the nucleus.[148]

In addition, ROS can act as second messengers to influence intracellular signal transduction mechanisms. These molecules could provide a link between extracellular signals received at the membrane level, and the modulation of gene expression at the nuclear level.[120] For example, treatment of vSMCs with H_2O_2 elevates intracellular stores of Ca^{2+} most likely through inhibition of normal ATP-dependent Ca^{2+} pumps in the endoplasmic reticulum.[49] Since Ca^{2+} signaling mechanisms are controlled by Ca^{2+} transport through these pumps, this infers an oxidant-mediated effect on signaling processes. In addition, oxidative stress inducers such as H_2O_2 and ionizing radiation modulate tyrosine kinase pathways, and activate downstream kinases involved in these pathways such as protein kinase C.[144,167,247] In vSMCs, H_2O_2 stimulates phosphorylation of the EGF receptor, thereby initiating a tyrosine kinase signaling cascade involving Shc, Grb2, Sos, and Ras.[202] Tyrosine phosphorylation and activation of MAP kinases (serine/threonine kinases) can also be influenced by treatment of vSMCs with PDGF, which increases intracellular H_2O_2 production to mediate these effects.[259] In these studies, kinase activation was inhibited upon increasing the cellular concentrations of catalase or N-acetyl cysteine, both antioxidants. MAP kinase activation can also be induced through the increase in intracellular ROS by key vascular injury agents such as OxLDL and angiotensin II.[8,268] Angiotensin II specifically increases intracellular H_2O_2 and subsequently contributes to rapid phosphorylation of p42/44 and p38 MAP kinases.[225,268] In addition, arachidonic acid, through Rac-1-dependent H_2O_2 production, can also activate c-Jun N-terminal kinase (JNK).[234]

Reactive Oxygen Species as Protein Modifiers and Phosphorylation Mediators

ROS can also play a key event in redox modulation of transcription factors, which can have positive or negative effects on transcriptional states. As reviewed by Stadtman and Berlett,[249] the outcomes of protein oxidation by ROS include oxidation of amino acid residue side chains, cleavage of peptide bonds and formation of covalent protein–protein cross-linked derivatives. Oxidative modifications and posttranslational modifications of transcription factors by ROS can greatly alter the DNA binding activity of the protein, affect its cellular localization, or influence its transcriptional activity. In regards to amino acid oxidation of proteins, cysteine residues are key regulators of the DNA binding capacity of transcription factors, and are significant targets for redox modification. The carbonyl content of proteins is also a widely known measure of oxidative damage to proteins. Carbonyl groups can be found in the form of aldehyde or ketone derivatives from protein reactions with ROS. Oxidative cleavage of the peptide backbone can generate fragments with N-terminal carbonyl moieties, while amino acids themselves can be modified via oxidative modifications of lysine, proline, arginine, and threonine residues. In a more physiological reaction, rather than direct oxidation, lipid peroxidation generates 4-hydroxy-2-nonenal, a compound that can react with proteins and add carbonyl groups to lysine, histidine, or cysteine residues.[66,164,266] Increases in carbonyl content, irrespective of the mechanism, have been shown in exposures to hypoxia, exercise, ischemia-reperfusion, oxidative burst, ozone, and tobacco smoke, and are key indicators of aging, physiological disorders, and disease (for a review see [249]).

Benzo[a]pyrene

Polycyclic aromatic hydrocarbons are ubiquitous environmental contaminants that originate from multiple sources, including vehicle exhaust emissions, heat and power generation, refuse burning, industrial processes, oil contamination by disposal or spills, cigarette smoke, and cooking of foods.[37] Of the many PAHs studied for their toxic effects in human populations, benzo[a]pyrene (BaP) has often been regarded as the prototypical PAH.

BaP is a five-membered ring generated as a byproduct of combustion of coal tar, petroleum, and tobacco. BaP is present at an average level of 100 ng/m^3 in heavily polluted air, 23 ng/L in drinking water, and 100 µg/kg in smoked foods,[11] and the average daily intake of BaP by the general U.S. population is approximately 2.2 µg/day.[81] The food chain is considered the dominant pathway for routine human exposure and accounts for about 97% of the total daily intake of BaP.[81] Inhalation and consumption of contaminated water are considered minor pathways of exposure for the general population, except for consumers of tobacco products or workers in the coal industry. PAH exposures often involve multiple sources and routes, and often involve co-exposure with other contaminants. As a result, the spectrum of toxic effects associated with single exposure to BaP may or may not reflect actual environmental exposures.

The inhalation of cigarette smoke has been strongly implicated as a causal factor in human cancers, as suggested by the high incidence of lung cancer among smokers,[226,267]. BaP has been estimated to be present at a level of 25 ng per cigarette,[228] and the average intake of BaP in smokers of one-pack of unfiltered or filtered cigarettes per day is 0.7 µg/day or 0.4 µg/day, respectively.[37] Many free radical species are also present in cigarette smoke, both in the gas-phase and inhaled particulate phase,[190] potentially contributing to increased incidence of cancer in smokers. Epidemiological data suggest that the amount of particulate matter, or "tar" that is inhaled correlates with increased rates of lung and larynx cancer.[82] Heavy smokers not only face a high risk for lung and larynx cancer, but also of upper digestive tract, pancreas, kidney, and urinary bladder cancers.[82]

Bay Region Hypothesis

Several PAHs contain a structural motif known as the "Bay Region." The bay region is defined as the area of a complex ring structure containing a single angular fused benzene ring adjacent to an aromatic ring (Fig. 8.4). The region encompassing carbons 9–12 is considered to be the bay region of BaP. The angular ring forms an area of steric hindrance, where oxidation or radical formation can easily occur, while detoxification and conjugation are impeded. The active center is located at the benzyl position (the carbon on the angular ring that is α to the aromatic ring).

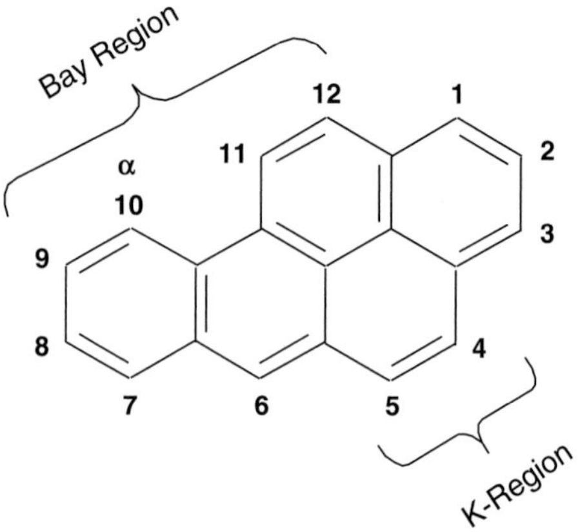

Fig. 8.4 Bay region and K-region reactive sites on benzo[a]pyrene

C^{10} of BaP is considered the active center (α-carbon) as its location is in the highly reactive benzylic position of the saturated, angular benzo-ring forming the bay region. The K-region represented by carbons at positions 4 and 5, represents an area of high electron density, and therefore high metabolic activity.

Molecular orbital calculations have shown that epoxides formed on these saturated benzo-rings undergo ring opening to form a carbonium ion more readily than non-bay-region epoxides, and are highly susceptible to nucleophilic attack, such as that by DNA.[182] Benzo[a]pyrene 7,8-diol-9,10-epoxide (BPDE), a putative carcinogenic metabolite of BaP, contains an epoxide ring at the tenth position and has been shown to form DNA adducts with the N^2 position of guanine. The strength of a carcinogenic PAH correlates with the formation of a carbonium ion within the bay region of the molecule. However, exceptions to this rule may exist since a highly toxic BaP metabolite (BaP 4,5-oxide) capable of adducting DNA has been reported to be formed on the K-region of the molecule.[182]

Metabolism of Benzo[a]pyrene, Enzyme Systems and Reactivity of Metabolites

BaP is a procarcinogen, and as such, requires metabolic activation to reactive intermediates to elicit toxic effects. Many enzymatic systems participate in the metabolism of BaP leading to enhancement of, or protection from toxicity.[73] The multiple metabolic products generated from oxidative metabolism of the parent compound exhibit varying reactivities, leading to complicated pathways of cytotoxicity, macromolecular damage, and overall deficits in cell function and integrity.

Both Phase I and II enzymes metabolize BaP to hydrophilic intermediates as a means of detoxification and elimination from the organism. Phase I metabolic enzymes involved in BaP metabolism include cytochrome P450 mixed function oxidases (MFOs), epoxide reductases, and epoxide hydrolases (which can also be considered as Phase II enzymes), as well as the Phase II conjugating enzymes glutathione transferases, UDP-glucuronyl transferases, and sulfotransferases.[73] Endoplasmic reticulum-based cytochrome P450 monooxygenase reactions begin the metabolic cascade, introducing oxygen at any number of positions on the parent compound to form epoxides, the major forms of which are the 4,5-, 7,8-, and 9,10-isomers (Fig. 8.5).

Simple oxidation of BaP upon exposure to air can also produce the epoxides 1,2-, 2,3-, 4,5-, 7,8-, 9,10-, and 11,12-epoxide isomers. The 4,5-, 7,8-, and 9,10-diols, all present as *trans* isomers, are formed through subsequent metabolism of epoxides by epoxide hydrolase.[73] BaP *trans*-dihydrodiol oxidation can occur by the action of dihydrodiol dehydrogenases in the cytosol. Dihydrodiols, such as BaP 7,8-diol can be converted to catechols via dihydrodiol dehydrogenase, and subsequently autooxidize to an electrophilic *ortho*-quinone, as in the case of BaP 7,8-quinone.[242]

Nonenzymatic rearrangement of epoxides can also result in phenolic intermediates, of which five have been isolated: 1-, 3-, 6-, 7-, and 9-OH BaP isomers. 3-OH BaP is considered to be the major phenolic metabolite of BaP, arising from an NIH shift mechanism in an unstable 2,3-epoxide. However, this is not considered to be the primary pathway of formation, since direct hydroxylation on the C-3 position of BaP is predominant in most cell types.[73] Mechanisms of phenol formation independent of an epoxide intermediate are also possible, notably in the case of oxygenation at C-6 with subsequent quinone formation at the 1,6-, 3,6-, and 6,12-positions.[84,86] 3-OH BaP can be metabolized to quinones upon air oxidation,[21] and convert to BaP 3,6-quinone upon incubation with heat-inactivated microsomes.[231] In general, PAHs of low ionization potential, such as BaP, can be converted by one-electron oxidation via peroxidases or cytochrome P450 to toxic radical cations, an intermediate in further metabolism to quinones.[29] BaP 3,6-quinone accounts for 44% of the oxidation of 6-OH BaP,[123] and binding of BaP to DNA at the 1, 3, and 6 positions is associated with a free-radical mechanism of toxic action.[206] 6-oxy BaP has also been identified as a metabolite, involved as an intermediate of 6-OH BaP formation.[73]

Autooxidation of 6-OH BaP leads to quinone formation with the subsequent production of radicals, including $O_2^{-\cdot}$ and $\cdot$OH radicals and OH$^-$ through redox cycling events. These oxygen radicals may react further to produce H_2O_2. A positive feedback mechanism involving direct action of hydroxy radicals with BaP to generate 6-oxy-BaP radicals and BaP quinones has also been described.[258] Surprisingly, the 6-oxy-BaP radical is unusually stable and is unreactive to hydrogen-donating solvents and antioxidants.[118,257] As a result, quinone formation is highly likely and can account for a large metabolic yield of BaP in a variety of tissues.[124] BaP quinones participate in one-electron redox cycles between their corresponding hydroquinones (BaP diols) and semiquinone radicals. Coupling these

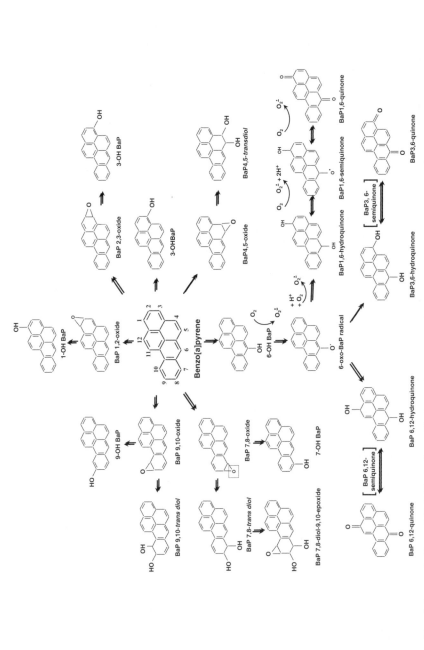

Fig. 8.5 Profile of the metabolism of BaP. Beginning with the parent compound, primary and secondary oxidative metabolites can be formed through metabolism by cytochrome P450 enzymes within cellular systems

NADPH-cytochrome P450 reductase catalyzed cycles with molecular oxygen produces ROS in the form of $O_2^{-\bullet}$ and H_2O_2.[132] Such redox cycles operate under physiological conditions and can be aided by cellular respiratory enzymes. The excessive generation of oxidants can ultimately alter redox status in target cells and induce cellular injury.

Secondary metabolites of BaP are formed following further enzyme attack of primary metabolites. Catechols are secondary metabolites formed by the dehydrogenation of dihydrodiols,[20,261] while additional epoxides form through monooxygenase attack of unoccupied positions in phenols and dihydrodiols.[21,27] Such is the case of BaP *trans*-7,8-diol, which is converted to two stereoisomers (anti and syn) of BPDE by recycling through the MFO system. The (+) isomer of anti-BPDE is the most active of all four diol epoxides (± anti and ± syn), acting as both a complete carcinogen and tumor initiator in mouse skin,[241] as well as a mutagen in Chinese hamster V79 cells.[88]

Factors controlling recycling through the MFO system include the amount of phenol or diol metabolites available for further action by MFOs, relative to the amount of competing BaP substrate available. Less recycling occurs when large amounts of BaP parent compound are available, and vice versa.[73] MFO recycling creates metabolites of far greater polarity that are not as easily extractable as the primary and secondary metabolites.[73] High levels of conjugating enzymes may also compete with the MFOs for the oxygenated primary or secondary metabolites, thus diminishing the availability of oxygenated metabolites for recycling.

In the case of lung microsomes, exposure to oxygen metabolites leads to a decreased rate of BaP metabolism, decreasing the potential for enzymatic detoxification reactions, and thereby increasing accumulation of potentially toxic BaP metabolites.[64] Levels of the detoxification enzymes superoxide dismutase (SOD) and catalase are also reduced in BaP-treated tissues and correlate with increased oxidative damage to DNA and protein.[110] In like manner, BaP increases the level of oxidative DNA damage in the form of 8-OHdG levels in liver, kidney, and lung.[110] Protein damage via oxidation, as reflected by protein carbonyl content, is also seen in cytosolic fractions of these tissues, though predominantly in the liver.[110]

Despite formation of potentially damaging intermediates that can promote cellular injury and toxicity, oxidative metabolism of BaP is a pathway of detoxification and elimination. Phenols and diols can be conjugated to water-soluble compounds by either sulfate or glucuronide conjugation,[73] with BaP phenols as the preferred substrates for UDP-glucuronyl transferases. Diminution of BaP and 6-OH BaP cytotoxicity by glucuronide conjugation is likely due to elimination of cytotoxic phenols and quinones.[203]

Metabolism of BaP can produce ROS in the form of $O_2^{-\bullet}$, $OH^\bullet$, OH^- and H_2O_2, all of which are capable of incurring some form of injury when present in high levels in the cell. BaP quinones and consequent generation of free radicals may mediate modulation of redox status in target cells by BaP. However, redox cycling may not be the primary mechanism of quinone cytotoxicity in all cell types. Zhu and coworkers[294] have shown that levels of cellular glutathione (GSH), quinone reductase (QR) activity, and ROS are not involved in BaP quinone-induced bone marrow stromal cell injury. Despite increases in GSH content and QR activity by pretreatment with 1,2-dithiole-3-thione (D3T), protection against BaP 1,6-quinone toxicity was not achieved. Interestingly, dicumarol, an inhibitor of QR, and buthionine sulfoximine (BSO), an inhibitor of GSH synthesis, did not alter BaP 1,6-quinone cytotoxicity either.[294] In actuality, BaP 1,6-quinone treatment of bone marrow stromal cells depleted cellular ATP content and induced mitochondrial morphology changes, leading to decreased cell survival.

Target Organs and Cellular Localization of Benzo[a]pyrene

Exposure to BaP by inhalation, oral or dermal exposure, results in distribution of the toxicant throughout the organism. The liver is often regarded as a primary target of BaP since this organ contains many of the enzymes involved in bioactivation of the parent molecule. Following intratracheal administration, 21% of a single BaP dose is available in the liver within 10 min.[278] High levels of BaP are found within 30 min in the liver, kidney, gastrointestinal tract, esophagus, small intestine, blood, and carcass.[278] In the lung and liver, quinone metabolites of BaP are present at high levels within 5 min after exposure. The intestinal concentration of BaP and its metabolites increases with time, suggesting the occurrence of biliary excretion and enterohepatic recirculation.[279] However, intestinal absorption of PAHs is highly dependent on the presence of bile in the stomach.[193] BaP can also be absorbed into liver, lung, and kidney after oral administration.[283]

BaP is highly lipophilic and readily taken up into cells through the plasma membrane. Once taken up into the cell, PAHs generally associate with hydrophobic molecules that participate in its distribution throughout intracellular compartments. Most PAHs preferentially accumulate in the mitochondrion and nucleus. Mitochondria themselves may be cellular targets of BaP, with quinone-induced cytotoxicity resulting from direct disruption of energy metabolism.[294] Barhoumi et al.[10] examined the partitioning of BaP into rat liver cells by fluorescence microscopy. In these cells, BaP was found to enter the cell within several minutes, and to rapidly localize in Golgi and cytoplasmic membranes, including the plasma membrane, endoplasmic reticulum, and nuclear envelope. Some accumulation was also found in the nucleus, mitochondrial matrix, and lysosomes. In addition, monooxygenases are believed to be present in the nucleus and nuclear envelope,[56,106,109,205,235] suggesting that BaP could in fact be metabolized in these compartments. In support of this, Bresnick and coworkers[25] showed that isolated nuclei could metabolize BaP to BPDE.

Benzo[a]pyrene Carcinogenicity

BaP is a key factor in promoting atherogenesis, however, its toxicity was first attributed to its carcinogenic properties. Understanding the mechanisms of BaP-induced carcinogenicity may aid in understanding its mechanisms of inducing atherogenesis, as some of these processes are similar. Miller and Miller[150,151] performed ground-breaking research in the 1950s with PAHs such as BaP showing that covalent binding of these chemicals to DNA was an initial critical step in carcinogenesis. Such modifications in DNA are handled by repair mechanisms within the cell nucleus and are subject to tight cellular regulation. Unrepaired genomic damage can slip through the pathway and go on to form preneoplastic lesions that give rise to neoplasia and malignant transformation. Factors such as solubility, distribution to target tissues, and intracellular localization relative to enzymes involved in biotransformation figure prominently in the expression of PAH carcinogenicity.

Initial studies of BaP carcinogenesis were performed by Levin and coworkers using a mouse skin model, whereby BaP and its metabolites were painted onto mouse skin over a period of 60 weeks.[126] At 0.4 µmol, parent compound, BaP 7,8-oxide, and 2-OH BaP showed the most prevalent incidences of tumors, with metabolites closely mimicking the response of BaP. The 2-OH BaP metabolite was shown to be the most carcinogenic, however it was disregarded as a major significant metabolite due to its high reactivity and instability.[240] At 0.15 µmol, BaP 7,8-diol showed a greater incidence of tumors than BaP 7,8-oxide. The carcinogenicity of these two latter metabolites was believed to involve conversion to BaP 7,8-diol-9,10-epoxide (BPDE).[125] Intraperitoneal injections of newborn mice with BaP, BaP 7,8-diol, and BPDE showed high incidences of malignant lymphomas of the thymus, spleen, bone marrow, lymph nodes, liver, and other organs, as well as lung adenomas, with a clear establishment of BaP 7,8-diol as the proximate carcinogenic metabolite of BaP.[105]

A number of factors determine human susceptibility to PAH-induced cancers. One is the heterogeneity of human genotypes regarding aryl hydrocarbon hydroxylase inducibility.[1] Although the average human lifetime exposure to BaP greatly exceeds the amount necessary to grow papillomas on the back of a mouse,[232] humans are generally less sensitive to BaP-induced carcinogenesis than other species. Kadlubar and Badawi[101] have shown that PAH-DNA adducts in human bladder correlate with polymorphism in the total metabolism of BaP by bladder microsomes and especially the formation of BaP 7,8-diol. Thus, the expression of metabolizing enzymes may be a critical determinant of carcinogen-DNA adduct formation and individual cancer susceptibility.[101] This paradigm may also influence other toxicity outcomes upon exposure to BaP.

Recycling of MFOs leads to further oxidation of BaP dihydrodiols and subsequent formation of highly toxic diol epoxides. BPDE is the most carcinogenic of all BaP metabolites tested. This compound contains an epoxide ring within the bay region of the molecule and is highly susceptible to nucleophilic attack. BaP-DNA adducts form on the 9,10-epoxide position, preferentially on the N^2 position of guanine, and lie in the minor groove of DNA.[277] BPDEs are easily converted into carbonium ions, which are alkylating agents, and thus mutagens and initiators of carcinogenesis. The proportion and amount of BaP binding to DNA (through BPDE) increases with time of exposure to BaP in culture. This is primarily due to induction of P450IA1 by BaP and increases in metabolism of the parent compound to the ultimate carcinogen.[51] In support of this, antibodies against P450IA1 reduce binding of BaP to DNA by over 90% in microsomal preparations of BaP-treated hepatocytes.[51] Long-term exposure of cells to BaP could result in activation of a higher proportion of BaP to the carcinogenic BPDE.[51] P450IIC11 can also metabolize BaP to 7,8- and 9,10-dihydrodiols, and further to BPDE. Antibodies against this enzyme and epitopically related P450s inhibit metabolism to these reactive metabolites and also inhibit enzyme catalyzed binding of BaP to DNA in the specific formation of BaP-N[7]Gua adducts detected by ^{32}P-postlabeling.[263] Yang et al.[284] provided evidence that BPDE is responsible for adduct formation in the *aprt* gene in CHO cells. Upon separate treatment with BaP and BPDE, the mutation spectra of this gene was analyzed and found to be similar between the two, suggesting that BPDE is responsible for some of the significant biological effects of the parent compound.

Macromolecular Adduction

Exposure to PAHs induces formation of various types of macromolecular adducts, of which DNA adducts have been most extensively characterized. DNA adduction profiles exhibit species-, strain-, and tissue-specific differences due to variations in metabolic activation and repair capability.[211] Studies using rat liver microsomes and mouse skin showed that binding of BaP at the C^6 position to DNA occurs. Although the major stable adduct of BaP identified was BPDE-10-N^2dG (a C^{10} adduct), DNA adduction primarily occurred at the C^6 position of BaP to the C^8 and N^7 positions of guanine, and N^7 of adenine. All of these latter adducts were lost from DNA by depurination. These results suggest that formation of PAH radical cations by one-electron oxidation plays a central role in activation of carcinogenic PAHs of low ionization potential and localization of charge in their radical cations.

In accord with this one-electron oxidation pathway, semiquinone intermediates formed during the redox cycling of quinones can directly bind DNA.[99,115,166] An end product of redox cycling, BaP 3,6-quinone, forms two DNA adducts with deoxyguanosine (dG), but not with deoxyadenosine, deoxycytosine, or deoxythymidine.[99] NAD(P)H quinone oxidoreductase$_1$ (NQO$_1$) can specifically reduce binding of quinone metabolites of BaP to DNA and protein. 6-OH BaP, a precursor to quinone formation, also binds DNA, most likely through participation of the 6-oxy BaP radical.[166] BaP 7,8-diol can also contribute to DNA adduct formation as seen in lung target cells co-incubated with activated neutrophils. The addition of phorbol myristate acetate (PMA)-activated neutrophils strongly enhanced BaP 7,8-diol adduct formation, while antioxidants added to co-incubations significantly reduced the number of adducts.[22] The K-region BaP 4,5-oxide forms DNA adducts, but does not fit into the minor groove of DNA as well as BPDE does, and consequently is more rapidly repaired by DNA repair systems.[59,181] Finally, 9-OH and 3-OH BaP can be further metabolized to covalently bind to DNA.[73] King et al.[111] suggested that metabolism of 9-OH BaP to the 4,5-epoxy-9-OH BaP metabolite is capable of DNA binding. In the case of 3-OH BaP, Kinoshita and Gelboin[112] showed DNA binding by a benzo[a]pyrene-3-glucuronide intermediate generated by the action of β-glucuronidase.

Nucleotide adduct formation by BaP leads to DNA mutations. Major mutations include G:C → T:A transversions, with mutations localized within runs of guanines.[284] Mutation by BaP is nonrandom, and preferentially targets runs of guanines flanked by adenine residues, such as those found in the hotspot region of codon 61 in human *c-Ha-ras1* proto-oncogene.

Deficient repair of DNA adducts formed by reactive BaP intermediates has been associated with increased rates of mutation in mammalian cells. In studies examining the mutagenicity of BaP in TA98 and TA100 Salmonella strains,[126] BaP 7,8-diol-9,10-epoxides and H_4-9,10-epoxides (9,10-epoxy-7,8,9,10-tetrahydroBaP) were identified as the most potent mutagenic metabolites. Mutagenic capacity is significantly decreased if the epoxide is located on the 7,8-position, as opposed to the 9,10-position. This follows the reactivity correlates predicted by the Bay Region Hypothesis. The 4,5-oxide of BaP is also mutagenic in these strains, but to a lesser degree than diol epoxides and H_4-9,10-epoxides. Of the multiple phenolic metabolites of BaP, only 1-, 3-, 6-, and 12-OH BaP isomers showed any mutagenic activity in bacterial or mammalian cells, with the 6-OH being the most mutagenic, though less so than BPDE. The six quinones (1,6-, 3,6-, 6,12-, 4,5-, 7,8-, and 11,12-isomers) and 4 dihydrodiols (4,5-, 7,8-, 9,10-, and 11,12-isomers) tested were all inactive as mutagens. In the presence of monooxygenase activity, many of the primary BaP metabolites (BaP 7,8-diol, and 1-, 2-, 3-, 6-, and 9-OH BaP) were activated to more mutagenic metabolites. Similar results were found upon examination of the mutagenicity of these metabolites in Chinese Hamster V79 cells.[126]

Different results were reported when the Salmonella TA104 tester strain was examined in separate investigations.[35] BaP 1,6-quinone and 3,6-quinone were both highly mutagenic, while the 6,12-quinone was only a weak mutagen. Two-electron reduction of BaP 3,6-quinone by NQO_1 to the hydroquinone was not mutagenic, whereas the one-electron reduction, catalyzed by NAD(P)H:cytochrome P450 reductase, was mutagenic. The mutagenicity of quinones by this pathway was attributable to the generation of oxygen radicals, particularly $O_2^{-•}$, and subsequently H_2O_2. In support of this view, SOD and catalase together inhibited reductase-mediated mutagenicity of BaP 3,6-quinone almost completely, while the two individually only show modest inhibition. As a result, oxygen radicals produced through redox cycling, rather than quinones themselves or their semiquinone intermediates, were implicated in this case as the mutagenic agents.

Quinone redox cycling is a predominant mechanism of ROS production upon exposure and subsequent metabolism of BaP within the cell. BaP quinones induce single-strand scissions in T7 bacteriophage DNA in vitro, an event most likely catalyzed by ROS participating in free-radical reactions within the cell.[124] Studies indicate that hydroxyl radicals produced in Fenton-type reactions can be responsible for strand scission.[124]

Benzo[a]pyrene and Atherosclerosis

BaP has been implicated in the initiation and progression of atherosclerotic disorders, particularly through modulation of growth and differentiation in aortic SMCs.[196] In vivo treatment of Sprague–Dawley rats with BaP is associated with development of aortic wall lesions with structural changes characteristic of the early stages of atherosclerosis, including loss of endothelial integrity, fragmentation of elastic laminae, expansion of the SMC mass, and orientation changes of medial SMCs.[291] A relationship also exists between induction of proliferative vSMCs involved in lesion formation and expression of *c-Ha-ras*, as shown by evidence that in vitro BaP challenge upregulates *ras* gene expression.[221] However, mutations are not detected in SMCs within the activating regions of c-Ha-, c-Ki-, or N-ras genes upon weekly in vivo BaP injections, indicating that such mutations are not responsible for BaP-induced alterations in SMC proliferation.[291] An epigenetic mechanism involving deregulation of *c-Ha-ras* expression has therefore been proposed.[197]

Biotransformation and metabolism of BaP during the course of atherogenesis is believed to occur mainly in the smooth muscle layers of the aorta,[233] although endothelial-mediated metabolism also occurs.[262] BaP is metabolized in SMCs by cytochrome P450 monooxygenases to intermediates that further oxidize to produce ROS. Specifically, 3-OH BaP, a precursor to quinone formation and generator of ROS, is a predominant BaP metabolite in SMCs,[18] and metabolism to quinones, namely the 3,6-isomer, can soon follow by air oxidation or further metabolism through the P450 system.[21,231] Quinone redox cycling is a common occurrence and can produce a multitude of oxygen radicals through the one- or two-electron reduction cycles. In vSMCs, this phenomenon has been shown upon treatment with BaP, evidenced by increases in the formation of ROS and depletion of antioxidant capacity within the cell.[108]

Additional support of a redox mechanism is provided in terms of protein oxidation and atherosclerotic plaque development. Reactive products of protein oxidation such as hydroxyleucine and hydrovaline are increased in advanced atherosclerotic plaques, indicating that oxy radicals, possibly along with the products of metal ion-catalyzed Fenton chemistry, and/or peroxyl and alkoxyl radicals, play a direct role in plaque formation.[262]

Albert and coworkers[2] were the first to show that PAHs increase the size of atherosclerotic lesions in chickens. These observations were confirmed by Bond et al.,[19] who also demonstrated a dose-dependent relationship between administration of BaP and dimethylbenzanthracene (DMBA) and the development of atherosclerosis in chickens. These studies likened the initiation and promotion of atherosclerotic lesions to that involved in carcinogenic tumor initiation and promotion, as was previously suggested by Benditt.[13] In other studies comparing long-term BaP treatment in atherosclerosis-susceptible White Carneau and atherosclerosis-resistant Show Racer pigeon models, the number and size of arterial lesions in the brachiocephalic arteries in females, but not males, of both species were enhanced.[85] Treatment with benzo[e]pyrene, a noncarcinogenic BaP analogue, did not enhance lesion development, therefore postulating that metabolic activation is required for BaP atherogenicity. BaP is a primary constituent of tobacco smoke, and many studies have focused on how BaP exposure by this route of administration affects the atherosclerotic process. Exposure to cigarette smoke increases the activity of the BaP metabolizing enzyme aryl hydrocarbon hydroxylase.[114] Correspondingly, the activity of aryl hydrocarbon hydroxylase (AHH) correlates with increased levels of atherosclerosis in avian species,[199] indicating that metabolites of BaP play a large role in atherosclerotic plaque development. In support of this, aortic microsomes from BaP-treated rats metabolize BaP to the 7R, 8S, 9,10-tetrahydrotetrol, 7,8-dihydrodiol, 1,6-quinone, 3,6-quinone, 6,12-quinone, 3-hydroxy, and 9-hydroxy-BaP moieties, suggesting that BaP present in cigarette smoke can be metabolized in the aorta to carcinogenic and toxic products, thereby initiating vessel injury and leading to accelerated atherosclerosis in cigarette smokers.[262]

Modulation of Gene Expression by Benzo[a]pyrene through the Aryl Hydrocarbon Receptor

The aryl hydrocarbon receptor (AHR) has been extensively characterized as the primary xenobiotic-regulated transcription factor involved in transcriptional regulation of drug metabolizing enzymes.[229] Through a ligand-inducible reaction, AHR binds to dioxin-responsive enhancer elements (DREs), also known as aryl hydrocarbon response elements (AHREs), in the regulatory regions of Phase I and II genes.[7,41,42,57,70,96,179] 2,3,7,8-Tetrachlorodibenzo-p-dioxin (TCDD) is often recognized as one of the most potent ligands of the AHR. AHR is a basic helix–loop–helix cytosolic protein that is present in the cytosol in complex with two heat shock protein 90 (HSP90) molecules and XAP2 (X associated protein 2). Binding of ligand to the receptor induces translocation to the nucleus where it releases the HSP90 and XAP2 proteins, and interacts with the aryl hydrocarbon nuclear translocator (ARNT). This AHR-ARNT heterodimer then binds DNA to transactivate or transrepress target genes (Fig. 8.6).

BaP is recognized as a ligand for AHR, and as such, in vivo and in vitro exposure to this chemical is often associated with activation of AHR-coupled signaling in mammalian and nonmammalian cells. Gene induction via BaP-AHR mechanisms often serves as a positive feedback regulatory loop that sustains metabolism of the parent compound.

Vaziri and Faller[270] have shown that BaP inhibits growth factor-stimulated DNA synthesis in cells expressing high levels of AHR. In these experiments, growth arrest by BaP is not seen in cells lacking AHR, nor cells treated with α-NF, an AHR antagonist.[270] BaP-treated cells also exhibited increased amounts of DNA adducts, while TCDD-treated cells did not, indicating that inhibition of cell growth by BaP may involve metabolism to genotoxic metabolites. Similar results are seen upon

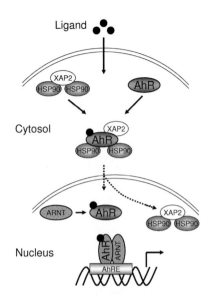

Fig. 8.6 Ah Receptor signaling pathway. Extracellular ligand is taken up by the cell, and binds to AHR, which is associated with two HSP90 proteins and XAP2. The new AHR complex translocates to the nucleus where it releases XAP2 and the two HSP90 proteins, and binds to ARNT. The AHR/ARNT heterodimer then binds to the AHRE to influence transcriptional events (modified from [149,281])

BaP treatment of rat hepatocytes.[292] In these experiments, pretreatment of cells with both α-NF and ellipticine antagonized BaP-induced inhibition of DNA synthesis, implicating AHR signal transduction mechanisms in the toxic response.

In follow-up studies, the time- and concentration-dependent effects of BaP on *c-fos*, *c-jun*, *c-myc*, and *c-Ha-ras* expression in cultured rat hepatocytes was evaluated.[293] BaP markedly inhibited the expression of *c-fos* and *c-jun*, with pronounced effects observed during the early part of the induction response. In contrast, the kinetics of *c-myc* and *c-Ha-ras* inducibility was increased by BaP leading to significant enhancement of mRNA levels relative to control counterparts. TCDD, an AHR agonist, elicited responses comparable to BaP for *c-jun* and *c-Ha-ras,* but not *c-fos or c-myc*. Interestingly, α-NF elicited *c-jun* and *c-Ha-ras* responses comparable to BaP, but reversed the modulatory effects of BaP on *c-fos* and *c-myc*. Diamide, a sulfhydryl oxidant, increased *c-fos*, *c-myc*, and *c-Ha-ras* gene expression, but did not influence the gene modulatory effects of BaP. Thus, the ability of BaP to influence growth-related gene expression in cultured rat hepatocytes involves both AHR signaling and oxidative stress.

In addition, Rushmore et al.[220] have found that α-NF transcriptionally activates GSTA1 through an antioxidant response element, also known as the electrophile response element (ARE/EpRE) in HepG2 cells, indicating that complex molecular mechanisms involving the AHR may be operative in the regulation of gene expression via the ARE/EpRE. Analogously, evidence by Ramos and coworkers has shown that AHR signaling participates in ARE/EpRE regulation of the *c-Ha-ras* oncogene and the rGSTA1 gene.[34,108] The full length rGSTA1 promoter is negatively regulated by aromatic hydrocarbons such as BaP and TCDD through a crosstalk mechanism between AHRE and ARE/EpRE.[33] Partially responsible for this is the presence of a C/EBP-like site located within the consensus ARE/EpRE of the rGSTA1 promoter.[33] When this C/EBP-like site is mutated, positive regulatory function of rGSTA1 in response to aromatic hydrocarbons is regained. Therefore, in this promoter, it has been suggested that in response to aromatic hydrocarbons, the AHR protein itself, or AHRE, participate in the negative regulation of rGSTA1 via the C/EBP-like site located within the ARE/EpRE.[33]

c-Ha-ras

Ras genes were first discovered and described as oncogenes present in the Harvey and Kirsten rat sarcoma viruses.[52] The *ras* gene family consists of three members found in all eukaryotic cell types: *Ha-ras*, *K-ras*, and *N-ras*. The gene sequences of the *ras* family are highly conserved, suggesting that *ras* plays a key role in cell proliferation. Of significance is that *ras* genes have been found to be present and activated in 20% of all human tumors, lending support to their predominant role in the processes of cell transformation and cancer progression.[9] *Ras* oncogenes are capable of immortalizing and causing morphological transformation, anchorage independence, tumorigenicity, and metastasis.[223,244] They can also play a dual role in blocking or inducing differentiation, or acting as either oncogenes or oncosuppressor genes.[71,243,246] Studies by Ramos and coworkers have identified that the induction of *c-Ha-ras* gene expression mediates the increase in cell proliferation of aortic SMCs after toxic injury.[221]

The *c-Ha-ras* promoter does not contain TATA or CAT boxes, but instead relies on its GC-rich content and the positioning of key response elements in the promoter to regulate transcription.[198] Some of these key elements include TPA-responsive elements (TRE), AHRE (arylhydrocarbon response element), Sp1, and antioxidant/electrophile response elements (ARE/EpRE). A basic representation of the *c-Ha-ras* transcriptional start site and promoter region is depicted in Fig. 8.7. The heavily

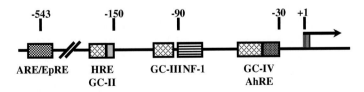

Fig. 8.7 Key transcriptional and regulatory elements in the human *c-Ha-ras* promoter that modulate its response to BaP (Modified from [198])

predominant GC boxes are characteristic of housekeeping genes such as *ras*, and are presumed to be involved in binding Sp1 proteins.[91] Two GC elements (GCII and GCIV) which span a 150-bp region from the major start site cluster are key in regulating the expression of human *c-Ha-ras*,[198] along with other sites within the promoter region including an HRE sequence element (CCGGAA) located 5′ of the GCII box, a functional NF-1/CTF binding site positioned between the GCIII and GCIV boxes (CCAAT) located at position −88, and a CACCC box downstream of GCIV.[165] From the start site cluster through position −75, there is no independent activity contributing to gene regulation due to absence of a TATA box.[198] GCIV is considered to mediate start site selection,[133] while GCII is necessary for full transient expression of the gene,[122] and HRE contributes to promoter activity.[133] The CCAAT site binds the NF-1/CTF protein, which has been previously identified as a DNA-binding protein necessary for the initiation of adenoviral DNA replication.[97]

The multiple transcriptional start sites of the *c-Ha-ras* gene span an area of 90 bp, in a major cluster 130 bp upstream from intron 1, notated as +1 to +11.[133] Minor start sites can also be located both upstream and downstream from this major cluster.[133] Nearly 80% of *c-Ha-ras* transcripts originate from the major start site cluster as shown in T24 and HeLa cells,[122] though two novel start sites at −122 and −263 have been found in vSMCs (Metz et al., unpublished results). Enhancer-like activity of the *c-Ha-ras* gene has been found within a variable tandem repeat sequence within the 3′ flanking sequences of human *c-Ha-ras*.[245] In addition, an initiator protein-binding element exists between +6 and +20, a region containing nine start sites.[133]

The *c-Ha-ras* growth regulatory gene encodes for a protein of 198 amino acids, and of approximately 21 kD in weight, with homology to the α-subunit of G-proteins. This protein is termed p21^{ras}, and has been shown to bind guanine nucleotides (GTP and GDP) and possess intrinsic GTPase activity.[140] In studies examining the role of the Ras protein in the regulation of the cell cycle it was found that p21^{ras} acts in late G_1 phase, just prior to initiation of S phase.[162] In addition, p21^{ras} promotes progression of cells through G_1 to initiate DNA synthesis without the requirement of growth factors in certain immortalized cell types.[60,248]

Signal Transduction through the Ras Pathway

Ras protein activation plays a key role in the mediation of cell signaling processes involving signal transduction from cellular membranes to the nucleus. These processes mediate a number of growth-related events including cell proliferation, differentiation, and transformation via the transduction of extracellular signals through tyrosine kinase and G-protein coupled receptors.[138] The signaling cascade involving Ras activation begins at the cellular membrane through binding of extracellular growth factors to the extracellular domains of tyrosine kinase receptors such as EGF or PDGF (Fig. 8.8). These receptors become autophosphorylated at their tyrosine residues and associate with the adaptor protein Grb2 on their intracellular domain. Grb2 then binds and activates Sos, recruiting it to the membrane level

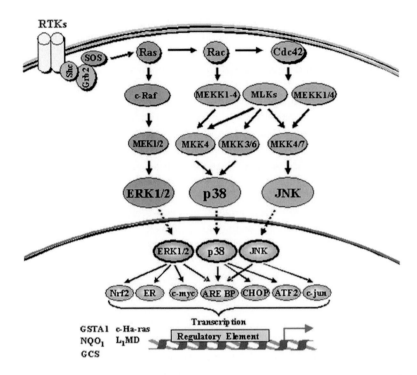

Fig. 8.8 Ras and intracellular kinase pathways. Activation of Ras through receptor binding to membrane-associated tyrosine kinases leads to activation of intracellular kinases and nuclear transcription factors, leading to transcriptional regulation of a number of genes.

where SOS then interacts with Ras, inducing replacement of GDP on Ras by GTP.[141] This places Ras in an active state that leads to Raf phosphorylation and downstream activation of serine/threonine phosphorylation signaling cascades.[160] Alternatively, Ras can activate Rac1/2 and Cdc42 proteins that then induce a phosphorylation signaling cascade to activate JNK and/or p38.[40] Phosphorylation cascades involving Rac and Cdc42 proteins have been shown to be independent of ERK activation,[155] however, others have shown that the Rac/Cdc42-activated kinase PAK1 can phosphorylate MEK1. The activity of MEK1 does not increase, but its interaction with Raf does, influencing progression through the MAPK and ERK cascade.[69] As a result, a crosstalk mechanism between the ERK, p38, and JNK signaling cascades is likely to be mediated through Rac and Cdc42 proteins. Implications of crosstalk between these three cascades are significant since each is responsible for independent outcomes regarding cellular responses.[72,227] The ERK cascade predominantly regulates cell growth and differentiation processes, while the p38 cascade regulates cytokine production and apoptosis. JNK cascades were originally identified as stress-activated protein kinases that had the ability to phosphorylate the c-Jun transcription factor.[43] As a result, the JNK cascade is primarily involved in regulating growth, differentiation, survival, apoptosis, inflammation, development, and stress responses. Many transcription factors are downstream elements of this signaling cascade, and their phosphorylation and activation have key effects on the initiation or repression of transcriptional events.

The Ras protein interacts with the cytoplasmic face of the cellular membrane by farnesylation at the C-terminus. Mutations that prevent farnesylation prevent Ras association at the membrane, and also abolish the oncogenicity of Ras. Furthermore, point mutations at position 12 have been shown to induce neoplastic transformation of NIH-3T3 cells,[204] while mutations at codons 12, 13, and 60 are found in colorectal cancers and acute myeloid leukemia.[65] Position 12 is located in loop 1 of the Ras protein, a region that controls the hydrolysis of GTP. Mutations at codon 12 therefore lead to an oncogenic form of Ras, since GTP can no longer be hydrolyzed and the protein remains constitutively active.[9] Ras proteins in a constitutively active state result in continuous signal transduction, leading to malignant transformation of the cell. Overexpression of Ras proteins also contributes to tumorigenic phenotypes.[145]

c-Ha-ras and Atherosclerosis

The processes of cell proliferation and plaque formation characteristic of atherosclerosis are analogous to that of benign neoplastic tumors,[198] implicating a correlation between atherosclerosis and carcinogenesis. Meanwhile, disorders of cell growth and tumor formation have been linked to the deregulation of *ras* protooncogene expression in humans[9] and other species.[131] Thus, protooncogene expression may support a mechanism of atherosclerotic plaque development. Studies by Penn and coworkers helped support this correlation by showing that DNA isolated from atherosclerotic plaques of both humans and cockerels is positive in the transfection-nude mouse tumor assay.[184,186]

Ras proteins, as key regulators of mitogenic signaling cascades, play a large role in the control of cell cycle events and subsequent cellular growth. Indolfi and coworkers[90] examined the role of Ras protein in cellular growth and proliferation characteristic of vascular injury. Proliferation of vSMCs is a key response to arterial injury, not in atherosclerosis, but also in restenosis after balloon angioplasty. Cellular Ras was inactivated in rats that were next subjected to balloon injury, using DNA vectors expressing Ras transdominant negative mutants. Neointimal formation after injury was reduced, implicating a possible therapeutic use of local delivery of Ras transdominant negative mutants in vivo to prevent vascular injury incurred by balloon angioplasty.

In vivo, vSMCs exist in a contractile, nonproliferative state, and regulate the vascular tone of the artery. Once these cells are injured, and the atherosclerotic process is initiated, vSMCs are transformed to a more proliferative/synthetic phenotype.[196] A similar phenotypic change has been observed in vitro upon transfection of aortic SMCs with *c-Ha-ras*[EJ]. An altered phenotype was observed in stable transfectants over a 6-week period, and was characterized by changes in morphology, anchorage-independent growth, and enhanced mitogenic responsiveness.[223] Other studies have shown that *c-Ha-ras*[EJ] transfection also affords a marked proliferative advantage of SMCs over nontransfected controls in both cell cycle regulated and randomly cycling cells.[276] Oncogenic *ras* also influenced growth-related signal transduction of SMCs, incurred enhanced serum-sensitivity and EGF-responsiveness, and induced loss of α-smooth muscle actin expression, all factors that characterize a highly proliferative SMC phenotype present in atherogenesis.[223]

Increased expression of ERK2 protein, a downstream kinase of the Ras:MAPK pathway, and its phosphorylated form, was evident in *c-Ha-ras*[EJ] transfected SMCs, supporting the constitutive activation of this signal transduction cascade by oncogenic Ras.[276] In addition, the protein kinase C (PKC) signal transduction pathway is upregulated in *c-Ha-ras*[EJ] transfected cells. PKC regulates mammalian cell growth and differentiation,[173] further implicating Ras in deregulating growth-related signaling.

c-Ha-ras and Benzo[a]pyrene

c-Ha-ras oncogene expression has been implicated in the progression of chemical-induced atherogenesis. BaP and related hydrocarbons have been shown to be chemical atherogens, inducing fibro-proliferative atherosclerotic plaques in a number of species.[2,85,177] Upon treatment of growth arrested rat aortic SMCs with BaP, serum-induced *c-Ha-ras* protooncogene expression was observed.[221] Though *c-Ha-ras* is a growth regulatory housekeeping gene that is constitutively expressed within the cell, cell cycle dependent expression has been shown in vSMCs and is associated with enhanced proliferation of these cells.[222]

Metabolism of BaP generates a number of different oxidative metabolites and byproducts. These species have the ability to adduct DNA, induce sequence mutations, and influence the transcription of a number of genes. Studies utilizing the BaP metabolite 7,8-dihydroxy-9,10-epoxy-7,8,9,10-tetrahydrobenzo[a]pyrene have shown that its reaction with a DNA fragment of *c-Ha-ras* generates a transforming oncogene with mutations in codons 12, 13, 61, or a combination of these.[273] In addition, mutations in *c-Ha-ras* codons 12 and 61 are also evident upon interaction of *c-Ha-ras* and oxygen radicals,[50] radicals produced upon metabolism of BaP. A highly carcinogenic PAH similar to BaP, DMBA, targets the second position of *Ha-ras* codon 61, inducing A→T mutations that lead to tumors in both the skin and liver of mice.[131] However, while BaP-induced proliferation of vSMCs involves increases in expression of the *c-Ha-ras* oncogene, this proliferative advantage is not due to mutations in any of the "hot spot" regions of *ras* genes (codons 12, 13, 60, and 61).[291]

c-Ha-ras and Redox Signaling Pathways

Phosphorylation through redox signaling cascades activates proteins that bind to key response elements in regulatory genes and modulate their transcription. The regulation of *c-Ha-ras* expression is certainly no exception. The induction of *c-Ha-ras* mRNA and DNA synthesis by BaP, as well as BaP-induced protein binding to AHRE sequences of *c-Ha-ras* is inhibited by α-naphthoflavone (α-NF), a cytochrome P450 inhibitor. Since α-NF has the potential to compete with BaP for intracellular protein-binding sites, a mechanism of action for BaP-induced expression of *c-Ha-ras* could involve protein binding to response elements in the *c-Ha-ras* promoter.[221] The AHR was implicated as a target protein in this mechanism since an AHRE sequence is present in the upstream promoter region of *c-Ha-ras*. However, activation of AHR binding to the *c-Ha-ras* AHRE alone is not sufficient to activate transcription of the *c-Ha-ras* gene.[24] Likely partners for the AHR include the proteins that bind to the ARE/EpRE.[24] A second mechanism explaining inhibition of *c-Ha-ras* expression by α-NF could involve inhibition of cytochrome P450 metabolism of BaP. α-NF has been shown to inhibit P450-mediated BaP metabolism within 1–6 h.[217] Therefore, metabolites of BaP may regulate BaP-induced *c-Ha-ras* expression. In fact, Kerzee and Ramos showed that oxidative metabolites and byproducts of BaP metabolism (BaP 3,6-quinone and hydrogen peroxide) are capable of enhancing serum-activated *c-Ha-ras* expression in vSMCs.[108] This expression is inhibited upon pretreatment with ellipticine, an AHR antagonist and cytochrome P450 inhibitor, and precluded upon upregulation of antioxidant capacity by *N*-acetylcysteine. Treatment of vSMCs with buthionine-(S,R)-sulfoximine, a cellular glutathione depletor, also enhanced expression of *c-Ha-ras*, further implicating a redox mechanism in *c-Ha-ras* expression.

Mitogenic Signaling Induced by Benzo[a]pyrene

BaP is also known to interfere with mitogenic signal transduction pathways within the cell, namely those involving Ca^{2+} and EGF. Disruption of Ca^{2+} homeostasis by PAHs inhibits activation of both B and T lymphocytes in rodents and humans.[207] In human peripheral blood mononuclear cell lymphocytes (HPBMCs) treated with BaP 4,5-epoxide and BPDE, a 20–30% depletion of reduced glutathione (GSH) is seen, along with an elevation of intracellular Ca^{2+} that can be reduced upon treatment with α-NF. These outcomes may be a result of sulfhydryl damage induced by these epoxide metabolites. As a result of alterations in Ca^{2+} homeostasis, cell activation and proliferation in these cells is also compromised.[207] A contribution by BaP metabolism is supported by the finding that cultures of epidermal keratinocytes also exhibit increased overall metabolism of BaP upon pre-incubation in high Ca^{2+} medium prior to BaP treatment.[47] These results indicate that in addition to the known effects of Ca^{2+} in the regulation of cellular differentiation, expression and inducibility of enzymes involved in BaP metabolism can be regulated by this ion.

BaP also exerts profound effects on PKC-mediated phosphorylation of mammalian cell proteins. PKC is a serine/threonine kinase that participates in mitogenic signal transduction cascades involved in growth and differentiation. Increases in diacylglycerol and intracellular Ca^{2+} activate PKC and initiate a series of phosphorylation-dependent events leading to transcriptional activation of immediate early genes.[23] During PKC-related signal transduction, *c-jun* and *c-fos* protooncogene transcription is activated during the G_0 to G_1 transition,[116] facilitating production of the AP-1 complex that binds to TPA-responsive elements, transactivating growth-related genes. Any interference with this pathway would result in deregulated cellular growth and differentiation. Previous studies in this laboratory have shown that BaP challenged vSMCs exhibit a concentration-dependent inhibition of PKC activity, occurring as early as 30 min and extending up to 24 h after treatment.[175] In these cells, 3-OH BaP elicited a comparable response, suggesting that modulation of PKC activity could be affected by oxidative metabolites of the parent compound. However, inhibition of PKC-related signal transduction was not related to generalized interference with cell cycle events,[176] suggesting that interference with mitogenic signaling by BaP is a complex process.

BaP can also mimic growth factor signaling pathways leading to alterations of cell growth and proliferation.[260] This point is best exemplified by BaP interference with EGF signaling cascades. The EGF receptor (EGFR) is a membrane-bound tyrosine kinase receptor that primarily activates the Ras-MAPK signaling pathway following receptor autophosphorylation. In human placental cell lines, BaP decreases EGF-binding as well as EGFR proteins, resulting in alterations in trophoblast proliferation and endocrine function.[290] Time-dependent decreases in EGF binding are also seen upon BaP treatment of mouse fibroblasts.[95] BPDE does not alter EGF binding, implying that metabolism of the parent compound does not mediate EGF signaling, or that DNA damage is not responsible for the inhibitory response. Other PAH inducers of P450 inhibit EGF binding, possibly through a pathway involving binding of AHR.[95]

However, EGF-mediated activation of tyrosine kinases can be affected by oxidative stress, a potential result of oxidative metabolism of BaP. H_2O_2 potentiates EGF-induced phosphorylation,[98] as well as phosphorylation of the EGF receptor after UVB-induced increases in intracellular H_2O_2 levels.[189] OxLDLs, major players in the progression of atherosclerosis, also induce tyrosine phosphorylation of EGFR and activate this signaling pathway.[256] Other signaling pathways can be influenced by BaP and related hydrocarbons. BaP and TCDD activate insulin-like growth factor (IGF-I) signaling pathways under insulin-deficient conditions in human mammary epithelial cells.[260] Upon BaP treatment, tyrosine phosphorylation of IGF-Irβ, IRS-1, and Shc is increased, indicating that signaling is mimicked through the IGF-I receptor (IGF-IR).[260] In these studies, BaP was also shown to significantly increase activity of phosphatidylinositol-3-kinase (PI3K).[260]

Oxidant-Regulated Signaling in vSMCs

In renal mesangial and corticotubular epithelial cells, as well as hepatocytes, induction of oxidative stress by BaP activates redox signaling.[3,292] In both HepG2 cells and vSMCs, oxidative stress leads to activation of ARE/EpRE, located in the 5' region of critical target genes.[24,33]

Antioxidant/Electrophile Response Element

Antioxidant/electrophile response elements (ARE/EpRE) are *cis*-acting regulatory sequences that mediate the basal and inducible expression of several genes, including the growth regulatory gene *c-Ha-ras* and those of the Phase II detoxifying enzymes glutathione-S-transferase A1,A2, and A3 (GSTA1, GSTA2, GSTA3), NADPH:quinone oxidoreductase (NQO_1) and γ-glutamyl cysteine synthetase (γGCS).[24,58,67,100,103,163,220,271] Located in the upstream promoter region of these genes, the ARE/EpRE regulates transcription through protein binding to its core sequence and complex assembly.

When first discovered by Rushmore et al.,[218] the ARE/EpRE was defined as the β-naphthoflavone (β-NF) response element. The sequence was identified in the 5' promoter region of the rat (r) GSTA1 gene (known then as GSTYa) as a unique xenobiotic response element involved in inducible expression by planar aromatic hydrocarbons such as β-NF and 3-methylcholanthrene (3-MC).[218] Shortly after, Rushmore and Pickett found that transcriptional activation of GSTA1 could be induced through the β-NF response element in response to phenolic antioxidants such as *t*-butylhydroquinone (tBHQ).[219] It was then that this unique regulatory element was renamed and defined as the antioxidant response element (ARE). Around the same time, Daniel and coworkers had defined a unique regulatory element in the mouse (m) GSTA1 gene that was responsive to planar aromatic compounds (3-MC, β-NF, and TCDD), as well as electrophiles (*trans*-4-phenyl-3-buten-2-one, and dimethyl fumarate).[67] Responsiveness to planar aromatic compounds required a functional AHR and cytochrome P450 1A1 activity, therefore it was concluded that inducibility by these compounds was due to metabolism to electrophilic intermediates. As such, this regulatory element was defined as an electrophile response element (EpRE), since transcriptional activation occurred through both electrophilic inducers and compounds that metabolized to electrophilic intermediates. After discovery by both Pickett and Daniel's groups, individuals have interchangeably used ARE or EpRE to define this regulatory element.

Soon after the ARE/EpRE was defined in both the rat and mouse GSTA1 genes, it was identified in the 5' flanking region of the rat NAD(P)H:quinone reductase gene ($rNQO_1$),[57] and also found to be responsive to both metabolizable planar aromatic hydrocarbons and phenolic antioxidants. Shortly thereafter, Pickett and coworkers defined the core sequence of the ARE/EpRE required for transcriptional activation as 5'-TGACNNNGC-3', where N represents any nucleotide.[220] Using analysis of CAT deletion constructs from the rGSTA1 promoter, they also demonstrated in this study that the ARE/EpRE is responsive to both hydrogen peroxide and phenolic antioxidants that undergo redox cycling, implicating that this element can be regulated during conditions of oxidative stress.

The ARE/EpRE has since been identified in the human (h) NQO_1 gene by Jaiswal and coworkers, the γGCS gene by Mulcahy and coworkers, and in the human *c-Ha-ras* (hHaras) gene by Ramos and coworkers.[24,128,163] In 1997, Wasserman and Fahl further characterized the ARE/EpRE core sequence of mGSTA1. Through systematic mutational analysis of the mGSTA1 ARE/EpRE, the initial core sequence identified by Rushmore et al.[218] was extended, and characterized as: 5'-TMAnnRTGAY nnnGCRwwww-3'.[275] Also in this study, data was provided for the presence of ARE/EpRE sequences matching this extended core in a variety of mammalian promoter sequences. These genes, in addition to those already mentioned, include β-globin, myoglobin, Alzheimer gene STM2, collagenase, P-450 aromatase, GST-Pi, ferritin-L, glutathione transporter, tyrosinase, and interleukin-6.[275] The ARE/EpRE was also later modified and extended in the NQO_1 promoter as 5'-GAGTCACAGTGAG TCGGCAAAATT-3' (Nioi et al. 2003).

   While the promoter sequences of all of the genes listed above contain a core ARE/EpRE sequence, the context in which it is found in each is very different. The ARE/EpRE of the $rNQO_1$ promoter consists of a palindromic sequence, 5'-TCTAG*AGTCACAGTGACT*TGGC-3', where both half sites act synergistically to induce high basal level gene expression.[58] The rGSTA1 promoter contains a consensus ARE/EpRE site that is sufficient for transcriptional activation, and a distal ARE/EpRE-like site: 5'-AAA*TGGCATTGC*TAA-TGG*TGACAAAGC*AAC-3'.[168] The mGSTA1 promoter ARE/EpRE is the same as rGSTA1 save for one base pair change in the distal flanking region (5'-AAA*TGACATTGC*TAATGG*TGACAAAGC*AAC-3').[68] These two sequences are also defined as AP-1-like binding sequences. While in mGSTA1 they individually have low enhancer activity and no inducibility, together they confer electrophile inducibility to this regulatory sequence.[68] Jaiswal and coworkers reported that basal and inducible expression in the hNQO1 promoter requires an ARE/EpRE containing two TREs (5'-*GCAGTCA*CAG*TGACTCAGCA*GAATC-3').[282] In the catalytic γGCS_h subunit gene, a single consensus site in the upstream promoter region mediates basal and inducible expression (5'-TCCCC*GTGACTCAGCG*CTTT-3'),[163] while induction of the regulatory γGCS_l subunit gene is mediated by a consensus ARE/EpRE and an AP-1 sequence 33 base pairs upstream.[157] In addition, the consensus ARE/EpRE sequences in both γGCS_h and γGCS_l contain an embedded AP-1 sequence. Finally, a single consensus ARE/EpRE located in the promoter region of *c-Ha-ras* mediates the transcriptional activation of this gene: 5'-AGCTCCTGG*GTGACAGAGC*-GAGAAGCT-3'.[24]

Protein Binding to ARE/EpRE

To derive the mechanism by which ARE/EpRE can mediate expression of these genes, a number of investigators, including our laboratory, have endeavored to characterize the proteins that assemble on this regulatory site. As a result, several proteins that interact with ARE/EpREs have been identified, including Nrf1;[83,271,272] Nrf2;[83,92,154,157,169,271,272,281] Nrf3;[224] Jun family proteins;[14,68,83,127,129,281,295] small Maf proteins;[67,281] Fra1;[281] c-Fos;[14,68,127,129,271] C/EBPβ;[34] AHR;[34,269] ERα and ERβ;[158] and hPMC2.[159] Wasserman and Fahl have also identified proteins of various molecular weights to bind to the ARE/EpRE.[274] Although the list is long and ever growing, many of the proteins that contribute to ARE/EpRE complex formation are still unknown.

   Mechanisms of protein activation to interact with ARE/EpREs have also been widely investigated, to gain insight as to how these proteins can be regulated. Regulation by signaling pathways involving ERK and p38 MAP kinases,[103,286,287,295] tyrosine kinase,[46] phosphatidylinositol 3-kinase,[103,104] and protein kinase C[87] have been implicated, as well as stress-regulated shuttling mechanisms involving Keap1;[93,48,146] and antioxidant/xenobiotic shuttling mechanisms involving Keap1 (or the similar protein INrf2).[93,44,171] However, regardless of the mechanism of activation, ARE/EpREs are universally responsive to planar aromatic compounds (PAHs, TCDD, 3-MC), β-NF, phenolic antioxidants (t-BHQ, 3,5-di-t-butylcatechol, butylated hydroxyanisole (BHA)), thiol-containing compounds, phorbol esters (12-O-tetradecanoylphorbol-13-acetate (TPA)), as well as H_2O_2 and t-butylhydroperoxide.[153,170]

The ARE/EpRE shows sequence similarity to a number of different regulatory elements. The TPA response element (TRE), also considered an AP-1 response element, is characterized by the sequence 5'-TGA(G/C)TCA.[121] This represents exactly the 5' end of the core ARE/EpRE sequence, and is found intact within the ARE/EpRE core of hNQO$_1$ and γGCS promoters. In addition, there is sequence similarity to the erythroid transcription factor NF-E2 binding sequence, which is characterized by the sequence 5'-(T/C)GCTGA(G/C)TCA(T/C)-3'.[6] High sequence homology to a TRE type-Maf recognition element (T-MARE) is also found, characterized by the sequence: 5'-TGCTGACTCAGCA-3'.[107] Finally, the heme responsive element characterized by the sequence (T/C)GCTGAGTCA, shows sequence similarity to the 5' end of the ARE/EpRE core.[89]

Proteins that bind to ARE/EpRE sequences in the various promoter regions were initially identified due to sequence similarities with these response elements above. TRE binding proteins, such as the Fos and Jun family proteins;[16,79,187] NF-E2 site binding proteins Nrf1,Nrf2, and Nrf3;[31,156,224] and Maf proteins that bind to MAREs[107] are all involved in protein complex binding to ARE/EpREs. Specific protein recognition is dictated in a context specific manner, and additional work to investigate the complexity of ARE/EpRE protein complex assembly in individual promoters and cell types is being conducted in a number of different laboratories.

Overall, protein binding to the ARE/EpRE in c-Ha-ras activates transcription of this gene, which in turn stimulates the uncontrolled proliferation and dedifferentiation of vSMCs leading to lesion formation characteristic of atherosclerosis. This molecular mechanism links oxidative stress and redox signaling to the onset of atherogenesis. The fact that a number of diverse factors bind the ARE/EpRE and that this element is present in the promoter regions of a number of different genes indicates that there could be many other mechanisms of action involving redox signaling in the atherosclerotic process.

Concluding Remarks

In closing, atherosclerosis is one of the leading causes of death in the United States, and its onset can be initiated by exposure to ubiquitous environmental contaminants such as BaP, which originate from vehicle exhaust emissions, industrial processes, oil contamination, and cigarette smoke. Exposure to BaP, and similar chemicals, may lead to the onset and progression of atherosclerosis by growth stimulation of cells lining the arterial wall. Metabolism of BaP in the body may generate byproducts that disrupt important growth processes in vascular cells, leading to increased proliferation and formation of atherosclerotic lesions. Indeed, through cytochrome P450-mediated metabolism, oxidative metabolites of BaP are produced in the form of free radicals, peroxides, quinones, and reactive intermediates, which activate redox signaling cascades. Arterial vSMCs therefore undergo oxidative stress as a result of BaP challenge and subsequent metabolism, thus leading to the transcriptional activation of growth regulatory genes, such as *c-Ha-ras*, and induced growth and proliferation characteristic of arterial lesion formation. These mechanisms are often cell-specific, protein-specific, and sequence-specific, adding to the complexity of research in this field. Elucidation of the pathways by which BaP, and other chemicals like it, induce the uncontrolled growth of vSMCs will lead to a better understanding of the atherosclerotic process, and the potential predisposition of certain individuals to the disease.

References

1. Agency for Toxic Substances and Disease Registry. Toxicological Profile for Polycyclic Aromatic Hydrocarbons. ATSDR, US Public Health Service, Atlanta, GA, 1990.
2. Albert RE, Vanderlaan M, Burns FJ, Nishizumi M. Effects of carcinogens on chicken atherosclerosis. Cancer Res 1977;37:2232–2235.
3. Alejandro NF, Parrish AR, Bowes III RC, Burghardt RC, Ramos KS. Phenotypic profiles of cultured glomerular cells following repeated cycles of hydrocarbon injury. Kidney Int 2000;57:1571–1580.
4. Alexander RW. Theodore Cooper Memorial Lecture. Hypertension and the pathogenesis of atherosclerosis. Oxidative stress and the mediation of arterial inflammatory response: a new perspective. Hypertension 1995;25:155–161.
5. American Heart Association. (2005) Heart Disease and Stroke Statistics — 2005 Update. American Heart Association, Dallas, Texas.
6. Andrews NC, Erdjument-Bromage H, Davidson MB, Tempst P, Orkin SH. Erythroid transcription factor NF-E2 is a haematopoietic-specific basic-leucine zipper protein. Nature 1993;362:722–727.
7. Asman DC, Takimoto K, Pitot HC, Dunn TJ, Lindahl R. Organization and characterization of the rat class 3 aldehyde dehydrogenase gene. J Biol Chem 1993;268:12530–12536.
8. Auge N, Escargueil-Blanc I, Lajoie-Mazenc I, Suc I, Andrieu-Abadie N, Peiraggi MT, Chatelut M, Thiers JC, Jaffrezou JP, Laurent G, Levade T, Negre-Salvayre A, Salvayre R. Potential role for ceramide in mitogen-activated protein kinase activation and proliferation of vascular smooth muscle cells induced by oxidized low density lipoprotein. J Biol Chem 1998;273:12893–12900.
9. Barbacid M. Ras genes. Annu Rev Biochem 1987;56:779–827.
10. Barhoumi R, Mouneimne Y, Ramos KS, Safe SH, Phillips TD, Centonze VE, Ainley C, Gupta MS, Burghardt RC. Analysis of benzo[a]pyrene partitioning and cellular homeostasis in a rat liver cell line. Toxicol Sci 2000;53:264–270.
11. Baum EJ. Occurrence and surveillance of polycyclic aromatic hydrocarbons. In Gelboin HV, Ts'o POP (Eds). Polycyclic Hydrocarbons and Cancer. Academic Press, New York: Academic Press, 1978, pp. 45–70.

12. Benditt EP, Benditt JM. Evidence for a monoclonal origin of human atherosclerotic plaques. Proc Natl Acad Sci USA 1973;70:1753–1756.

13. Benditt EP. Evidence for a monoclonal origin of human atherosclerotic plaques and some implications. Circulation 1974;50:650–652.

14. Bergelson S, Daniel V. Cooperative interaction between ETS and AP-1 transcription factors regulates induction of glutathione S-transferase Ya gene expression. Biochem Biophys Res Comm 1994;200:290–297.

15. Beutler E, Yeh M, Fairbanks VF. The normal human female as a mosaic of X-chromosome activity: studies using the gene for G-6-PD deficiency as a marker. Proc Natl Acad Sci USA 1962;48:9–16.

16. Bohmann D, Bos TJ, Admon A, Nishimura T, Vogt PK, Tjian R. Human proto-oncogene c-jun encodes a DNA binding protein with structural and functional properties of transcription factor AP-1. Science 1987;238:1386–1392.

17. Bolli R. Oxygen-derived free radicals and postischemic myocardial dysfunction ('stunned myocardium'). J Am Coll Cardiol 1988;12:239–249.

18. Bond JA, Omiecinski CJ, Juchau MR. Kinetics, activation, and induction of aortic mono-oxygenases – Biotransformation of benzo[a]pyrene. Biochem Pharmacol 1979;28:305–311.

19. Bond JA, Gown AM, Yang HL, Benditt EP, Juchau MR. Further investigation of the capacity of polynuclear aromatic hydrocarbons to elicit atherosclerotic lesions. J Toxicol Environ Health 1981;7:327–335.

20. Booth J, Sims P. Different pathways involved in the metabolism of the 7,8- and 9,10-dihydrodiols of benzo[a]pyrene. Biochem Pharmacol 1976;25:979–980.

21. Borgen A, Darvey H, Castagnoli N, Crocker TT, Rasmussen RE, Wang IT. Metabolic conversion of benzo[a]pyrene by Syrian hamster liver microsomes and binding metabolites to deoxyribonucleic acid. J Med Chem 1973;16:502–506.

22. Borm PJ, Knaapen AM, Schins RP, Godschalk RW, Schooten FJ. Neutrophils amplify the formation of DNA adducts by benzo[a]pyrene in lung target cells. Environ Health Perspect 1997;105(Suppl 5):1089–1093.

23. Boyle WJ, Smocal T, Defize LHK, Angel P, Woodgett JR, Karin M, Hunter T. Activation of protein kinase C decreases phosphorylation of c-Jun at sites that negatively regulate its DNA-binding activity. Cell 1991;64:573–584.

24. Bral CM, Ramos KS. Identification of benzo[a]pyrene-inducible cis-acting elements within c-Ha-ras transcriptional regulatory sequences. Mol Pharmacol 1997;52:974–982.

25. Bresnick E, Stoming TA, Vaught JB, Thakkar DR, Jerina DM. Nuclear metabolism of benzo[a]pyrene and (±)-trans-7,8-dihydroxy-7,8-dihydro-benzo[a]pyrene. Arch Biochem Biophys 1977;183:31–37.

26. Burton KP, McCord JM, Ghai G. Myocardial alterations due to free radical generation. Am J Physiol 1984;246:H776–H783.

27. Capdevila J, Estabrook RW, Prough RA. The microsomal metabolism of benzo[a]pyrene phenols. Biochem Biophys Res Commun 1978;82:518–525.

28. Carew TE, Schwenke DC, Steinberg D. Antiatherogenic effect of probucol unrelated to its hypocholesterolemic effect: Evidence that antioxidants in vivo can selectively inhibit low density lipoprotein degradation in macrophage-rich fatty streaks and slow the progression of atherosclerosis in the Watanabe heritable hyperlipidemic rabbit. Proc Natl Acad Sci USA 1987;84:7725–7729.

29. Cavalieri EL, Rogan EG. The approach to understanding aromatic hydrocarbon carcinogenesis: The central role of radical cations in metabolic activation. Pharmacol Ther 1992;55:183–199.

30. Cavarocchi NC, England MD, O'Brien JF, Solis E, Russo P, Schaff HV, Orszulak TA, Pluth JR, Kaye MP. Superoxide generation during cardiopulmonary bypass: Is there a role for vitamin E? J Surg Res 1986;40:519–527.

31. Chan JY, Han X, Kan YW. Cloning of Nrf1, and NF-E2-related transcription factor, by genetic selection in yeast. Proc Natl Acad Sci USA 1993;90:11371–11375.

32. Chen X-L, Medford RM. Oxidation–reduction sensitive regulation of vascular inflammatory gene expression. In: Pearson JA (Ed). Vascular Adhesion Molecules and Inflammation. Basel: Birkhauser Verlag, 1999; pp. 161–178.
33. Chen Y-H, Ramos KS. Negative regulation of rat GST-Ya via antioxidant/electrophile response element is directed by a C/EBP-like site. Biochem Biophys Res Commun 1999;265: 18–23.
34. Chen Y-H, Ramos KS. A CCAAT/Enhancer-binding protein site within antioxidant/electrophile response element along with CREB-binding protein participate in the negative regulation of rat GST-Ya gene in vascular smooth muscle cells. J Biol Chem 2000;275: 27366–27376.
35. Chesis PL, Levin DE, Smith MT, Ernster L, Ames BN. Mutagenicity of quinones: Pathways of metabolic activation and detoxification. Proc Natl Acad Sci USA 1984;81:1696–1700.
36. Chin JH, Azhar S, Hoffman BB. Inactivation of endothelium-derived relaxing factor by oxidized lipoproteins. J Clin Invest 1992;89:10–18.
37. Committee on Biologic Effects of Atmospheric Pollutants. Particulate Polycyclic Organic Matter. Div Med Sci Natl Res Council, Washington, DC: National Academy of Science, 1972.
38. Cornhill JF, Barrett WA, Herderick EE, Mahley RW, Fry DL. Topographic study of sudanophilic lesions in cholesterol-fed minipigs by image analysis. Arteriosclerosis 1985;5:415–426.
39. Cosentino F, Sill JC, Katusic ZS. Role of superoxide anions in the mediation of endothelium-dependent contractions. Hypertension 1994;23:229–235.
40. Coso OA, Chiariello M, Yu J-C, Teramoto H, Crespo P, Xu N, Miki T, Gutkind JS. The small GTP-binding proteins Rac1 and Cdc42 regualte the activity of the JNK/SAPK signaling pathway. Cell 1995;81:1137–1146.
41. Denison MS, Fisher JM, Whitlock JP Jr. Inducible, receptor-dependent protein-DNA interactions at a dioxin-responsive transcriptional enhancer. Proc Natl Acad Sci USA 1988a;85: 2528–2532.
42. Denison MS, Fisher JM, Whitlock Jr JP. The DNA recognition site for the dioxin-Ah receptor complex. J Biol Chem 1988b;263:17221–17224.
43. Dérijard B, Hibi M, Wu I-H, Barrett T, Su B, Deng T, Karin M, Davis RJ. JNK1: A protein kinase stimulated by UV light and Ha-ras that binds and phosphorylates the c-Jun activation domain. Cell 1994;76:1025–1037.
44. Dhakshinamoorthy S, Jaiswal AK. Functional characterization and role of Inrf2 in antioxidant response element-mediated expression and antioxidant induction of NAD(P)H:quinone oxidoreductase1 gene. Oncogene 2001;20:3906–3917.
45. Diamond JR, Karnovsky MJ. Focal and segmental glomerulosclerosis: analogies to atherosclerosis. Kidney Int 1988;33:917–924.
46. Dieter MZ, Freshwater SL, Solis WA, Nebert DW, Dalton TP. Tyrphostin AG879, a tyrosine kinase inhibitor: Prevention of transcriptional activation of the electrophile and the aromatic hydrocarbon response elements. Biochem Pharmacol 2001;61:215–225.
47. DiGiovanni J, Gill RD, Nettikumara AN, Colby AB, Reiners Jr JJ. Effect of extracellular calcium concentration on the metabolism of polycyclic aromatic hydrocarbons by cultured mouse keratinocytes. Cancer Res 1989;49:5567–5574.
48. Dinkova-Kostova AT, Holtzclaw WD, Cole RN, Itoh K, Wakabayashi N, Katoh Y, Yamamoto M, Talalay P. Direct evidence that sulfhydryl groups of Keap 1 are the sensors regulating induction of phase 2 enzymes that protect against carcinogens and oxidants. Proc Natl Acad Sci USA 2002;99:11908–11913.
49. Doan TN, Gentry DL, Taylor AA, Elliott SJ. Hydrogen peroxide activates agonist-sensitive Ca^{2+}-flux pathways in canine venous endothelial cells. Biochem J 1994;297:209–215.
50. Du MQ, Carmichael PL, Phillips DH. Induction of activating mutations in the human c-Ha-ras1 proto-oncogene by oxygen free radicals. Mol Carcinog 1994;11:170–175.
51. Eberhart J, Coffing SL, Anderson JN, Marcus C, Kalogeris TJ, Baird WM, Park SS, Gelboin HV. The time-dependent increase in the binding of benzo[a]pyrene to DNA through (+)-anti-benzo[a]pyrene-7,8-diol-9,10-epoxide in primary rat hepatocyte cultures results from induction of cytochrome P450IA1 by benzo[a]pyrene treatment. Carcinogenesis 1992;13:297–301.

52. Ellis RW, DeFeo D, Shih TY, Gonda MA, Young HA, Tsuchida N, Lowy DR, Scolnick EM. The p21 src genes of Harvey and Kirsten sarcoma viruses originate from divergent members of a family of normal vertebrate genes. Nature 1981;292:506–511.

53. Esterbauer H, Quehenberger O, Jürgens G. Oxidation of human low density lipoprotein with special attention to aldehydic lipid peroxidation products. In: Rice-Evans C, Halliwell B (Eds). Free Radicals: Methodology and Concepts. London: Richelieu Press, 1988;pp. 243–268.

54. Faggiotto A, Ross R. Studies of hypercholesterolemia in the nonhuman primate. II. Fatty streak conversion to fibrous plaque. Arteriosclerosis 1984;4:341–356.

55. Faggiotto A, Ross R, Harker L. Studies of hypercholesterolemia in the nonhuman primate. I. Changes that lead to fatty streak formation. Arteriosclerosis 1984;4:323–340.

56. Fahl WE, Jefcoate CR, Kasper CB. Characteristics of benzo[a]pyrene metabolism and cytochrome P-450 heterogeneity in rat liver nuclear envelope and comparison to microsomal membrane. J Biol Chem 1978;253:3106–3113.

57. Favreau LV, Pickett CB. Transcriptional regulation of the rat NAD(P)H:quinone reductase gene. Identification of regulatory elements controlling basal level expression and inducible expression by planar aromatic compounds and phenolic antioxidants. J Biol Chem 1991;266:4556–4561.

58. Favreau LV, Pickett CB. The rat quinone reductase antioxidant response element. J Biol Chem 1995;270:24468–24474.

59. Feldman G, Remsen J, Shinohara K, Cerutti P. Excisability and persistence of benzo[a]pyrene DNA adducts in epithelioid human lung cells. Nature 1978;274:796–798.

60. Feramisco JR, Gross M, Kamata T, Rosenberg M, Sweet RW. Microinjection of the oncogene form of the human H-ras (T-24) protein results in rapid proliferation of quiescent cells. Cell 1984;38:109–117.

61. Ferrari R, Ceconi C, Curello S, Guarnieri C, Caldarera CM, Alberini A, Visioli O. Oxygenmediated myocardial damage during ischaemia and reperfusion: Role of the cellular defenses against oxygen toxicity. J Mol Cell Cardiol 1985;17:937–945.

62. Ferrari R, Agnoletti L, Comini L, Gaia G, Bachetti T, Cargnoni A, Ceconi C, Curello S, Visioli O. Oxidative stress during myocardial ischemia and heart failure. Eur Heart J 1998;19:B2–B11.

63. Fialkow PJ. The origin and development of human tumors studed with cell markers. N Engl J Med 1974;291:26–35.

64. Flowers NL, Miles PR. Alterations of pulmonary benzo[a]pyrene metabolism by reactive oxygen metabolites. Toxicology 1991;68:259–274.

65. Forrester K, Almoguera C, Han K, Grizzle WE, Perucho M. Detection of high incidence of K-ras oncogenes during human carciongenesis. Nature 1987;327:298–303.

66. Friguet B, Stadtman ER, Szweda L. Modification of glucose-6-phosphate dehydrogenase by 4-hydroxy-2-nonenal. J Biol Chem 1994;269:21639–21643.

67. Friling RS, Bensimon A, Tichauer Y, Daniel V. Xenobiotic-inducible expression of murine glutathione S-transferase Ya subunit gene is controlled by an electrophile-responsive element. Proc Natl Acad Sci USA 1990;87:6258–6262.

68. Friling RS, Bergelson S, Daniel V. Two adjacent AP-1-like binding sites form the electophile-responsive element of the murine glutathione S-transferase Ya subunit gene. Proc Natl Acad Sci USA 1992;9:668–672.

69. Frost J, Xu S, Hutchison M, Marcus S, Cobb MH. Actions of Rho family small G proteins and p21-activated protein kinases on mitogen-activated protein kinase family members. Mol Cell Biol 1996;16:3707–3713.

70. Fujisawa-Sehara A, Yamane M, Fujii-Kuriyama Y. A DNA-binding factor specific for xenobiotic responsive elements of P-450c gene exists as a cryptic form in cytoplasm: Its possible translocation to the nucleus. Proc Natl Acad Sci USA 1988;5:5859–5863.

71. Gambari R, Spandidos DA. Chinese hamster lung cells transformed with the human Ha-ras-1 oncogene: 5-azacytidine mediated induction to adipogenic conversion. Cell Biol Int Rep 1986;10:173.

72. Garrington TP, Johnson GL. Organization and regulation of mitogen-activated protein kinase signaling pathways. Curr Opin Cell Biol 1999;11:211–218.

73. Gelboin HV. Benzo[a]pyrene metabolism, activation, and carcinogenesis: Role and regulation of mixed-function oxidases and related enzymes. Physiol Rev 1980;60:1107–1166.

74. Gottlieb RA, Burleson KO, Kloner RA, Babior BM, Engler RL. Reperfusion injury induces apoptosis in rabbit cardiomyocytes. J Clin Invest 1994;4:1621–1628.

75. Grech E, Jack CI, Bleasdale C, Jackson MJ, Baines M, Faragher EB, Hind CR, Perry RA. Differential free radical activity after successful and unsuccessful thrombolytic treperfusion in acute myocardial infarction. Coron Artery Dis 1993;4:769–774.

76. Gregus Z, Klaassen CD. Mechanisms of toxicity. In: Klaassen C (Ed). Casarett and Doull's Toxicology, The Basic Science of Poisons, 6th edition. Chap. 3 New York: McGraw-Hill, 2001; pp. 35–82.

77. Gupta M, Singal PK. Time course of structure, function and metabolic changes due to an exogenous source of oxygen metabolites in rat heart. Can J Physiol Pharmacol 1989;67:1549–1559.

78. Haberland ME, Steinbrecher UP. Modified low-density lipoproteins: Diversity and biological relevance in atherogenesis. In: Lusis AJ, Rotter JI, Sparkes RS (Eds). Molecular Genetics of Coronary Artery Disease: Candidate Genes and Processes in Atherosclerosis. Monographs in Human Genetics, Vol. 14. Basel: Karger, 1992; pp. 35–61.

79. Halazonetis TD, Georgopoulos K, Greenberg ME, Leder P. c-Jun dimerizes with itself and with c-Fos, forming complexes of different DNA binding affinities. Cell 1988;5:917–924.

80. Harrison DG. Cellular and molecular mechanisms of endothelial cell dysfunction. J Clin Invest 1997;100:2153–2157.

81. Hattemer-Frey HA, Travis CC. Benzo-a-pyrene: Environmental partitioning and human exposure. Toxicol Ind Health 1997;7:141–157.

82. Hoffmann D, Schmeltz I, Hecht SS, Wynder EL. Tobacco carcinogenesis. In: Gelboin HV, Ts'o POP (Eds). Polycyclic Hydrocarbons and Cancer. New York: Academic Press, 1978; pp. 85–117.

83. Holderman MT, Miller KP, Dangott LJ, Ramos KS. Identification of albumin precursor protein, phi AP3, and α-smooth muscle actin as novel components of redox sensing machinery in vascular smooth muscle cells. Mol Pharmacol 2002;61:1–9.

84. Hollstein M, McCann J, Angelosanto FA, Nichols WW. Short-term tests for carcinogens and mutagens. Mutat Res 1979;65:133–226.

85. Hough JL, Baird MB, Sfeir GT, Pacini CS, Darrow D, Wheelock C. Benzo[a]pyrene enhances atherosclerosis in White Carneau and Show Racer pigeons. Arterioscler Thromb 1993;13:1721–1727.

86. Huang AL, Berard D, Hager GL. Glucocorticoid regulation of the HaMuSV p21 gene conferred by sequences from mouse mammary tumor virus. Cell 1981;27:245–255.

87. Huang H-C, Nguyen T, Pickett CP. Regulation of the antioxidant response element by protein kinase C-mediated phosphorylation of NF-E2-related factor 2. Proc Natl Acad Sci USA 2000;97:12475–12480.

88. Huberman E, Sachs L, Yang SK, Gelboin HV. Identification of mutagenic metabolites of benzo[a]pyrene in mammalian cells. Proc Natl Acad Sci USA 1976;3:607–611.

89. Inamdar NM, Ahn YI, Alam J. The heme-responsive element of the mouse heme oxygenase-1 gene is an extended AP-1 binidng site that resembles the recognition sequences for MAF and NF-E2 transcription factors. Biochem Biophys Res Commun 1996;221:570–576.

90. Indolfi C, Avvedimento EV, Rapacciuolo A, Di Lorenzo E, Esposito G, Stabile E, Feliciello A, Mele E, Giuliano P, Condorelli G. Inhibition of cellular ras prevents smooth muscle cell proliferation after vascular injury in vivo. Nat Med 1995;1:541–545.

91. Ishii S, Kadonaga JT, Tjian R, Brady JN, Merlino GT, Pastan I. Binding of the Sp1 transcription factor by the human Harvey ras 1 proto-oncogene promoter. Science 1986;232:1410–1413.

92. Itoh K, Chiba T, Takahashi S, Ishii T, Igarashi K, Katoh Y, Oyake T, Hayashi N, Satoh K, Hatayama I, Yamamoto M, Nabeshima Y. An Nrf2/Small Maf heterodimer mediates the

induction of phase II detoxifying enzyme genes through antioxidant response elements. Biochem Biophys Res Commun 1997;236:313–322.

93. Itoh K, Wakabayashi N, Katoh Y, Ishii T, Igarashi K, Engel JD, Yamamoto M. Keap1 represses nuclear activation of antioxidant responsive elements by Nrf2 through binding to the amino-terminal Neh2 domain. Genes Dev 1999;13:76–86.

94. Itoh K, Wakabayashi N, Katoh Y, Ishii T, O'Connor T, Yamamoto M. Keap1 regulates both cytoplasmic-nuclear shuttling and degradation of Nrf2 in response to electrophiles. Genes Cells 2003;8:379–391.

95. Ivanovic V, Weinstein IB. Benzo[a]pyrene and other inducers of cytochrome P1-450 inhibit binding of epidermal growth factor to cell surface receptors. Carcinogenesis 1982;3:505–510.

96. Jaiswal AK. Human NAD(P)H:quinone oxidoreductase2: Gene structure, activity, and tissue specific expression. J Biol Chem 1994;269:14502–14508.

97. Jones KA, Kadonaga JT, Rosenfeld PJ, Kelly TJ, Tjian R. A cellular DNA-binding protein that activates eukaryotic transcription and DNA replication. Cell 1987;48:79–89.

98. Jope RS, Song L, Grimes CA, Zhang L. Oxidative stress oppositely modulates protein tyrosine phosphorylation stimulated by muscarinic G protein-coupled and epidermal growth factor receptors. J Neurosci Res 1999;55:329–340.

99. Joseph P, Jaiswal AK. NAD(P)H:quinone oxidoreductase1 (DT diaphorase) specifically prevents the formation of benzo[a]pyrene quinone-DNA adducts generated by cytochrome P450IA1 and P450 reductase. Proc Natl Acad Sci USA 1994;91:8413–8417.

100. Jowsey IR, Jiang Q, Itoh K, Yamamoto M, Hayes JD. Expression of the aflatoxin B1-8,9-epoxide-metabolizing murine glutathione S-transferase A3 subunit is regulated by the Nrf2 transcription factor through an antioxidant response element. Mol Pharmacol 2003;64:1018–1028.

101. Kadlubar FF, Badawi AF. Genetic susceptibility and carcinogen-DNA adduct formation in human urinary bladder carcinogenesis. Toxicol Lett 1995;82–83:627–632.

102. Kajstura J, Cheng W, Reiss K, Clark WW, Sonnenblick EH, Krajewski S, Reed JC, Olivetti G, Anversa P. Apoptotic and necrotic myocyte cell deaths are independent contributing variables of infarct size in rats. Lab Invest 1996;74:86–107.

103. Kang KW, Ryu JH, Kim SG. The essential role of phosphatidylinositol 3-kinase and of p38 mitogen-activated protein kinase activation in the antioxidant response element-mediated rGSTA2 induction by decreased glutathione in H4IIE hepatoma cells. Mol Pharmacol 2000;58:1017–1025.

104. Kang KW, Cho MK, Lee CH, Kim SG. Activation of phosphatidylinositol 3-kinase and Akt by tert-butylhydroquinone is responsible for antioxidant response element-mediated rGSTA2 induction in H4IIE cells. Mol Pharmacol 2001;59:1147–1156.

105. Kapitulnik J, Levin W, Conney AH, Yagi H, Jerina DM. Benzo[a]pyrene 7,8-dihydrodiol is more carcinogenic than benzo[a]pyrene in newborn mice. Nature 1977;266:378–380.

106. Kasper C. Biochemical distinctions between the nuclear and microsomal membranes from rat hepatocytes. J Biol Chem 1971;246:577–581.

107. Kataoka K, Noda M, Nishizawa M. Maf nuclear oncoprotein recognizes sequences related to an AP-1 site and forms heterodimers with both Fos and Jun. Mol Cell Biol 1994;14:700–712.

108. Kerzee JK, Ramos KS. Activation of c-Ha-ras by benzo[a]pyrene in vascular smooth muscle cells involves redox stress and aryl hydrocarbon receptor. Mol Pharmacol 2000;58:152–158.

109. Khandwala AS, Kasper CB. Preferential induction of aryl hydroxylase activity in rat liver nuclear envelope by 3-methylcholanthrene. Biochem Biophys Res Commun 1973;54:1241–1246.

110. Kim KB, Lee BM. Oxidative stress to DNA, protein, and antioxidant enzymes (superoxide dismutase and catalase) in rats treated with benzo[a]pyrene. Cancer Lett 1997;113:205–212.

111. King HW, Thompson MH, Brookes P. The role of 9-hydroxy-benzo[a]pyrene in the microsome mediated binding of benzo[a]pyrene to DNA. Int J Cancer 1976;18:339–344.

112. Kinoshita N, Gelboin HV. Beta-glucuronidase catalyzed hydrolysis of benzo[a] pyrene-3-glucuronide and binding to DNA. Science 1978;199:307–309.

113. Kita T, Nagano Y, Yokode M, Ishii K, Kume N, Ooshima A, Yoshida H, Kawai C. Probucol prevents the progression of atherosclerosis in Watanabe heritable hyperlipidemic rabbit, an animal model of familial hypercholesterolemia. Proc Natl Acad Sci USA 1987;84:5928–5931.

114. Kitamura S. Effects of cigarette smoking on metabolic events in the lung. Environ Health Perspect 1987;72:283–296.

115. Kodama M, Ioki Y, Nagata C. Binding of benzo[a]pyrene semiquinone radicals with DNA and polynucleotides. Gann 1977;68:253–254.

116. Kovary K, Bravo R. Expression of different Jun and Fos proteins during the G_0-to-G_1 transition in mouse fibroblasts: In vitro and in vivo associations. Mol Cell Biol 1991;11:2451–2459.

117. Kramer JH, Arroyo CM, Dickens BF, Weglicki WB. Spin-trapping evidence that graded myocardial ischemis alters post-ischemic superoxide production. Free Radic Biol Med 1987;3:153–159.

118. Krzywanska E, Piekarski L. Benzo[a]pyrene free radicals formation in the presence of butylated hydroxyanisole and their possible importance in carcinogenesis. Neoplasma 1977;24:395–400.

119. Kunsch C, Luchoomun J, Grey JY, Olliff LK, Saint LB, Arrendale RF, Wasserman MA, Saxena U, Medford RM. Selective inhibition of endothelial and monocyte redox-sensitive genes by AGI-1067: a novel antioxidant and anti-inflammatory agent. J Pharmacol Exp Ther 2004;308:820–829.

120. Kunsch C, Medford RM. Oxidative stress as a regulator of gene expression in the vasculature. Circ Res 1999;85:753–766.

121. Lee W, Haslinger A, Karin M, Tjian R. Two factors that bind and activate the human metallothionein II$_A$ gene in vitro also interact with the SV40 promoter and enhancer regions. Nature 1987;325:368–372.

122. Lee W, Keller EB. Regulatory elements mediating transcription of the human Ha-ras gene. J Mol Biol 1991;220:599–611.

123. Lesko S, Caspary W, Lorentzen R, Ts'o POP. Enzymic formation of 6-oxobenzo[a]pyrene radical in rat liver homogenates from carcinogenic benzo[a]pyrene. Biochemistry 1975;14:3978–3984.

124. Lesko SA, Lorentzen RJ. Benzo[a]pyrene dione-benzo[a]pyrene diol oxidation-reduction couples: Involvement in DNA damage, cellular toxicity, and carcinogenesis. J Toxicol Environ Health 1985;16:679–691.

125. Levin W, Wood AW, Wislocki PG, Kapitulnik J, Yagi H, Jerina DM, Conney AH. (±)-Trans-7,8-dihydroxy-7,8-dihydrobenzo[a]pyrene: A potent skin carcinogen when applied topically to mice. Proc Natl Acad Sci USA 1976;73:3867–3871.

126. Levin W, Wood AW, Wislocki PG, Chang RL, Kapitulnik J, Mah HD, Yagi H, Jerina DM, Conney AH. Mutagenicity and carcinogenicity of benzo[a]pyrene derivatives. In: Gelboin HV, Ts'o POP, (Eds). Polycyclic Hydrocarbons and Cancer. New York: Academic Press, 1978; pp. 189–202.

127. Li Y, Jaiswal AK. Identification of Jun-B as third member in human antioxidant response element-nuclear proteins complex. Biochem Biophys Res Commun 1992a;188:992–996.

128. Li Y, Jaiswal AK. Regulation of human NAD(P)H:quinone oxidoreductase gene. Role of AP-1 binding site contained within human antioxidant response element. J Biol Chem 1992b;267:15097–15104.

129. Li Y, Jaiswal AK. Human antioxidant-response-element-mediated regulation of type 1 NAD(P)H:quinone oxidoreductase gene expression: effect of sulfhydryl modifying agents. Eur J Biochem 1994;226:31–39.

130. Linder D, Gartler SM. Glucose-6-phosphate dehydrogenase mosaicism: Utilization as a cell marker in the study of leiomyomas. Science 1965;150:67–69.

131. Loktionov A, Hollstein M, Martel N, Galendo D, Cabral JRP, Tomatis L, Yamasaki H. Tissue-specific activating mutations of Ha- and Ki-ras oncogenes in skin, lung, and liver

tumors induced in mice following transplacental exposure to DMBA. Mol Carcinog 1990;3:134–140.

132. Lorentzen RJ, Ts'o POP. Benzo[a]pyrenedione/benzo[a]pyrenediol oxidation-reduction couples and the generation of reactive reduced molecular oxygen. Biochemistry 1977;16:1467–1473.

133. Lu J, Lee W, Jiang C, Keller EB. Start site selection by Sp1 in the TATA-less human Ha-ras promoter. J Biol Chem 1994;269:5391–5402.

134. Lyon MF. Chromosomal and subchromosomal inactivation. Annu Rev Genet 1968;2:31–51.

135. Mackness MI, Abbott CA, Arrol S, Durrington PN. The role of high-density lipoprotein and lipid-soluble antioxidant vitamins in inhibiting low-density lipoprotein oxidation. Biochem J 1993a;294:829–834.

136. Mackness MI, Arrol S, Abbott CA, Durrington PN. Is paraoxonase related to atherosclerosis. Chem Biol Interact 1993b;87:161–171.

137. Mackness MI, Durrington PN. Lipid transport and lipoprotein metabolism. In: Rice-Evans C, Bruckdorfer KR (Eds). Oxidative Stress, Lipoproteins and Cardiovascular Dysfunction. London: Portland Press Ltd, 1995; pp. 33–53.

138. Malarkey K, Belham CM, Paul A, Graham A, McLees A, Scott PH, Plevin R. The regulation of tyrosine kinase signaling pathways by growth factor and G-protein-coupled receptors. Biochem J 1995;309:361–375.

139. Malinow MR. Plasma homocysteine and arterial occlusive diseases: A mini-review. Clin Chem 1995;41:173–176.

140. Marshall MS. Ras target proteins in eukaryotic cells. FASEB J 1995;9:1311–1318.

141. Marx J. Forging a path to the nucleus. Science 1993;260:1588–1590.

142. Masuda J, Ross R. Atherogenesis during low level hypercholesteolemia in the nonhuman primate. I. Fatty streak formation. Arteriosclerosis 1990a;10:164–177.

143. Masuda J, Ross R. Atherogenesis during low level hypercholesteolemia in the nonhuman primate. II. Fatty streak conversion to fibrous plaque. Arteriosclerosis 1990b;10:178–187.

144. Maziere C, Floret S, Santus R, Morliere P, Marcheux V, Maziere JC. Impairment of the EGF signaling pathway by the oxidative stress generated with UVA. Free Radic Biol Med 2003;34:629–636.

145. McKay IA, Marshall CJ, Cales C, Hall A. Transformation and stimulation of DNA synthesis in NIH-3T3 cells are a titratable function of normal p21N-ras expression. EMBO J 1986;5:2617–2621.

146. McMahon M, Itoh K, Yamamoto M, Hayes JD. Keap 1-dependent proteasomal degradation of transcription factor Nrf2 contributes to the nagative regulation of antioxidant response element-driven gene expression. J Biol Chem 2003;278:21592–21600.

147. McMillan BJ, Bradfield CA. The aryl hydrocarbon receptor is activated by modified low-density lipoprotein. Proc Natl Acad Sci USA 2007;104:1412–1417.

148. Mendelson KG, Contois L-R, Tevosian SG, Davis RJ, Paulson KE. Independent regulation of JNK/p38 MAP kinases by metabolic oxidative stress in the liver. Proc Natl Acad Sci USA 1996;93:12908–12913.

149. Meyer BK, Perdew GH. Characterization of the AhR-Hsp90-XAP2 core complex and the role of the immunophilin-related protein XAP2 in AhR stabilization. Biochemistry 1999;38:8907–8917.

150. Miller EC, Miller JA. Searches for ultimate chemical carcinogens and their reactions with cellular macromolecules. Cancer 1981;47:2327–2345.

151. Miller JA. Carcinogenesis by chemicals: An overview – G.H.A. Clowes Memorial Lecture. Cancer Res 1970;30:559–576.

152. Miller JA, Surh Y-J. Sulfonation in chemical carcinogenesis. In: Kauffman FC (Ed). Conjugation-Deconjugation Reactions in Drug Metabolism and Toxicity. Berlin: Springer-Verlag, 1994; pp. 429–457.

153. Miller KP, Chen Y-H, Hastings VL, Bral CM, Ramos KS. Profiles of antioxidant/electrophile response element (ARE/EpRE) nuclear protein binding and c-Ha-ras transactivation in vascular smooth muscle cells treated with oxidative metabolites of benzo[a]pyrene. Biochem Pharmacol 2000;60:1285–1296.

154. Miller KP, Ramos KS. DNA sequence determinants of nuclear protein binding to the c-Ha-ras antioxidant/electrophile response element in vascular smooth muscle cells: Identification of Nrf2 and HSP90β as heterocomplex components. Cell Stress Chaperones 2005;10:114–125.

155. Minden A, Lin A, Claret F-X, Abo A, Karin M. Selective activation of the JNK signaling cascade and c-Jun transcriptional activity by the small GTPases Rac and Cdc42Hs. Cell 1995;81:1147–1157.

156. Moi P, Chan K, Asunis I, Cao A, Kan YW. Isolation of NF-E2-related factor 2 (Nrf2), a NF-E2-like basic leucine zipper transcriptional activator that binds to the tandem NF-E2/AP-1 repeat of the beta-globin locus control region. Proc Natl Acad Sci USA 1994;91:9926–9930.

157. Moinova HR, Mulcahy RT. Up-regulation of the human γ-glutamylcysteine synthetase regulatory subunit gene involves binding of Nrf-2 to an electrophile response element. Biochem Biophys Res Commun 1999;261:661–668.

158. Montano MM, Jaiswal AK, Katzenellenbogen BK. Transcriptional regulation of the human quinone reductase gene by antiestrogen-liganded estrogen receptor-α and estrogen receptor-β. J Biol Chem 1998;273:25443–25449.

159. Montano MM, Wittmann BM, Bianco NR. Identification and characterization of a novel factor that regulates quinone reductase gene transcriptional activity. J Biol Chem 2000;275: 34306–34313.

160. Moodie SA, Willumsen BM, Weber MJ, Wolfman A. Complexes of ras GTP with raf-1 and mitogen-activated protein kinase kinase. Science 1993;260:1658–1661.

161. Morel DW, Chisholm GM. Antioxidant treatment of diabetic rats inhibits lipoprotein oxidation and cytotoxicity. J Lipid Res 1989;30:1827–1834.

162. Mulcahy LS, Smith MR, Stacey DW. Requirement for ras proto-oncogene function during serum-stimulated growth of NIH 3T3 cells. Nature 1985;313:241–243.

163. Mulcahy RT, Wartman MA, Bailey HH, Gipp JJ. Constitutive and beta-naphthoflavone-induced expression of the human gamma-glutamylcysteine synthetase heavy subunit gene is regulated by a distal antioxidant response element/TRE sequence. J Biol Chem 1997;272: 7445–7454.

164. Nadkarni DV, Sayre LM. Structural definition of early lysine and histidine adduction chemistry of 4-hydroxynonenal. Chem Res Toxicol 1995;8:284–291.

165. Nagase T, Ueno Y, Ishii S. Transcriptional control of the human Harvey ras proto-oncogene: Role of multiple elements in the promoter region. Gene 1990;94:249–253.

166. Nagata C, Kodama M, Ioki Y. Electron spin resonance study of the binding of the 6-oxybenzo[a]pyrene radical and benzo[a]pyrene semiquinone radicals with DNA and polynucleotides. In: Gelboin HV, Ts'o POP (Eds). Polycyclic Hydrocarbons and Cancer. New York: Academic Press, 1978; pp. 247–260.

167. Nakamura K, Hori T, Sato N, Sugie K, Kawakami T, Yodoi J. Redox regulation of a src family protein tyrosine kinase p56lck in T cells. Oncogene 1993;8:3133–3139.

168. Nguyen T, Rushmore TH, Pickett CB. Transcriptional regulation of a rat liver glutathione S-transferase Ya subunit gene. J Biol Chem 1994;269:13656–13662.

169. Nguyen T, Huang HC, Pickett CB. Transcriptional regulation of the antioxidant response element: Activation by Nrf2 and repression by MafK. J Biol Chem 2000;275:15466–15473.

170. Nguyen T, Sherratt PJ, Pickett CB. Regulatory mechanisms controlling gene expression mediated by the antioxidant response element. Annu Rev Pharmacol Toxicol 2003;43: 233–260.

171. Nguyen T, Yang CS, Pickett CB. The pathways and molecular mechanisms regulating Nrf2 activation in response to chemical stress. Free Radic Biol Med 2004;37:433–441.

172. Nioi P, McMahon M, Itoh K, Yamamoto M, Hayes JD. Identification of a novel Nrf2-regulated antioxidant response element (ARE) in the mouse NAD(P)H:quinone oxidoreductase 1 gene: reassessment of the ARE consensus sequence. Biochem J 2003;374: 337–348.

173. Nishizuka Y. Studies and perspectives of protein kinase C. Science 1986;233:305–312.

174. Nygard O, Nordrehaug JE, Refsum H, Ueland PM, Farstad M, Vollset SE. Plasma homocysteine levels and mortality in patients with coronary artery disease. N Engl J Med 1997;337:230–236.

175. Ou X, Ramos KS. Benzo[a]pyrene inhibits protein kinase C activity in subcultured rat aortic smooth muscle cells. Chem Biol Interact 1994;93:29–40.

176. Ou X, Weber TJ, Chapkin RS, Ramos KS. Interference with protein kinase C-related signal transduction in vascular smooth muscle cells by benzo[a]pyrene. Arch Biochem Biophys 1995;318:122–130.

177. Paigen B, Havens MB, Morrow A. Effect of 3-methylcholanthrene on the development of aortic lesions in mice. Cancer Res 1985;45:3850–3855.

178. Parkinson A. Biotransformation of xenobiotics. In: Klaassen CD (Ed). Casarett and Doull's Toxicology, The Basic Science of Poisons, 6th edition. Chap. 6. New York: McGraw-Hill, 2001;pp. 133–224.

179. Paulson KE, Darnell Jr JE, Rushmore T, Pickett CB. Analysis of the upstream elements of the xenobiotic compound-inducible and positionally regulated glutathione S-transferase Ya gene. Mol Cell Biol 1990;10:1841–1852.

180. Pearson TA, Wang A, Solez K, Heptinstall RH. Clonal characteristics of fibrous plaques and fatty streaks from human aortas. Am J Pathol 1975;81:379–387.

181. Pelkonen O, Boobis AR, Levitt RC, Kouri RE, Nebert DW. Genetic differences in the metabolic activation of benzo[a]pyrene in mice. Attempts to correlate tumorigenesis with mutagenesis in vitro. Pharmacology 1979;18:281–293.

182. Pelkonen O, Nebert DW. Metabolism of polycyclic aromatic hydrocarbons: Etiologic role in carcinogenesis. Pharmacol Rev 1982;34:189–222.

183. Peng HB, Libby P, Liao JK. Induction and stabilization of IκB-α by nitric oxide mediates inhibition of NF-κB. J Biol Chem 1995;270:14214–14219.

184. Penn A, Garte SJ, Warren L, Nesta D, Mindich B. Transforming gene in human atherosclerotic plaque DNA. Proc Natl Acad Sci USA 1986;83:7951–7955.

185. Penn A, Snyder C. Arteriosclerotic plaque development is "promoted" by polynuclear aromatic hydrocarbons. Carcinogenesis 1988;9:2185–2189.

186. Penn A, Hubbard FC Jr, Parkes JL. Transforming potential is detectable in arteriosclerotic plaques of young animals. Arterioscler Thromb 1991;11:1053–1058.

187. Perkins KK, Dailey GM, Tjian R. Novel Jun- and Fos-related proteins in Drosophila are functionally homologous to enhancer factor AP-1. EMBO J 1988;7:4265–4273.

188. Perry MH, Erlanger MW, Gustafsson TO, Perry EF. Reversal of cadmium-induced hypertension by D-myo-inositol-1,2,6-triphosphate. J Toxicol Environ Health 1989;28:151–159.

189. Peus D, Vasa RA, Meves A, Pott M, Beyerle A, Squillance K, Pittelkow MR. H_2O_2 is an important mediator of UVB-induced EGF-receptor phosphorylation in cultured keratinocytes. J Invest Dermatol 1998;110:966–971.

190. Pryor WA. Cigarette smoke radical and the role of free radicals in chemical carcinogenicity. Environ Health Perspect 1997;105:875–882.

191. Przyklenk K, Kloner RA. Superoxide dismutase plus catalase improve contractile function in the canine model of the 'stunned myocardium'. Circ Res 1986;58:148–156.

192. Puhl H, Waeg G, Esterbauer H. Inhibition of LDL oxidation by vitamin E and other anitoxidants. Atheroscler Rev 1993;25:277–285.

193. Rahman A, Barrowman JA, Rahimtula A. The influence of bile on the bioavailability of polynuclear aromatic hydrocarbons from the rat intestine. Can J Physiol Pharmacol 1986;64:1214–1218.

194. Ramos KS, McMahon KK, Alipui C, Demick D. Modulation of smooth muscle cell prolliferation by dinitrotoluene. In: Witner CM, Snyder RR, Jollow DJ et al. (Eds). Biologic Reductive Intermediates. Vol 5, New York: Plenum Press, 1990; pp. 805–807.

195. Ramos KS, Bowes RC III, Ou X, Weber TJ. Responses of vascular smooth muscle cells to toxic insult: Cellular and molecular perspectives for environmental toxicants. J Toxicol Environ Health 1994;43:419–440.

196. Ramos KS, Parrish AR. Growth-related signaling as a target of toxic insult in vascular smooth muscle cells: Implications in atherogenesis. Life Sci 1995;57:627–635.

197. Ramos KS, Zhang Y, Sadhu DN, Chapkin RC. The induction of proliferative phenotypes in vascular smooth muscle cells by benzo[a]pyrene is characterized by upregulation of

phosphatidylinositol metabolism and c-Ha-ras gene expression. Arch Biochem Biophys 1996;332:213–222.

198. Ramos KS. Redox regulation of c-Ha-ras and osteopontin signaling in vascular smooth muscle cells: Implications in chemical atherogenesis. Annu Rev Pharmacol Toxicol 1999;39:243–265.

199. Ramos KS, Melchert RB, Chacon E, Acosta D Jr. Toxic responses of the heart and vascular systems. In: Klaassen CD (Ed). Casarett and Doull's Toxicology, The Basic Science of Poisons, 6th edition. Chap. 18. New York: McGraw-Hill, 2001; pp. 597–652.

200. Ramos KS, Partridge CR. Atherosclerosis and cancer: flip sides of the neoplastic response in mammalian cells? Cardiovasc Toxicol 2005;5:245–255.

201. Rao GN, Berk BC. Active oxygen species stimulate vascular smooth muscle cell growth and proto-oncogene expression. Circ Res 1992;70:593–599.

202. Rao GN. Hydrogen peroxide induces complex formation of SHC-Grb2-SOS with receptor tyrosine kinase and activates ras and extracellular signal-regulated protein kinases group of mitogen activated protein kinases. Oncogene 1996;13:713–719.

203. Recio L, Hsie AW. Glucuronide conjugation reduces the cytotoxicity but not the mutagenicity of benzo[a]pyrene in the CHO/HGPRT assay. Teratog Carcinog Mutagen 1984;4:391–402.

204. Reddy EP, Reynolds RK, Santos E, Barbacid M. A point mutation is responsible for the acquisition of transforming properties by the T24 human bladder carcinoma oncogene. Nature 1982;300:149–152.

205. Rogan E, Roth R, Cavalieri E. Enzymology of polycyclic hydrocarbon binding to nucleic acids In: Jones PW, Freudenthal R (Eds). Carcinogenesis. New York: Raven Press, 1978a; pp. 265–271.

206. Rogan E, Roth R, Katomski P, Benderson J, Cavalieri E. Binding of benzo[a]pyrene at the 1, 3, 6 positions to nucleic acids in vivo on mouse skin and in vitro with rat liver microsomes and nuclei. Chem Biol Interact 1978b;22:35–51.

207. Romero DL, Mounho BJ, Lauer FT, Born JL, Burchiel SW. Depletion of glutathione by benzo[a]pyrene metabolites, ionomycin, thapsigargin, and phorbol myristate in human peripheral blood mononuclear cells. Toxicol Appl Pharmacol 1997;144:62–69.

208. Rosenfeld ME, Tsukada T, Chait A, Bierman EL, Gown AM, Ross R. Fatty streak expansion and maturation in Watanabe heritable hyperlipidemic and comparably hypercholesterolemic fat-fed rabbits. Arteriosclerosis 1987a;7:24–34.

209. Rosenfeld ME, Tsukada T, Gown AM, Ross R. Fatty streak initiation in Watanabe heritable hyperlipidemic and comparably hypercholesterolemic fat-fed rabbits. Arteriosclerosis 1987b;7:9–23.

210. Rosenfeld ME, Palinski W, Ylä-Herttuala S, Carew TE. Macrophages, endothelial cells, and lipoprotein oxidation in the pathogenesis of atherosclerosis. Toxicol Pathol 1990;18: 560–571.

211. Ross JA, Nesnow S. ^{32}P-postlabeling in studies of polycyclic aromatic hydrocarbon activation. IARC Scientif Public (Lyon) 1993;124:71–78.

212. Ross R, Masuda J, Raines EW, Gown AM, Katsuda S, Sasahara M, Malden LT, Masuko H, Sato H. Localization of PDGF-β-protein in macrophages in all phases of atherogenesis. Science 1990;248:1009–1012.

213. Ross R. Atherosclerosis: A defense mechanism gone awry. Am J Pathol 1993a;143: 987–1002.

214. Ross R. Cellular mechanisms of atherosclerosis. Atheroscler Rev 1993b;25:195–200.

215. Ross R. The pathogenesis of atherosclerosis: A perspective for the 1990s. Nature 1993c;362: 801–809.

216. Ross R. Atherosclerosis–an inflammatory disease. N Engl J Med 1999;340:115–126.

217. Rudiger HW, Marxen J, Kohl FV, Melderis H, von Wichert PV. Metabolism and formation of DNA adducts of benzo[a]pyrene in human diploid fibroblasts. Cancer Res 1979;39: 1083–1088.

218. Rushmore TH, King RG, Paulson KE, Pickett CB. Regulation of glutathione S-transferase Ya subunit gene expression: Identification of a unique xenobiotic-responsive element

controlling inducible expression by planar aromatic compounds. Proc Natl Acad Sci USA 1990;87:3826–3830.

219. Rushmore TH, Pickett CB. Transcriptional regulation of the rat glutathione S-transferase Ya subunit gene. Characterization of a xenobiotic-responsive element controlling inducible expression by phenolic antioxidants. J Biol Chem 1990;265:14648–14653.

220. Rushmore TH, Morton MR, Pickett CB. The antioxidant responsive element. J Biol Chem 1991;266:11632–11639.

221. Sadhu DN, Merchant M, Safe SH, Ramos KS. Modulation of protooncogene expression in rat aortic smooth muscle cells by benzo[a]pyrene. Arch Biochem Biophys 1993;300: 124–131.

222. Sadhu DN, Ramos KS. Modulation by retinoic acid of spontaneous and benzo[a]pyrene-induced c-Ha-ras expression. Antimutagen Anticarcinogen Mech 1993;3:263–268.

223. Sadhu DN, Lundberg MS, Burghardt RB, Ramos KS. c-Ha-ras[EJ] transfection of rat aortic smooth muscle cells induces epidermal growth factor responsiveness and characteristics of a malignant phenotype. J Cell Physiol 1994;161:490–500.

224. Sankaranarayanan K, Jaiswal AK. Nrf3 negatively regulates ARE-mediated expression and antioxidant induction of NAD(P)H:Quinone oxidoreductase1 gene. J Biol Chem 2004;279:50810–50817.

225. Sano M, Fukuda K, Sato T, Kawaguchi H, Suematsu M, Matsuda S, Koyasu S, Matsui H, Yamauchi-Takihara K, Harada M, Saito Y, Ogawa S. ERK and p38 MAPK, but not NF-kappaB, are critically involved in reactive oxygen species-mediated induction of IL-6 by angiotensin II in cardiac fibroblasts. Circ Res 2001;89:661–669.

226. Sasco AJ, Secretan MB, Straif K. Tobacco smoking and cancer: a brief review of recent epidemiological evidence. Lung Cancer 2004;45:S3–S9.

227. Schaeffer HJ, Weber MJ. Mitogen-activated protein kinases: Specific messages from ubiquitous messengers. Mol Cell Biol 1999;19:2435–2444.

228. Schmeltz I, Hoffmann D, Wynder EL. Toxic and tumorigenic agents in tobacco smoke. Analytical methods and modes of origin. Trace Subst Environ Health 8, Symp 1974;281–295.

229. Schmidt JV, Bradfield CA. Ah Receptor signaling pathways. Annu Rev Cell Dev Biol 1996;12:55–89.

230. Scragg R, Jackson R, Holdaway I, Woollard G, Woollard D. Changes in plasma vitamin E levels in the first 48 hr after onset of acute myocardial infarction. Am J Cardiol 1989;64: 971–974.

231. Selkirk JK, Croy RG, Roller PP, Gelboin HV. High-pressure liquid chromatographic analysis of benzo(a)pyrene metabolism and covalent binding and the mechanism of action of 7,8-benzoflavone and 1,2-epoxy-3,3,3-trichloropropane. Cancer Res 1974;34:3474–3480.

232. Selkirk JK. Benzo[a]pyrene carcinogenesis: A biochemical selection mechanism. J Toxicol Environ Health 1977;2:1245–1258.

233. Serabjit-Singh CJ, Bend JR, Philpot RM. Cytochrome P-450 monooxygenase system localization in smooth muscle of rabbit aorta. Mol Pharmacol 1985;28:72–79.

234. Shin EA, Kim KH, Han SI, Ha KS, Kim JH, Kang KI, Kim HD, Kang HS. Arachidonic acid induces the activation of the stress-activated protein kinase membrane ruffling and H_2O_2 production via a small GTPase Rac1. FEBS Lett 1999;452:355–359.

235. Sikstrom R, Lanoix J, Bergeron JJM. An enzymatic analysis of a nuclear envelope fraction. Biochim Biophys Acta 1976;448:88–102.

236. Simic D, Mimic-Oka J, Pljesa M, Milanovic D, Radojevic S, Ivanovic B, Kalimanovska-Ostric D, Matic D, Simic T. Time course of erythrocyte antioxidant activity in patients treated by thrombolysis for acute myocardial infarction. Jpn Heart J 2003;44:823–832.

237. Simionescu M, Simionescu N. Proatherosclerotic events: pathobiochemical changes occurring in the arterial wall before monocyte migration. FASEB J 1993;7:1359–1366

238. Singal PK, Khaper N, Palace V, Kumar D. The role of oxidative stress in the genesis of heart disease. Cardiovasc Res 1998;40:426–432.

239. Sky-Peck HH. Trace metals, neoplasia. Clin Physiol Biochem 1986;4:99–111.

240. Slaga TJ, Bracken WM, Dresner S, Levin W, Yagi H, Jerina DM, Conney AH. Skin tumor-initiating activities of the twelve isomeric phenols of benzo[a]pyrene. Cancer Res 1978;38:678–681.

241. Slaga TJ, Bracken WM, Gleason G, Levin W, Yagi H, Jerina DM, Conney AH. Marked differences in skin tumor-initiating activities of the optical enantiomers of the diastereomeric benzo[a]pyrene 7,8-diol-9,10-epoxides. Cancer Res 1979;39:67–71.

242. Smithgall TE, Harvey RG, Penning TM. Spectroscopic identification of ortho-quinones as the products of polycyclic aromatic trans-dihydrodiol oxidation catalyzed by dihydrodiol dehydrogenase. A potential route of proximate carcinogen metabolism. J Biol Chem 1988;263:1814–1820.

243. Spandidos DA, Wilkie NM. Malignant transformation of early passage rodent cells by a single mutated human oncogene. Nature 1984;310:469–475.

244. Spandidos DA, Anderson MLM. A study of mechanisms of carcinogenesis by gene transfer of oncogenes into mammalian cells. Mutat Res 1987;185:271–291.

245. Spandidos DA, Holmes L. Transcriptional enhancer activity in the variable tandem repeat DNA sequence downstream of the human Ha-ras 1 gene. FEBS Lett 1987;218:41–46.

246. Spandidos DA. The effect of exogenous human ras and myc oncogenes in morphological differentiation of the rat pheochromocytoma PC12 cells. Int J Dev Neurosci 1989b;7:1–4.

247. Staal FJ, Anderson MT, Staal GEJ, Herzenberg LA, Gitler C, Herzenberg LA. Redox regulation of signal transduction: Tyrosine phosphorylation and calcium influx. Proc Natl Acad Sci USA 1994;91:3619–3622.

248. Stacey DW, Jung HG. Transformation of NIH 3T3 cells by microinjection of Ha-ras p21 protein. Nature 1984;310:508–511.

249. Stadtman ER, Berlett BS. Reactive oxygen-mediated protein oxidation in aging and disease. Chem Res Toxicol 1997;10:485–494.

250. Stary HC. Evolution and progression of atherosclerotic lesions in coronary arteries of children and young adults. Arteriosclerosis 1989;9:I19–I32.

251. Stary HC, Chandler AB, Dinsmore RE, Fuster V, Glagov S, Insull Jr W, Rosenfeld ME, Schwartz CJ, Wagner WD, Wissler RW. A definition of advanced types of atherosclerotic lesions and a histological classification of atherosclerosis. A report from the Committee on Vascular Lesions of the Council on Arteriosclerosis, American Heart Association. Arterioscler Thromb Vasc Biol 1995;15:1512–1531.

252. Steinberg D, Carew TE, Fielding C, Fogelman AM, Mahley RW, Sniderman AD, Zilversmit DB. Lipoproteins and the pathogenesis of atherosclerosis. Circulation 1989a;80:719–723.

253. Steinberg D, Parthasarathy S, Carew TE, Khoo JC, Witztum JL. Beyond cholesterol. Modifications of low-density lipoprtoein that increases its atherogenicity. N Engl J Med 1989b;320:915–924.

254. Steinberg D. Role of oxidized LDL and antioxidants in atherosclerosis. Adv Exp Med Biol 1995;369:39–48.

255. Steinberg D. A critical look at the evidence for the oxidation of LDL in atherogenesis. Atherosclerosis 1997;131:S5–S7.

256. Suc I, Meilhac O, Lajoie-Mazenc I, Vandaele J, Jurgens G, Salvayre R, Negre-Salvayre A. Activation of EGF receptor by oxidized LDL. FASEB J 1998;12:665–671.

257. Sullivan PD, Calle LM, Shafer K, Nettleman M. Effect of antioxidants on benzo[a]pyrene free radicals. In: Jones PW, Freudenthal RI (Eds). Carcinogenesis: A Comprehensive Survey. New York: Raven Press, 1978; pp. 1–8.

258. Sullivan PD. Free radicals of benzo[a]pyrene and derivatives. Environ Health Perspect 1985;64:283–295.

259. Sundaresan M, Yu ZX, Ferrans VJ, Irani K, Finkel T. Requirement for generation of H_2O_2 for platelet-derived growth factor signal transduction. Science 1995;270:298–301.

260. Tannheimer SL, Ethier SP, Caldwell KK, Burchiel SW. Benzo[a]pyrene- and TCDD-induced alterations in tyrosine phosphorylation and insulin-like growth factor signaling pathways in the MCF-10A human mammary epithelial cell line. Carcinogenesis 1998;19:1291–1297.

261. Thakker DR, Yagi H, Lehr RE, Kevin W, Buening M, Lu AYH, Chang RL, Wood AW, Conney AH, Jerina DM. Metabolism of trans-9,10-digydroxy-9,10-dehydrobenzo[a]pyrene occurs primarily by arylhydroxylation rather than formation of a diol epoxide. Mol Pharmacol 1978;14:502–513.
262. Thirman MJ, Albrecht JH, Krueger MA, Erickson RR, Cherwitz DL, Park SS, Gelboin HV, Holtzman JL. Induction of cytochrome CYPIA1 and formation of toxic metabolites of benzo[a]pyrene by rat aorta: A possible role in atherogenesis. Proc Natl Acad Sci USA 1994;91:5397–5401.
263. Todorovic R, Devanesan PD, Cavalieri EL, Rogan EG, Park SS, Gelboin HV. A monoclonal antibody to rat liver cytochrome P450 IIC11 strongly and regiospecifically inhibits constitutive benzo[a]pyrene metabolism and DNA binding. Mol Carcinog 1991;4:308–314.
264. Touyz RM, Schiffrin EL. AngII-stimulated superoxide production is mediated via phopholipase D in human vascular smooth muscle cells. Hypertension 1999;34:976–982.
265. Touyz RM. Oxidative stress and vascular damage in hypertension. Curr Hypertens Rep 2000;2:98–105.
266. Uchida K, Stadtman ER. Covalent modification of 4-hydroxynonenal to glyceraldehyde-3-phosphate. J Biol Chem 1993;268:6388–6393.
267. US Department of Health Education and Welfare. Smoking and Health (Report of the Advisory Committee to the Surgeon General of the Public Health Service). Public Health Service Publ. No. 1103. Washington, DC: US Govt. Printing Office, 1967.
268. Ushio-Fukai M, Alexander RW, Akers M, Griendling KK. p38 mitogen-activated protein kinase is a critical component of the redox-sensitive signaling pathways activated by angiotensin II: Role in vascular smooth muscle cell hypertrophy. J Biol Chem 1998;273:15022–15029.
269. Vasiliou V, Puga A, Chang C-Y, Tabor MW, Nebert DW. Interaction between the Ah receptor and proteins binding to the AP-1-like electrophile response element (EpRE) during murine phase II [Ah] battery gene expression. Biochem Pharmacol 1995;50:2057–2068.
270. Vaziri C, Faller DV. A benzo[a]pyrene-induced cell cycle checkpoint resulting in p53-independent G_1 arrest in 3T3 fibroblasts. J Biol Chem 1997;272:2762–2769.
271. Venugopal R, Jaiswal AK. Nrf1 and Nrf2 positively and c-Fos and Fra1 negatively regulate the human antioxidant response element-mediated expression of NAD(P)H:quinone oxidoreductase1 gene. Proc Natl Acad Sci USA 1996;93:14960–14965.
272. Venugopal R, Jaiswal AK. Nrf2 and Nrf1 in association with Jun proteins regulate antioxidant response element-mediated expression and coordinated induction of genes encoding detoxifying enzymes. Oncogene 1998;17:3145–3156.
273. Vousden KH, Bos JL, Marshall CJ, Phillips DH. Mutations activating human c-Ha-ras1 protooncogene (HRAS1) induced by chemical carcinogens and depurination. Proc Natl Acad Sci USA 1986;83:1222–1226.
274. Wasserman WW, Fahl WE. Comprehensive analysis of proteins which interact with the antioxidant responsive element: Correlation of ARE-BP-1 with the chemoprotective induction response. Arch Biochem Biophys 1997a;344:387–396.
275. Wasserman WW, Fahl WE. Functional antioxidant response elements. Proc Natl Acad Sci USA 1997b;94:5361–5366.
276. Weber TJ, Ramos KS. c-Ha-ras^{EJ} transfection in vascular smooth muscle cells circumvents PKC requirement during mitogenic signaling. Am J Physiol 1997;273:H1920–H1926.
277. Weinstein IB, Jeffrey AM, Leffler S, Pulkrabek P, Yamasaki H, Grunberger D. Interactions between polycyclic aromatic hydrocarbons and cellular macromolecules. In: Gelboin HV, POP Ts'o (Eds). Polycyclic Hydrocarbons and Cancer. New York: Academic Press, 1978; pp. 4–36.
278. Weyand EH, Bevan DR. Benzo[a]pyrene disposition and metabolism in rats following intratracheal instillation. Cancer Res 1986;46:5655–5661.
279. Weyand EH, Bevan DR. Benzo[a]pyrene metabolism in vivo following intratracheal administration. In: Cooke M, Dennis AJ (Eds). Polynuclear Aromatic Hydrocarbons: A Decade of Progress. Proceedings of the 10th International Symposium. Columbus, OH: Batelle Press, 1988; pp. 913–923.

280. Whitlock Jr JP. Induction of cytochrome P4501A1. Annu Rev Pharmacol Toxicol 1999;39: 103–125.

281. Wild AC, Moinova HR, Mulcahy RT. Regulation of γ-glutamylcysteine synthetase subunit gene expression by the transcription factor Nrf2. J Biol Chem 1999;274:33627–33636.

282. Xie T, Belinsky M, Xu Y, Jaiswal AK. ARE-, TRE-mediated regulation of gene expression: Response to xenobiotics and antioxidants. J Biol Chem 1995;270:6894–6900.

283. Yamazaki H, Terada M, Tsuboi A, Matsubara C, Hata T, Kakiuchi Y. Distribution and binding pattern of benzo[a]pyrene in rat liver, lung and kidney constituents after oral administration. Toxicol Environ Chem 1987;15:71–81.

284. Yang H, Mazur-Melnyk M, de Boer JG, Glickman BW. A comparison of mutational specificity of mutations induced by S9-activated B[a]P and benzo[a]pyrene-7,8-diol-9,10-epoxide at the endogenous aprt gene in CHO cells. Mutat Res 1999;423:23–32.

285. Ytrehus K, Myklebut R, Mjos OD. Influence of oxygen radicals generated by xanthine oxidase in the isolated perfused rat heart. Cardiovasc Res 1986;20:597–603.

286. Yu R, Lei W, Mandlekar S, Weber MJ, Der CJ, Wu J, Kong A-NT. Role of a mitogen-activated protein kinase pathway in the induction of phase II detoxifying enzymes by chemicals. J Biol Chem 1999;274:27545–27552.

287. Yu R, Mandlekar S, Lei W, Fahl WE, Tan T-H, Kong A-NT. p38 mitogen-activated protein-kinase negatively regulates the induction of phase II drug-metabolizing enzymes that detoxify carcinogens. J Biol Chem 2000;275:2322–2327.

288. Zafari AM, Ushio-Fukai M, Akers M, Yin Q, Shah A, Harrison DG, Taylor WR, Griendling KK. Role of NADH/NADPH oxidase-derived H_2O_2 in angiotensin II-induced vascular hypertrophy. Hypertension 1998;32:488–495.

289. Zalba G, Beaumont J, San Jose G, Fortuno A, Fortuno MA, Diez J. Vascular oxidant stress: Molecular mechanisms and pathophysiological implications. J Physiol Biochem 2000;56: 57–64.

290. Zhang L, Connor EE, Chegini N, Shiverick KT. Modulation by benzo[a]pyrene of epidermal growth factor receptors, cell proliferation, and secretion of human chorionic gonadotropin in human placental cell lines. Biochem Pharmacol 1995;50:1171–1180.

291. Zhang Y, Ramos KS. The induction of proliferative vascular smooth muscle cell phenotypes by benzo[a]pyrene does not involve mutational activation of ras genes. Mutat Res 1997;373:285–292.

292. Zhao W, Ramos KS. Inhibition of DNA synthesis in primary cultures of adult rat hepatocytes by benzo[a]pyrene and related aromatic hydrocarbons: Role of Ah receptor-dependent events. Toxicology 1995;99:179–189.

293. Zhao W, Ramos KS. Modulation of hepatocyte gene expression by the carcinogen benzo[a]pyrene. Toxicol In Vitro 1998;12:395–402.

294. Zhu H, Li Y, Trush MA. Characterization of benzo[a]pyrene quinone-induced toxicity to primary cultured bone marrow stromal cells from DBA/2 mice: Potential role of mitochondrial dysfunction. Toxicol Appl Pharmacol 1995;130:108–120.

295. Zipper LM, Mulcahy RT. Inhibition of ERK and p38 MAP kinases inhibits binding of Nrf2 and induction of GCS genes. Biochem Biophys Res Commun 2000;278:484–492.

296. Zweier JL. Measurement of superoxide-derived free radicals in the reperfused heart. Evidence for a free radical mechanism of reperfusion injury. J Biol Chem 1988;263: 1353–1357.

297. Zwijsen RM, Japenga SC, Heijen AM, van den Bos RC, Koeman JH. Induction of platelet-derived growth factor chain A gene expression in human smooth muscle cells by oxidized low density lipoproteins. Biochem Biophys Res Commun 1992;186:1410–1416.

Chapter 9
The Role of Glutathione Pathways in the Prevention of Atherosclerosis

Jordan L. Holtzman

The Role of Oxidized Serum Lipids in the Chronic Vascular Inflamation Associated with the Development of Atherosclerosis

Our current concept of the etiology of atherosclerosis is that it is a chronic inflammatory process. In support of this model serum markers of inflammation, such as high levels of C-reactive protein[4,96] and fibrinogen, [61,151,212] have been observed in numerous studies to be sensitive predictors of future cardiovascular adverse events. These markers are a group of serum proteins that are termed "acute phase reactants." Their serum levels increase in the presence of any inflammatory process, the most common of which are infections. And indeed it has been suggested that atherosclerosis may be due to a focus of infection, such as periodontal disease.[197] The infection then presumably spreads to the vascular tissues to initiate a local inflammatory process. Against this model it has been found in clinical trials that antibiotics do not prevent adverse vascular events.[65] Furthermore, agents, such as statins, which have no antibacterial activity, have been shown in innumerable studies to be highly effective in the reduction of number of vascular events occuring in a vulnerable population. The apparent association between periodontal and vascular disease may be due to the fact that both conditions are much more common in smokers.

Alternatively, in recent years there has been a growing body of evidence suggesting that the inflammation may be initiated by oxidized, serum lipids. This mechanism is clearly chemically plausible, since the serum is a highly oxidizing medium. It contains high concentrations of molecular oxygen, ascorbic acid and protein bound iron. These are the essential ingredients of Fenton's reagent, a strong oxidizing system which produces the hydroxyl radical through the Haber-Weiss reaction.[64] This radical extracts hydrogen atoms from unsaturated lipids to produce lipid radicals. These in turn react with molecular oxygen to form lipid peroxy radicals leading to a cascade in which the lipid radical abstracts a hydrogen atom from a second molecule of lipid to form a lipid hydroperoxide and a new radical molecule. The plausibility of this mechanism for the development of atherosclerotic lesions is supported by the observation that increased serum iron levels, which would increase the rate of formation of the hydroxyl radical, is associated with increased oxidant damage.[108,210]

J.L. Holtzman (ed.), *Atherosclerosis and Oxidant Stress: A New Perspective*.
© Springer 2008

Furthermore, there are extensive data in the literature indicating that this peroxidation does occur.[42,164] Unfortunately, many of these studies were based on the detection of thiobarbituric acid reactive substrates (TBAS), which presumably is primarily malondialdehyde (MDA). MDA is produced during the decompostion of the peroxylipids. Unfortunately, this assay does have problems with cross reactivity with other compounds, but high levels of TBAS does suggest that there is the lipid peroxidation in the serum. Yet, other investigators have detected the lipid hydroperoxides by more specific methodology, such as chemiluminescence, either after HPLC separation[56,91,132,159,203,206] or directly without prior separation (Miyazawa 1989).[25,68,123–125,165,211]

Similarly, a number of workers have found that the oxidized lipids can be detected immunologically in both atherosclerotic plaques[195,209] and in the serum.[72,195]

Finally, indiviuals with severe cardiovascular disease have antibodies to oxidized LDL suggesting that they have been exposed to high levels of these oxidized lipids.[160] Some workers have reported that there is even a direct correlation between the levels of oxidized lipids present in the serum and the severity of cardiovascular disease.[50,117,134] Similarly, Minekura et al.[122] have demonstrated that 4-hydroxy-2-nonenal, another product of lipid peroxidation, inhibits endothelial function. In a similar vein, Shen and Sevanian[166] reported that oxidized lipid directly stimulated the GSH pathways which are known to be enhanced in the presence of oxidant stress. Clearly, together these data support a role for oxidant injury in the development of atherosclerosis.

In a review of the association between various genetic variants of both prooxidant and antioxidants Leopold and Loscalzo[105] have summarized a vast body of data indicating that there is an increased level of lipid peroxides in individuals with significant vascular disease.

Mechanisms for the Initiation of Vessel Injury by Oxidized Lipids

The oxidized lipids are highly cytotoxic and could directly lead to endothelial damage. For example, Rangaswamy et al.[150] reported that the infusion of oxidized LDL leads directly to endothelial injury. The area of injury can in turn form a nidus for the development of atherosclerosis.

A more widely accepted mechanism for the role of oxidized lipids in the initiation of vessel injury is that they activate blood macrophages.[142,143,173] These cells have receptors for oxidized LDL. On binding to these receptors, the cells are activated, infiltrate into the vessel wall and initiate an inflammatory process within the intima. The infilitrating macrophages contain high concentrations of the oxidized lipids and become foam cells, a characteristic finding in atherosclerotic lesions. As these cells die they release the lipids into the palque. The lipids are isolated from the circulation by a fibrous lid on the plaque. If this lid ruptures, the lipids are released into the blood stream leading to the formation of a clot and arterial occlusion, thereby initiating an acute myocardial infarction (AMI).

The Role of Antioxidant Systems in the Protection of the Vessel Wall from Oxidant Injury

The levels of the oxidized lipids are a function of their rate of formation and the rate at which the body can reduce them to their nontoxic, alcoholic metabolites. Since the blood is a highly oxidizing medium, the rate of production of the peroxy-lipids is primarily a function of the concentration of the plasma lipids. As a result, if oxidant injury is a major factor in the development of atherosclerosis, then the steady state levels of the lipid hydroperoxides is going to be primarily determined by the rate at which they are detoxified by various protective pathways.[15,16,71] There are three systems involved in their detoxification. These include the paroxonases and two families of glutathione dependent enzymes, the glutathione peroxidases (GPxs) and the glutathione-S-transfereases (GSTs).[15,16,101,167]

The primary role of the paroxonases appears to be to cleave the oxidized fatty acids from the serum phospholipids. On the other hand, the GPxs and GSTs serve to catalyze the reduction of the free, oxidized fatty acids. GSH is the largest reservoir of reducing equivalents in the cell with free concentrations in the mM range. Depletion of cellular GSH by severe oxidant stress leads to cell death.

In the serum, the free GSH concentration is much lower with reported levels being between 3 and $20\,\mu M$.[8,81,120] Since the serum GSH is readily oxidized to give mixed protein disulfides, about 90% is present in the oxidized form. Hence, when one is seeking to determine its free, serum concentration, it is necessary to either promptly determine it within minutes[8,120] or immediately alkylate the free GSH sulfhydryl to prevent its oxidation.[81] When this is not done, then the apparent free, serum, GSH concentration has been reported to be as low as $0.5\,\mu M$.[196]

The Correlation between the GSH and Cysteine Levels and Vascular Disease

Several workers have examined the correlation between the serum GSH levels and vascular disease. Belch et al.[18] reported that patients with evidnece of vascular disease had lower, acid soluble, total serum thiols, but increased levels of erythrocyte thiols. The latter would suggest that since GSH is the most pleniful intracellular thiol, there was an increase in its synthesis in response to oxidant injury. Similary, Nuttall et al.[131] reported that in normal volunteers, there was a decline in serum GSH with age and an associated increase in lipid peroxides. On the other hand, Cals et al.[29] found that in community living, elderly, healthy subjects the levels of GSH and TBAS were the same as in young adults while the GSH was lower and the TBAS were higher in the infirmed elderly.

In another study, Morrison et al.[129] compared the total serum GSH levels in the adolescent children of patients with cardiovascular disease to the levels in children of matched controls. They found that the children of the controls had significantly higher total serum GSH levels than the children of the cases ($p > 0.002$). These data indicate that the serum GSH levels are under genetic control and that long term, high levels protect against vascular disease.

A similar association has been reported in adults. For example, Ashfaq et al.[13] reported that carotid artery, intimal thickening was associated with lower levels of GSH. Similarly, Kinscherf et al.[89] found that oxidized LDL levels and severe vascular disease were associated with low levels of serum thiols. This was a follow-up study of a report by Franceschini et al.[54] demonstrating that the administration of N-acetylcysteine, a source of cysteine for the synthesis of GSH, increased the plasma HDL levels.

Cigarette smokers have also been found to have lower levels of GSH,[163] while smoking cessation led to increased levels.[98] Together, these data suggest that the low serum GSH levels may be one factor leading to the early onset of atherosclerosis in smokers.

On the other hand, Mills et al.[121] and Go and Jones[59] have reported that vascular injury was more appropriately associated with the cysteine/cystein ratio rather than the GSH/GSSG ratio. Since the level of cysteine is the limiting factor in the synthesis of GSH, it would suggest that the intracellular concentrations of GSH may be decreased in the presence of low levels of this amino acid. In line with these observations Vento et al.[190] and Koramaz et al.[93] reported that N-acetylcysteine was cardioprotective when administered during coronary artery bypass. Furthermore, Darley-Usmar et al.[36] reported that the activation of macrophages by oxidized LDL increased cytosolic GSH, suggesting that such increases do have a role in protecting cells from oxidant damage.

A similar result was observed in a double blind study of the effect of the infusion of GSH into patients with peripheral arterial vascular disease (PAVD).[10] The treated patients had marked increases in various measures of perfusion, including increased walking distance and increased macro- and microcirulatory flow. Since hydrogen peroxide is a vasoconstrictor, it is likely that this improved performance was due to a reduction of the peroxide leading to significant vasodilitation.

One of the most interesting aspects of the epidemiological studies has been the observation that increased levels of the enzyme catalyzing the destruction of serum GSH, γ-glutamyltransferase, is a sensitive marker for future cardiovascular events.[51,102,103,158] These data might suggest that this enzyme destroys the serum GSH leading to the lower levels and thereby promoting vascular disease.

In conclusion, the relatively scant data published to date would suggest that low levels of serum and intracellular GSH may be a risk factor for vascular disease.

The Selenium Dependent GSH-Peroxidases and Paraoxonases

There are four well characterized selenium dependent GPxs in mammalian organisms which are designated as GPx1–4.[11] In all four the selenium is present as a selenocysteine. The forms GPx1–3 are homotetramers while GPx4 is monomeric.[185] GPx1 and GPx2 are highly homologous, cytosolic enzymes that can reduce the hydroperoxides of free fatty acids, cholesterol and cholesterol esters, but not fatty acids bound to either phospholipids or triglycerides. On the other hand, GPx3, the serum form, and GPx4, another cytosolic enzyme, can reduce the phospholipid hydroperoxides without prior cleavage of the fatty acid.[52,185,204] It is not clear whether the reduction of the phospholipid hydroperoxides by GPx3 is enhanced by prior cleavage of the fatty acid peroxide from the phospholipid. Although knocking out GPx4 is a early lethal mutant,[75] there are no epidemiological studies on the role of this GPx in the prevention of disease. Yet, it has been shown in vitro to be increased by the cytokines that are involved in the acute phase reaction, suggesting that it may play a role in protecting the endothelium from oxidant injury.[171,202]

There is also a cytosolic GPx which does not contain a selenocysteine (NSGPX).[55] Like GPx3 and GPx4, it can catalyze the reduction of phospholipid hydroperoxides without prior cleavage of the oxidized fatty acid. As with GPx4, there are no epidemiological data concerning its possible role in the protection against vascular disease.

In the serum the cleavage of the oxidized fatty acids from the phospholipids and triglycerides is catalyzed by a family of esterases bound to the HDL fraction, the paraoxonases.[101,167] Serdar et al.[164] have shown that there is a correlation between the paraoxanse activity and the degree of vascular injury. Further, in support of their role in the prevention of vascular disease, knockout mice on a high cholesterol diet have an accelerated development of atherosclerosis when compared to their normal, liter mates.[167] Similarly, there are two common polymorphic forms at position 191 which have significant differences in their capacity to protect against the oxidation of LDL.[5,14] Furthermore, Rozenberg et al.[154] reported that the tranfection of paraoxanase into mice decreases the level of oxidant damage. On the other hand, although there is an extensive literature suggesting that the paraoxnases may have a role in protecting vessels against oxidant damage, population studies have not observed any consistent correlation between the levels of this enzyme and cardiovascular adverse events.[101]

The Role of GPx1 in the Prevention of Vascular Injury

GPx1 is the classic, cytosolic form of the GPxs. It is found in all cells. The highly homologous form, GPx2 is also cytosolic, but is primarily found in the gastrointestinal tract where it may have a role in the prevention of colon cancer. GPx1 was cloned and sequenced by Mullenbach et al.[130] GPx1 knockout mice show an increased suceptibility to oxidant injury but they do not have a significant reduction in life span.[188] Similarly, de Haan[39] found that knocking out GPx1 had no effect on the development of atherosclerosis in mice fed with a high fat diet. Since atherosclerosis is the leading cause of death in humans, these results might suggest that GPx1 does not have a role in the prevention of arterial disease. Yet, such may not be the case, since, unlike humans, the primary cause of death in both mice and rats is cancer rather than atherosclerosis. This may be due to the fact that their ratio of

HDL to total cholesterol is much higher than in humans, possibly because they lack a transfer protein, cholesterol ester transfer protein (CETP), which tranfers lipids from the HDL to LDL.

In line with a possible role for GPx1 in the prevention of atherosclerosis, a number of studies have reported that there is an inverse correlation between the degree of vascular disease and the activity of erythrocyte GPx1.[21,24,109,110,113,164] Simlary, Winter et al.[200] found that a genetic variant of GPx1, in which there is a repeat region of only six instead of seven alanines, was over represented in a group of patients with vascular disease when conpared to controls. This finding suggests that the decreased GPx activity associated with this variant could represent an important factor in the development of atherosclerosis. Furthermore, Siemianowicz et al.[169] have reported that children from families with a high incidence of cardio-vascular disease had lower levels of erythrocyte GPx1 and catalase when compared to controls. This has also been reported in patients with hypertension, a risk factor for atherosclerosis.[84] This evidence of increased oxidant stress in patients with hypertension has also been observed in their polymorphonuclear leukocytes.[94] Hapyn et al.[66] did not find a similar correlation with the antioxidant pathways in the erythrocytes of childern from families prone to early atherosclerosis. Inspite of these discrepancies, I feel that the preponderance of evidence would suggest that low levels of GPx1 is associated with an increased risk of vascular disease.

Yet, since the erythrocytes are not likely to be a significant target for the toxic effects of oxidized LDL, the results of these studies would imply that this correlation is a surrogate marker for the GPx1 activity within the endothelial cells.[90] It would further suggest that GPx1 serves a vital role in protecting the endothelium from injury by the oxidized LDL. This is consistent with the observations of Mezzetti et al.[119] who reported that there were lower levels of GPx1 in the aorta than in the internal mammary artery. This latter artery is unusually resistant to the development of atherosclerosis. This resistance could result from these higher levels of GPx1. In a follow-up study, they observed a similar difference between the levels of GPx1 in diseased carotid arteries taken at surgery when compared to that found in internal mammary arteries taken during coronary artery bypass surgery.[100] In light of these interesting results, it is unfortunate that these workers did not not examine this same question in normal arteries taken at autopsy from young individuals.

Interestingly, the in vitro exposure of platelets to N-3-unsaturated fatty acids, agents known to prevent vascular events by increasing platelet stability, were reported to lead to an increase in GPx1 activity[104] Since platelets do not synthesize proteins, this effect on these cell fragments would suggest that the fatty acids acti-vate GPx1 rather than increase its synthesis. A similar effect has been observed with blood monocytes.[82]

It has also been reported that platelet GPx1 declines with age[189] and is lower in smokers compared to nonsmokers.[172] These data suggest that the association of lower levels of GPx1 in platelets may be one factor in their increased susceptibility to activation seen in both the elderly and smokers.

The Role of GPx3 in the Prevention of Vascular Disease

GPx3 is a serum glycoprotein associated with the plasma HDL fraction.[31] It was initially thought that the serum GPx activity was catalyzed by GPx1 that had leaked from the liver. This proved to be incorrect when both Maddipati and Marnett[112] and Takahashi et al.[176] purified the enzyme from serum. It was cloned and sequenced from humans by Takahashi et al.[177] and from mice by Maser et al.[114] Both groups reported that the kidney is the primary site of GPx3 synthesis. The sequences in the two species are 100% identical, suggesting that this enzyme is highly conserved and hence, that it serves a vital role in survival. To date the only activity observed for GPx3 has been the reduction of lipid hydroperoxides.

Yet, work from Holmgren's laboratory had suggested that GPx3 was not catalytically active because its Km for GSH was two orders of magnitude higher than the previously reported free, serum GSH concentration.[8,20,196] We found that this apparent discrepancy between the serum GSH concentration and the concentraion required for significant GPx3 activity was due to the presence of Tris buffer in the assay mixture.[31] When we substituted phosphate buffer for Tris, we were able to demonstrate significant activity with as little as 4.5 µM GSH, a concentration within the range reported for the free, serum GSH (Fig. 9.1).

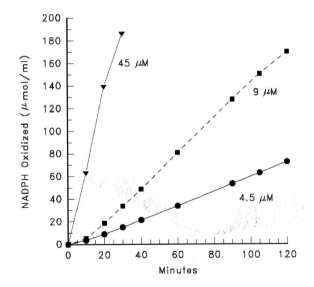

Fig. 9.1 The effect of varying GSH concentrations on the reduction of tert.-Butylhydroperoxide by purified, plasma, GPx3. The assay was performed in phosphate buffered saline (Data taken from Chen et al.[31])

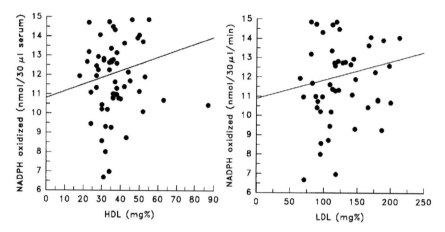

Fig. 9.2 The correlation between the GPx3 activity and the plasma (A) HDL and (B) LDL concentrations (Data taken from Chen et al.[31])

We also found that GPx3 was present solely in the HDL fraction. In light of this result, we next examined whether there was a correlation between the HDL and LDL levels and the GPx3 activity in samples obtained from the clinical laboratory. We found that there was a small, but statistically nonsignificant positive correlation between the GPx3 activity and the HDL (Fig. 9.2A) (slope = 0.0182; $p > 0.5$; $N = 45$). On the other hand, there was a small, but significant negative correlation between the GPx3 activity and the LDL (Fig. 9.2B) (slope =-0.00733; $p < 0.05$; $N = 31$). These data suggest that a portion of the protective effect of the HDL may be due to the presence of both GPx3 and paraoxanase in this fraction.

Finally, we examined the effect of homocysteine on the GPx3 activity. Homocysteine is produced by the S-demethylation of S-adenosylmethionine. A large number of epidemiological studies have suggested that hyperhomocysteinemia is an independent risk factor for atherosclerosis.[62,127] Furthermore, it has been found in prospective studies of patients with coronary artery disease, that those with hyperhomocysteinemia had more rapid progression of their disease.[115,133] Even though some investigators have not found an association between hyperhomo-cysteinemia and vascular disease,[6,187,191] it is still widely accepted as an independent risk factor for the development of early atherosclerosis.[127] Our studies might suggest a biochemical basis for this effect. We observed that at physiological, free, serum, GSH concentrations and physiological, free, serum, homocysteine concentrations, GPx3 was markedly inhibited (Fig. 9.2).

These data would suggest that high, free homocysteine levels could accelerate the development of atherosclerosis by blocking the GPx3 reduction of oxidized lipids. This is in line with the observations of Voutilainen et al.[193] who reported that there was an increase in plasma lipid oxidation products in subjects with hyperhomocysteinemia. On the other hand, Huerta et al.[73] found that there was no correlation between homo-cysteine levels and various indices of oxidant stress. Unfortunately, neither of these

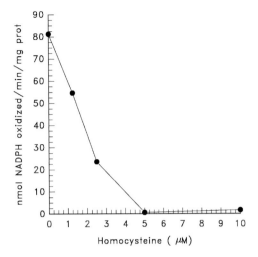

Fig. 9.3 The effect of homocysteine on the activity of purified GPx3 in the presence of 9 μM GSH (Data taken from Chen et al.[31])

authors determined the plasma GSH and GPx3 levels. If, as our data indicate, homocysteine is a competative inhibitor of GPx3, then the ratio of GSH to homocyteine, along with the GPx3 level, would be a potentially better index for the prediction adverse vascular events rather than the homocysteine levels alone.

In support of the role of GPx3 in the protection of individuals from vascular injury, there are two reports of an observational study by Blann and coworkers[22,149] suggesting that the activity of the GPx3 is lower in patients with extensive cardiovascular disease than in healthy controls. Unfortunately, it is not clear from their reports whether they controlled for other risk factors in their data analysis or from the statistical problems that arise from multiple comparisons. If they did, then it would suggest that low serum activity of the GPx3 is a major risk factor for the development of cardiovascular disease.

Our data suggesting that all three components should be determined in order to access the risk of disease is in agreement with the studies noted above in which it was found that low levels of serum GSH were associated with early occurrence of vascular events.[13,29,89,98,129,131,163]

Another observation suggesting that GPx3 may serve to protect the vessels from oxidant damage is the finding that the kidney is a major site of GPx3 synthesis.[114,177] Patients with renal failure typically have accelerated atherosclerosis. This could be due in part to decreased levels of this enzyme. Compounding the decreased GPx3 levels, renal patients also frequently have hyperhomocysteinemia and hyperlipidemia.

Interestingly, Moat et al.[126] observed that GPx3 was significanly higher in patients with a genetic form of hyperhomocysteinemia, suggesting that high levels of this amino acid may induce GPx3. This would further confound the interpretation of the epidemiological studies, since this induction could partially compensate for the inhibition of the peroxidase activity. Clearly, it would be important to determine all three components to ascertain whether this system has a significant role in decreasing vascular injury.

Finally, Voetsch et al.[192] reported that the presence of several genetic variants in the promoter region of GPx3 was associated with a significant increase in the incidence of arterial ischemic strokes. These data lend strong evidence to the role of this peroxidase in the protection of the vascular wall. In summary, these observations would suggest that the reported association between increased vascular disease and hyperhomocysteinemia may be due to inhibition of GPx3.[31,71] Yet, these findings also suggest a possible reason for the discrepant results among the various epidemiological studies. The problem may be that homocysteine only accelerates the progression of athersclerosis when the individual has a low serum GSH or GPx3 activity. Yet, to date, no investigators have examined all three components in the same subjects.

The Role of the Gluthathione S-Transferases Polymorphinsms in the Development of Vascular Disease

The GSTs are a family of enzymes found in the cytosol and endoplasmic reticulum. They catalyze the covalent binding of GSH to electrophyllic compounds.[9,63,67,99] Several forms have also been found to have peroxidase activity. These enzymes are found in all aerobic organisms. In mammalian species there are four major classes of the cytosolic forms, forms A, M, P, and theta, and two forms in the endoplasmic reticulum. Furthermore, within families of the cytosolic forms, GSTA has four subforms and GSTM has five.[67] The active GSTs are homodiamers. The activity of the cytosolic forms, except GSTT1, can be determined by their conjugation of 1-chloro-2,4-dinitrobenzene.[67] Unfortunately, there is no definitive metabolic pattern for the various substrates of the GSTs which can unequivocally distinguish them from each other, except for the failure of GSTT1 to catalyze the metabolism of 1-chloro-2,4-dinitrobenzene and the exclusive metabolism of trans-stilbene oxide by GSTM.[161] Hence, their genotype is usually detemined rather than their phenotype. In population studies this does limit our ability to correlate their catalytic activities with outcomes. Fortunately, all of the GSTs have been cloned, sequenced, and their chromosomal locations determined.[67] Hence, this has permitted at least some evaluation of their role in preventing oxidant injury.

Like GPx3, GPx4, and NSGPx, the GSTs can also catalyze the reduction of phospholipid hydroperoxides without prior cleavage of the oxidized fatty acid.[74]

The first evidence suggesting that GST polymorphisms may increase susceptibility to disease was the observation that a significantly higher proportion of the leukocytes in smokers with lung cancer (65%) than smokers without tumors (40%) was GSTM null.[162] This observation has been replicated in a number of studies of tobacco related lung and bladder cancers and possibly head and neck cancers.[26–28,32,57,88,95,87,111,118,135,137,146,152] Similarly, the null genotype of GSTM has been reported to be associated with an increased incidence of colon cancer.[35,37,77] It is presumed that these tumors arise as a result of exposure of the colonic epithelium to high levels of the various toxins produced by the gut bacteria. On the other hand, an excess prevalence of the null genotypes has not been observed in patients with tumors which are not thought to be induced by exposure to environmental carcinogens, including breast[7] and ovarian cancers.[97]

Several groups have examined whether similar polymorphisms are associated with the accelerated vascular disease seen in smokers. These studies are based on the observation that the vascular disease in this population could result from the same biochemical reactions which lead to an increased incidence of cancer.[19,23,182] It has long been known that the carcinogenic components of tobacco smoke are procarcinogens which first have to be metabolized by the cell to give the ultimate carcinogen.[69,70] This reactive metabolite then forms adducts with the DNA, leading to the mutations that are associated with the initiation of tumorgenesis. Studies on the aortas of various species, including humans, have demonstrated that this tissue can catalyze these same metabolic processes that lead to the initiation of cancer[23,38,182,186](Holtzman et al. MS in prep).

Further support for this paradigm comes from the observations of Izzotti et al.[78,79] who found that the smooth muscle cells obtained from the atherosclerotic lesions of GSTM nul smokers had more adducted DNA than those from individuals with at least one allel of GSTM. Similarly, de Waart et al.[41] observed a more rapid progression of intimal thickening in smokers who were GSTM1 nul than in those who were not GSTM1 nul. On the other hand, Olshan et al.[136] in a report from the ARIC group, a longterm cohort study, and Wang et al.,[194] in a study of patients undergoing cardiac catheterization for an acute ischemic event, failed to find any association between GSTM1 null and vascular disease in smokers.

To further add to the confusion, in three publications from the ARIC group, they reported that indiviuals who had the nul genotype for another GST, GSTT1, had evidence of less vascular injury than those with at least one GSTT1 allel.[106,107,136] On the other hand, Tamer et al.[179] and Abu-Amero et al.[1] found in case-control studies of patients with an AMI that there was an increased prevelance of GSTM1 nul and GSTT1 nul in the cases who also smoked, while Girisha et al.[58] found an effect only of GSTT1 nul. Doney et al.[45] found a similar effect of GSTT1 nul in diabetic patients.

These conflicting observations on the effect of GST genotypes in smokers on the incidence of vascular disease may be due to a variety of factors; the most important of which may be that these studies generally had small sample sizes and therefore under powered. Another problem is that these studies were forced to use the genotype, whereas any deleterious or benefical effect of a specific GST will depend upon its actual activity in the endothelium. This can only be ascertained by determining its actual enzymatic activity. Unfortunately, this is not possible at present.

Since the GSTs can catalyze the reduction of phospholipid hydroperoxides, they could also protect against oxidant stress in nonsmokers. And indeed, Stickel et al.[174] observed that in patients with a genetic iron overload disease, hemochromatosis, which presuably leads to severe oxidant injury, the incidence of cirrhosis was greater in a C282Y polymorphism of GSTP1 than in those without this allel. These data would suggest that this GST could protect the cell against oxidant injury.

On the other hand, Pessah-Rasmussen et al.[147] reported that in a substudy of 80-year-old men in Malmo who had no history of symptomatic, cardiovascular disease, there was a positive correlation rather than an inverse correlation between the extent of PAVD and their leukocyte GSTM activity. Clearly this is a skewed population since 80-year-old men without cardiovascular disease represent a highly selected population. The presence of GSTM could have been one factor leading to their survival to this ripe old age.

In line with this, in a population of middle aged men they observed the expected inverse correlation between the leukocyte GSTM activity and the presence of PAVD.[148] This would suggest that middle aged men who lack GSTM may be at an increased risk for this condition. Yet, they did not observe a correlation in patients undergoing coronary artery bypass surgery, suggesting that coronary artery disease has several different etiologies which may have masked the effect of the GSTM phenotype, including the possibility that other genotypes may be important in this process. Evans et al.[53] found a similar lack of association between the GSTM phenotype and ischemic heart disease. A major problem with both of these studies is that in their analysis they did not distinguish between smokers and nonsmokers. Since the increased incidence of atherosclerosis seen in individuals with other risk factors, such as hypertension or hyperlipidemias, may not be related to the formation of the toxic metabolites, such individuals may have diluted out any genetic deficiency in GSTM which might be associated with the arterial disease seen only in smokers.

This possibility is born out in a study by Wilson et al.[198] who examined the frequency of GSTM1 nul in patients undergoing coronary angiography for evaluation of a presumptive AMI. They categorized the patients according to whether they have had an AMI and also whether they were found to have significant coronary artery stenosis (>50%) (Table 9.1).

In this population there was no correlatin between the GSTM1 genotype and cardiovascular disease in nonsmokers or former smokers. On the other hand, in smokers the GSTM1 nul genotype appeared to have a protective effect on the incidence of significant arterial stenosis. They reported a similar finding in a subsequent study in a different population.[199]

One possible explanation for the discrepancies between the induction of cancer and the development of vascular disease is that the GSTs may be catalyzing the formation of more toxic metabolites of carcinogens in tobacco smoke instead of

Table 9.1 The frequency of GSTM1 null in controls and patients undergoing coronary angiography

Acute MI	Stenosis	All subjects (%)	Nonsmokers (%)	Former smokers (%)	Current smokers (%)
–	–	57	55	61	67
+	–	59	56	62	60
+	+	48	53	46	32

Data taken from Wilson et al.[198]

detoxifying them. Such enhanced toxicity of GSH conjugates has been shown for some of the haloalkanes.[67]

Another possible problem with all of these studies on subjects with an AMI is that they all examined only patients who made it to catheterization. It is generally accepted that only about half of the patients survive long enough to get medical care. Hence, these investigators were dealing with a biased population of those who survived long enough to be catheterized. It may well be that those individuals with a null genotype for GSTM1 and/or GSTT1 have a higher initial mortality than individuals with the normal genotype and therefore would not have been included in their sample. To further confuse these findings, they reported that the prevelance of the GSTM1 nul was much higher in their control populations than has generally been reported[67] or that was reported by Pessah-Rasmussen et al.[148] In fact, the ratios observed in the previous studies have generally been exactly the opposite of those observed in these studies.

Effect of Ischemic Heart Disease, Diabetes Mellitus and Chronic Renal Failure on the GSH Peroxidases

Ischemic Heart Disease

Early reports indicated that ischemic heart disease was associated with high levels of lipid peroxides.[46,80] Similarly, several groups have found that patients with an acute ischemic event have decreased levels of GPx1 in their erythrocytes,[43,92,170,207] neutrophils,[48] and platelets.[85,141] Similar changes have been observed in chronic ischemia with an increase in markers of lipid peroxidation[47] and erythrocyte GSH levels.[178] Interestingly, Simic et al.[170] also reported that at 6 days post reperfusion after an AMI, there was as much as a 60% increase in GPx1 activity. This is surprising since mature erythrocytes do not synthesize new proteins, suggesting that there is a pool of inactive enzyme in these cells which is activated by the reperfusion.

Diabetes Mellitus

As is well known, diabetes mellitus, both the insulin dependent (IDDM; type 1) and noninsulin dependent (NIDDM; type 2) are associated with a marked increase in the incidence of vascular disease. Even though these two forms of diabetes mellitus have different etiologies, in both conditions there is evidence of enhanced oxidant injury with a decrease in the antioxidant systems. IDDM results from a loss of insulin production due to destruction of the beta cells of the pancreas. On the other hand, at least in the early stages of NIDDM, there are high levels of circulating insulin with a decreased response to this hormone.

NIDDM is part of a complex of risk factors which includes obesity, hypertension, hyperlipidemia, vascular disease, and insulin resistance. This complex is termed the "metabolic syndrome." Unlike IDDM, NIDDM is characterized in its early stages by an increase in both production and serum levels of insulin. A number of studies have shown that this syndrome is associated with decreases in the antioxidant pathways. For example, Pasaoglu et al.[144] found that there was increased TBAS in both the serum and erythrocytes with decreased level of GSH in both compartments. An early report has suggested that GPx1 was unaltered in NIDDM while GPx3 was actually elevated.[83] On the other hand, more recent studies from one group[60,140] have indicated that there is a significant decrease in GPx3 activity with an increase in the plasma TBAS. Similarly, Zaltzberg et al.[213] found that there was an increase in plasma TBAS, decreased levels of plasma but not erythrocyte GSH and decreased erythrocyte GPx1, GST, and GSH reductase activities. Yet, these reductions in the antioxidant pathways appear to be associated with the hyperlipidemia rather than the NIDDM[34,49,86] On the other hand, De Mattia et al.[40] and Telci et al.[180] reported that patients with NIDDM had evidence of oxidant stress in the absence of hyperlipidemia. This stress was partially reversed by the chronic administration of N-acetylcysteine.[40] Finally, Shurtz-Swirski et al.[168] presented evidence that in NIDDM peripheral polymorphonuclear leukocytes were activated in the presence of decreased levels of plasma GSH, lending support to the role of oxidant stress in the vascular injury.

Child et al.[33] reported that many of the indices of oxidant stress and lipid abnormalities in NIDDM could be reversed by the administration of oral folate. Since tetrahydrofolate is the methyl donor involved in the conversion of homocysteine to methionine, this improvement in the risk factors associated with the metabolic syndrome could be due to the reduction in the observed homocysteine levels.

These effects of NIDDM do not appear to be due to the hyperlgycemia since treatment of patients with an oral antidiabetic agent, glimepride, showed increased evidence of oxidant stress in the presence of good glycemic control.[2] This agent is a member of the sulfonylurea family which works by increasing insulin secretion. Furthermore, although this family of agents can control the hyperglycemia characteristic of NIDDM, they have not been shown to significantly decrease the incidence of cardiovascular events during chronic administration.[184] This might suggest that decreasing oxidant stress may be critical to the prevention of the long-term effects of this disease.

One of the well documented, epidemiological observations is that black patients show a higher incidence of complications from NIDDM. In line with this Zitouni et al.[214] reported that the levels of GPx1 were significantly lower in African subjects with NIDDM compared to caucasians. But the levels in both groups were lower than that found in controls. As would be expected the levels of GPx3 were correlated with albumin excretion, a measure of renal impairment. Since the African subjects had a greater decrease of renal function, the lower levels of GPx3 could be due to lower capacity of the kidneys to synthesize this enzyme.

There have been few studies on the effect of IDDM on the antioxidant pathways. Both Yaqoob et al.[205] and Ruiz et al.[156] reported that there were lower levels of

GPx1 and higher levels of serum TBAS and lipid peroxides in individuals with IDDM. The decrease in GPx1 and increases in indices of oxidant stress were accentuated in individuals with poorer control of their diabetes and with cardiovascular disease. Both groups reported that these defects were observed early in the disease process.[44] Interestingly, Matteucci and Giampietro[116] reported that there was evidence of oxidative stress in unaffected siblings and parents of IDDM patients.

The Effect of Renal Failure on the Antioxidant Pathways

Renal failure is associated with a marked increase in the incidence of both vascular disease and oxidant stress. Asayama et al.[12] reported that uremic children and adolescents had increased plasma TBAS. Ceballos-Picot et al.,[30] Lim et al.,[108] Roxborough et al.,[153] and Ozden et al.[139] found that in renal failure patients there was a decrease in GPx3, but essentially no effect on GPx1. This decrease in GPx3 would be expected in these patients, since it is primarily synthesized in the kidneys. Yet, Roxborough et al.[153] found by immunoassay that the total GPx3 in the serum was the same in patients with renal failure as in controls, suggesting that the lower activity in patients was primarily due to denaturation of the enzyme rather than to a lower rate of synthesis.

In another study in renal transplant patients 1 year after transplantaion, Ruiz et al.[157] found that the level of GPx3 was significanly higher in patients with little vascular pathology.

The Effect of Drugs on the GSH Dependent Pathways

Hormone Replacement Therapy

One of the most controversial areas of therapeutics in recent years has been the question of whether the administration of estrogens and progestins to postmenopausal women reduces the incidnece of vascular disease. This concept was based on the observation that premenopausal women have a significantly lower incidence of vascular events than age matched men. This lower incidence was attributed to a protective effect of estrogens. Furthermore, observational and cohort studies had suggested that estrogen replacement therapy did reduce the incidence of both strokes and AMI. Furthermore, in support of the potential benefit of hormone replacement therapy, Bednarek-Tupikowska et al.[17] reported that in early menopause there was a direct correlation between GPx1 levels and serum estradiol and an inverse correlation with TBAS levels. On the other hand, in a large placebo controlled trial of hormone replacement therapy in more elderly women in the Women's Health Initiative, it was reported that progestens and to a lesser extent estrogen actually increased the incidence of vascular events.[201] This has been a very controversial finding because many investigators contend that this study may not be relevant to early menopausal women who may benefit from replacement therapy. Prior to the publication of this study three groups had examined the effect of replacement therapy on oxidant stress[3,76,138] While Inal et al.[76] and Akcay et al.[3] found that replacement therapy had no effect, Ozden et al.[138] reported that therapy increased GPx1 activity and reduced plasma TBAS. Since these data would suggest that replacement therapy had either a neutral or positive effect on oxidant stress, the observed deleterious effect observed in the Women's Health Initiative would suggest that either the older studies were examining a younger population with a different response to estrogen or that the adverse effects of the hormones were unrelated to changes in the antioxidant systems.

Statins and Fibrates

Currently, the HMGCoA reductase inhibitors, the statins, are the most widely prescribed medication for the primary and secondary treatment of patients at a risk for vascular events. Their primary effect is to decrease the intracellular hepatic levels of cholesterol. This leads to increased levels of the LDL receptor and uptake and degradation of the LDL. The net effect is to lead to decreased plasma LDL concentrations. With lower levels of LDL there is a decrease in its oxidaiton products because of the reduced substrate concentration.

Yilmaz et al.[208] reported that one statin, fluvastatin increased GPx1 activity in erythrocytes after 3 months of treatment. Similarly, Molcanyiova et al.[128] found that simvastatin administration led to both a significant increase in GPx1 and a concommitant decrease in plasma TBAS. In another report, Pereira et al.[145] found that this effect was not due to an increase in plasma thiols. These data suggest that one of the beneficial effects of statins could be the induction of GPx1. Clearly, this avenue of investigation will require more studies to determine whether this is correct.

The fibric acid derivatives are another class of agents which have recently been found to decrease the incidence of vascular events.[155,181] These agents are PARPα agonist which have been used to lower serum triglycerides and raise HDL. Yet, in these two studies their effect on the HDL concentrations was not clinically significant. Another fibric acid derivative, fenofibrate, has been shown after 12 weeks of treatment to significantly decrease an indicator of oxidant stress, serum conjugated dienes, and at the same time to nearly double GPx1.[183] On the other hand, Sutken et al.[175] found that after treatment for 1 month, gemfibrozil had no effect on GPx1. Since erythrocytes have a 3-month life span and do not synthesize protein once in the circulation, this study may have been too short to observe an effect.

Together, these data suggest that both the statins and fibric acid derivatives may decrease oxidant stress both by decreasing the substrate available for oxidation and by inducing GPx1. Both actions could be important in their protection of endothelial cells from injury.

Conclusions

I feel that the preponderance of evidence would appear to lend credence to the widely held concept that oxidant injury may be a major factor in the development and progression of atherosclerosis. Furthermore, these data would also indicate that the GPxs may play a major role in delaying the develoment of this pathological condition.

References

1. Abu-Amero KK, Al-Boudari OM, Mohamed GH, Dzimiri N. T null and M null genotypes of the glutathione S-transferase gene are risk factor for CAD independent of smoking. BMC Med Genet 2006;7:38–45.
2. Abou-Seif MA. Youssef AA. Evaluation of some biochemical changes in diabetic patients. Clin Chim Acta 2004;346:161–170.
3. Akcay T, Dincer Y, Kayali R, Colgar U, Oral E, Cakatay U. Effects of hormone replacement therapy on lipid peroxides and oxidation system in postmenopausal women. J Toxicol, Environ Health 2000;59:1–5.
4. Albert MA, Ridker PM. The role of C-reactive protein in cardiovascular disease risk. Curr Cardiol Rep 1999;1:99–104.
5. Agachan B, Yilmaz H, Ergen HA, Karaali ZE, Isbir T. Paraoxonase (PON1) 55 and 192 polymorphism and its effects to oxidant-antioxidant system in turkish patients with type 2 diabetes mellitus. Physiol Res 2005;54:287–93.
6. Alfthan G, Pekkanen J, Jauhiainen M, Pitkaniemi J, Karvonen M, Tuomilehto J, Salonen JT, Ehnholm C. Relation of serum homocysteine and lipoprotein(a) concentrations to atherosclerotic disease in a prospective Finnish population based study. Atherosclerosis 1994;106:9–19.
7. Ambrosone CB, Coles BF, Freudenheim JL, Shields PG. Glutathione-S-transferase (GSTM1) genetic polymorphisms do not affecthuman breast cancer risk, regardless of dietary antioxidants. J Nutr 1999;129(2S Suppl):565S–568S.
8. Anderson ME, Meister A. Dynamic state of glutathione in blood plasma. J Biol Chem 1980;255:9530–9533.
9. Armstrong RN. Glutathione S-transferase: Reaction mechanism, structure and function. Chem Res Toxicol 1991;4:131–140.
10. Arosio E, De Marchi S, Zannoni M, Prior M, Lechi A. Effect of glutathione infusion on leg arterial circulation, cutaneous microcirculation, and pain-free walking distance in patients with peripheral obstructive arterial disease: a randomized, double-blind, placebo-controlled trial. Mayo Clinic Proc 2002;77(8):754–759.
11. Arthur JR. The glutathione peroxidases. Cell Mol Life Sci 2000;57:1825–1835.
12. Asayama K, Shiki Y, Ito H, Hasegawa O, Miyao A, Hayashibe H, Dobashi K, Kato K. Antioxidant enzymes and lipoperoxide in blood in uremic children and adolescents. Free Rad Biol Med 1990;9:105–109.
13. Ashfaq S, Abramson JL, Jones DP, Rhodes SD, Weintraub WS, Hooper WC, Vaccarino V, Harrison DG, Quyyumi AA. The relationship between plasma levels of oxidized and reduced thiols and early atherosclerosis in healthy adults. J Am College Cardiol 2006;47: 1005–1011.
14. Aviram M, Billecke S, Sorenson R, Bisgaier C, Newton R, Rosenblat M, Erogul J, Hsu C, Dunlop C, La Du B. Paraoxonase active site required for protection against LDL oxidation involves its free sulfhydryl group and is different from that required for its arylesterase/

paraoxonase activities: selective action of human paraoxonase allozymes Q and R. Arterioscler Thromb Vasc Biol 1998;18:1617–1624.

15. Aviram M, Fuhrman B. LDL oxidation by arterial wall macrophages depends on the oxidative status in the lipoprotein and in the cells: role of prooxidants vs. antioxidants. Molec Cellular Biochem 1998;188:149–159.

16. Aviram M. Macrophage foam cell formation during early atherogenesis is determined by the balance between pro-oxidants and anti-oxidants in arterial cells and blood lipoproteins. Antioxidants Redox Signal 1999;1:585–594.

17. Bednarek-Tupikowska G, Bohdanowicz-Pawlak A, Bidzinska B, Milewicz A, Antonowicz-Juchniewicz J, Andrzejak R. Serum lipid peroxide levels and erythrocyte glutathione peroxidase and superoxide dismutase activity in premenopausal and postmenopausal women. Gynec Endocrin 2001;15:298–303.

18. Belch JJF, Chopra M, Hutchison S, Lorimer R, Sturrock RD, Forbes CD, Smith WE. Free radical pathology in chronic arterial disease. Free Radical Biol Med 1989;6:375–378

19. Benditt EP, Benditt JM. Evidence for a monoclonal origin of human atherosclerotic plaques. Proc Nat Acad Sci USA 1973;70:1753–1756.

20. Bjornstedt M, Xue J-Y, Huang W-H, Akesson B, Holmgren A. The thioredoxin and glutaredoxin systems are efficient electrons donors to human plasma glutathione peroxidase. J Biol Chem 1994;269:29382–29384.

21. Blankenberg S, Rupprecht HJ, Bickel C, Torzewski M, Hafner G, Tiret L, Smeija M, Cambien F, Meyer J, Lackner KJ. Glutathione peroxidase 1 activity and cardiovascular events in patients with coronary artery disease. N Eng J Med 2003;349:1605–1613.

22. Blann AD, Maxwell SR, Burrows G, Miller JP. Antioxidants, von Willebrand factor and endothelial cell injury in hypercholesterolaemia and vascular disease. Atherosclerosis 1995;116:191–198.

23. Bond JA, Yang H-YL, Majesky MW, Benditt Juchau MR. Metabolism of benzo[a]pyrene and 7,12-dimethylbenz[a]anthracene in chicken aortas: monooxygenation, bioactivation to mutagens, and covalent binding to DNA in vitro. Toxicol Appl Pharmacol 1980;52:323–335.

24. Bor MV, Cevik C, Uslu I, Guneral F, Duzgun E. Selenium levels and glutathione peroxidase activities in patients with acute myocardial infarction. Acta Cardiol 1999;54:271–276.

25. Bowry VW, Stanley KK, Stocker R. High density lipoprotein is the major carrier of lipid hydroperoxides in human blood plasma from fasting donors. Proc Natl Acad Sci USA 1992;89:10316–10320.

26. Brockmoller J, Kerb R, Drakoulis N, Staffeldt B, Roots I. Glutathione S-transferase M1 and its variants A and B as host factors of bladder cancer susceptibility: A case-control study. Cancer Res 1994;54:4103–4111.

27. Brockmoller J, Cascorbi I, Kerb R, Sachse C. Roots I. Polymorphisms in xenobiotic conjugation and disease predisposition. Toxicol Lett 1998;102–103:173–183

28. Brockmoller J, Cascorbi I, Henning S, Meisel C, Roots I. Molecular genetics of cancer susceptibility. Pharmacology 2000;61:212–227.

29. Cals MJ, Succari M, Meneguzzer E, Ponteziere C, Bories PN, Devanlay M, Desveaux N, Gatey M, Luciani L, Blonde-Cynober F, Coudray-Lucas C. Markers of oxidative stress in fit, health-conscious elderly people living in the Paris area. The Research Group on Ageing. Nutrition 1997;13:319–326.

30. Ceballos-Picot I, Witko-Sarsat V, Merad-Boudia M, Nguyen AT, Thevenin M, Jaudon MC, Zingraff J, Verger C, Jungers P, Descamps-Latscha B. Glutathione antioxidant system as a marker of oxidative stress in chronic renal failure. Free Rad Biol Med 1996;21:845–853.

31. Chen N-Q, Liu Y-X, Greiner CD, Holtzman JL. Physiological Concentrations of Homocysteine Inhibit the Human, Plasma GSH-Peroxidase Which Reduces Organic Hydroperoxides. J Lab Clin Med 2000;136:58–65.

32. Cheng L, Sturgis EM, Eicher SA, Char D, Spitz MR, Wei Q. Glutathione-S-transferase polymorphisms and risk of squamous-cell carcinoma of the head and neck. Int J Cancer (Pred Oncol) 1999;84:220–224.

33. Child DF, Hudson PR, Jones H, Davies GK, De P, Mukherjee S, Brain AM, Williams CP, Harvey JN. The effect of oral folic acid on glutathione, glycaemia and lipids in Type 2 diabetes. Diab Nutr Metab 2004;17:95–102.
34. Colak E, Majkic-Singh N, Stankovic S, Sreckovic-Dimitrijevic V, Djordjevic PB, Lalic K, Lalic N. Parameters of antioxidative defense in type 2 diabetic patients with cardiovascular complications. Ann Med 2005;37:613–620.
35. Cotton SC, Sharp L, Little J, Brockton N. Glutathione S-transferase polymorphisms and colorectal cancer: a HuGE review. Am J Epidemiol 2000;151:7–32.
36. Darley-Usmar VM, Severn A, O'Leary VJ, Rogers M. Treatment of macrophages with oxidized low-density lipoprotein increases their intracellular glutathione content. Biochem J 1991;278:429–434.
37. de Bruin WCC, Wagenmans MJM, Board PG, Peters WHM. Expression of glutathione S-transferase r class isoenzymes in human colorectal and gastric cancers. Carcinogenesis 1999;20:1453–1457.
38. De Flora S, Izzotti A, Walsh D, Degan P, Petrilli GL, Lewtas J. Molecular epidemiology of atherosclerosis. FASEB J 1997;11:1021–1031.
39. de Haan JB, Witting PK, Stefanovic N, Pete J, Daskalakis M, Kola I, Stocker R, Smolich JJ. Lack of the antioxidant glutathione peroxidase-1 does not increase atherosclerosis in C57BL/J6 mice fed a high-fat diet. J Lipid Res 2006;47:1157–1167.
40. De Mattia G, Bravi MC, Laurenti O, Cassone-Faldetta M, Proietti A, De Luca O, Armiento A, Ferri C. Reduction of oxidative stress by oral N-acetyl-L-cysteine treatment decreases plasma soluble vascular cell adhesion molecule-1 concentrations in non-obese, non-dyslipidaemic, normotensive, patients with non-insulin-dependent diabetes. Diabetologia 1998;41:1392–1396.
41. de Waart FG, Kok FJ, Smilde TJ, Hijmans A, Wollersheim H, Stalenhoef AF. Effect of glutathione S-transferase M1 genotype on progression of atherosclerosis in lifelong male smokers. Atherosclerosis 2001;158:227–231.
42. Diaz MN, Frei B, Vita JA, Keaney Jr. JF. Antioxidants and atherosclerotic heart disease. N Engl J Med 1997;337:408–414.
43. Dogru-Abbasoglu S, Kanbagli O, Bulur H, Babalik E, Ozturk S, Aykac-Toker G, Uysal M. Lipid peroxides and antioxidant status in serum of patients with angiographically defined coronary atherosclerosis. Clin Biochem 1999;32:671–672.
44. Dominguez C, Ruiz E, Gussinye M, Carrascosa A. Oxidative stress at onset and in early stages of type 1 diabetes in children and adolescents. Diabetes Care 1998;21:1736–1742.
45. Doney AS, Lee S, Leese GP, Morris AD, Palmer CN. Increased cardiovascular morbidity and mortality in type 2 diabetes is associated with the glutathione S transferase theta-null genotype: a Go-DARTS study. Circulation 2005;111:2927–2934.
46. Dubois-Rande JL, Artigou JY, Darmon JY, Habbal R, Manuel C, Tayarani I, Castaigne A, Grosgogeat Y. Oxidative stress in patients with unstable angina. Eur Hrt J 1994;15: 179–183.
47. Dwivedi VK, Chandra M, Misra PC, Misra A, Misra MK. Status of some free radical scavenging enzymes in the blood of myocardial infarction patients. J Enzyme Inhib Med Chem 2006;21:43–46.
48. Efe H, Deger O, Kirci D, Karahan SC, Orem A, Calapoglu M. Decreased neutrophil antioxidative enzyme activities and increased lipid peroxidation in hyperlipoproteinemic human subjects. Clinica Chimica Acta 1999;279:155–165.
49. Efe H, Kirci D, Deger O, Yildirmis S, Uydu HA, Orem C. Erythrocyte antioxidant enzyme activities and lipid peroxidation in patients with types IIb and IV hyperlipoproteinemias. Tohoku J Exp Med 2004;202:163–172.
50. Ehara S, Ueda M, Naruko T, Haze K, Itoh A, Otsuka M, Komatsu R, Matsua T, Itabe H, Takano T, Tsukamoto Y, Yoshiyama M, Takeuchi K, Yoshikawa J, Becker A.E. Elevated levels of oxidized low density lipoprotein show a positive relationship with the severity of acute coronary syndromes. Circulation 2001;103:1955–1960.

51. Emdin M, Pompella A, Paolicchi A. Gamma-glutamyltransferase, atherosclerosis, and cardiovascular disease: triggering oxidative stress within the plaque. Circulation 2000;112: 2078–2080.

52. Esworthy RS, Chu FF, Geiger P, Girotti AW, Doroshow JH. Reactivity of plasma glutathione peroxidase with hydroperoxide substrates and glutathione. Arch Biochem Biophys 1993;307:29–34.

53. Evans DA, Seidegard J, Narayanan N. The GSTM1 genetic polymorphism in healthy Saudi Arabians and Filipinos, and Saudi Arabians with coronary atherosclerosis. Pharmacogenetics 1996;6:365–367.

54. Franceschini G, Werba JP, Safa O, Gikalov L, Sirtori CR. Dose-related increase of HDL-cholesterol after N-acetylcysteine in man. Pharmacol Res 1993;2:213–218.

55. Fisher AB, Dodia C, Manevich Y, Chen JW, Feinstein SI. Phospholipid hydroperoxides are substrates for non-selenium glutathione peroxidase. J Biol Chem 1999;274:21326–21334.

56. Frei B, Yamamoto Y, Niclas D, Ames BN. Evaluation of an isoluminol chemiluminescence assay for the detection of hydroperoxides in human blood plasma. Anal Biochem 1988;175:120–130.

57. Georgiou I, Filiadis IF, Alamanos Y, Bouba I, Giannakopoulos X, Lolis D. Glutathione S-transferase null genotypes in transitional cell bladder cancer: A case-control study. Eur Urol 2000;37:660–666.

58. Girisha KM, Gilmour A, Mastana S, Singh VP, Sinha N, Tewari S, Ramesh V, Sankar VH, Agrawal S. T1 and M1 polymorphism in glutathione S-transferase gene and coronary artery disease in North Indian population. Indian J Med Sci 2004;58:520–526.

59. Go YM, Jones DP. Intracellular proatherogenic events and cell adhesion modulated by extracellular thiol/disulfide redox state. Circulation 2005;111:2973–2980.

60. Gokkusu C, Palanduz S, Ademoglu E, Tamer S. Oxidant and antioxidant systems in niddm patients: influence of vitamin E supplementation. Endocrine Res. 2001;27:377–386..

61. Gotlieb A. Systemic and nontraditional markers of endothelial dysfunction. Can J Cardiol 2000;16(Suppl E):27E–31E.

62. Graham IM, Daly LE, Refsum HM, Robinson K, Brattstrom LE, Ueland PM, Palma-Reis RJ, Boers GH, Sheahan RG, Israelsson B, Uiterwaal CS, Meleady R, McMaster D, Verhoef P, Witteman J, Rubba P, Bellet H, Wautrecht JC, de Valk HW, Sales Luis AC, Parrot-Rouland FM, Tan KS, Higgins I, Garcon D, Andria G, Medrano MJ, Candito M, Evans AE, Andria G. Plasma homocysteine as a risk factor for vascular disease. The European Concerted Action Project. J Amer Med Assoc 1997;277:1775–1781..

63. Gulick AM, Fahl WE. Mammalian glutathione S-transferase: Regulation of an enzyme system to achieve chemotherapeutic efficacy. Pharmac Ther 1995;66:237–257.

64. Haber F, Weiss J. The catalytic decomposition of hydrogen peroxide by iron salts. Proc R Soc Lond 1934;147:332–351.

65. Haberbosch W, Jantos C. Chlamydia pneumoniae infection is not an independent risk factor for arterial disease. Herz 2000;25:79–83.

66. Hapyn E, Czerwionka-Szaflarska M, Drewa G. Enzymatic efficiency of erythrocyte antioxidant barrier and lipid peroxidation in children from families with high risk of early atherosclerosis. Med Sci Monit 2001;6:112–116.

67. Hayes JD, Pulford DJ. The glutathione S-transferase supergene family: Regulation of GST and the contribution of the isoenzymes to cancer chemoprotection and drug resistance. Crit Rev Biochem Mol Biol 1995;30:445–600.

68. Holley AE, Slater TF. Measurement of lipid hydroperoxides in normal human blood plasma using HPLC-chemiluminescence linked to a diode array detector for measuring conjugated dienes. Free Radic Res Commun 1991;15:51–63.

69. Holtzman JL, Gillette JR, Milne GWA. The incorporation of 18O2 into naphthalene in the enzymatic formation of 1,2- dihydronaphthalene-1,2-diol. J Biol Chem 1967;242: 4386–4387.

70. Holtzman JL, Gillette JR, Milne GWA. The metabolic products of naphthalene in mammalian systems. J Am Chem Soc 1967;89:6341–6343.

71. Holtzman JL. The role of low levels of the serum glutathione-dependet peroxidase and glutathione and high levels of serum homocysteine in the development of cardiovascualar disease. Clin Lab 2002;48:129–130.
72. Holvoet P, Perez G, Zhao Z, Brouwers E, Bernar H, Collen D. Malondialdehyde-modified low density lipoproteins in patients with atherosclerotic disease. J Clin Invest 1995;95: 2611–2619.
73. Huerta JM, Gonzalez S, Fernandez S, Patterson AM, Lasheras C. No evidence for oxidative stress as a mechanism of action of hyperhomocysteinemia in humans. Free Radical Res 2004;38:1215–21.
74. Hurst R, Bao Y, Jemth P, Mannervik B, Williamson G. Phospholipid hydroperoxide glutathione peroxidase activity of human glutathione transferases. Biochem J 1998;332: 97–100.
75. Imai H, Hirao F, Sakamoto T, Sekine K, Mizukura Y, Saito M, Kitamoto T, Hayasaka M, Hanaoka K, Nakagawa Y. Early embryonic lethality caused by targeted disruption of the mouse PHGPx gene. Biochem Biophys Res Commun 2003;305:278–286.
76. Inal M, Sunal E, Kanbak G, Zeytinoglu S. Effects of postmenopausal hormone replacement and alpha-tocopherol on the lipid profiles and antioxidant status. Clinica Chimica Acta 1997;268:21–9.
77. Inoue H, Kiyohara C, Shinomiya S, Marugame T, Tsuji E, Handa K, Hayabuchi H, Eguchi H, Fukushima Y, Kono S. Glutathione S-transferase polymorphisms and risk of colorectal adenomas. Cancer Lett 2001;163:201–206.
78. Izzotti A, De Flora S, Petrilli GL, Gallagher J, Rojas M, Alexandrov K, Bartsch H, Lewtas J. Cancer biomarkers in human atherosclerotic lesions: Detection of DNA adducts. Cancer Epidemiol Prevent 1995;4:105–110.
79. Izzotti A, Cartiglia C, Lewtas J, De Flora S. Increased DNA alterations in atherosclerotic lesions of individuals lacking the GSTM1 genotype. FASEB J 2001;15:752–727.
80. Jayakumari N, Ambikakumari V, Balakrishnan KG, Iyer KS. Antioxidant status in relation to free radical production during stable and unstable anginal syndromes. Atherosclerosis 1992;94:183–190.
81. Jones DP, Carlson JL, Samiec PS, Sternberg P, Jr, Mody Jr VC, Reed RL, Brown LA. Glutathione measurement in human plasma. Evaluation of sample collection, storage and derivatization conditions for analysis of dansyl derivatives by HPLC. Clin Chim Acta 1998;275:175–184.
82. Joulain C, Prigent AF, Nemoz G, Lagarde M. Increased glutathione peroxidase activity in human blood mononuclear cells upon in vitro incubation with n-3 fatty acids. Biochem Pharmacol 1994;47:1315–1323.
83. Kaji H, Kurasaki M, Ito K, Saito T, Saito K, Niioka T, Kojima Y, Ohsaki Y, Ide H, Tsuji M, Kondo T, Kawakami Y. Increased lipoperoxide value and glutathione peroxidase activity in blood plasma of type 2 (non-insulin-dependent) diabetic women. Klinische Wochenschrift 1985;63:765–768.
84. Kashyap MK, Yadav V, Sherawat BS, Jain S, Kumari S, Khullar M, Sharma PC, Nath R. Different antioxidants status, total antioxidant power and free radicals in essential hypertension. Mole Cell Biochem 2005;277:89–99.
85. Kaur G, Misra MK, Sanwal GG, Shanker K, Chandra M. Levels of glutathione reductase and glutathione peroxidase of human platelets in unstable angina and myocardial infarction. Bollettino Chimico Farmaceutico 1999;138:437–439.
86. Kaviarasan K, Arjunan MM, Pugalendi KV. Lipid profile, oxidant-antioxidant status and glycoprotein components in hyperlipidemic patients with/without diabetes. Clinica Chimica Acta 2005;362:49–56.
87. Kihara M, Kihara M, Noda, K. Lung cancer risk of GSTM1 null genotype is dependent on the extent of tobacco smoke exposure. Carcinogenesis 1994;15:415–418.
88. Kihara M, Kihara M, Noda K. Risk of smoking for squamous and small cell carcinomas of the lung modulated by combinations of CYP1A1 and GSTM1 gene polymorphisms in a Japanese population. Carcinogenesis 1995;16:2331–2336.

89. Kinscherf R, Cafaltzis K, Roder F, Hildebrandt W, Edler L, Deigner HP, Breitkreutz R, Feussner, G, Kreuzer J, Werle E, Michel G, Metz J, Droge W. Cholesterol levels linked to abnormal plasma thiol concentrations and thiol/disulfide redox status in hyperlipidemic subjects. Free Rad Biol Med 2003;35:1286–1292.

90. Kobayashi S, Inoue N, Azumi H, Seno T, Hirata K, Kawashima S, Hayashi Y, Itoh H, Yokozaki H, Yokoyama M. Expressional changes of the vascular antioxidant system in atherosclerotic coronary arteries. J Atheroscler Thromb 2002;9:184–190.

91. Kontush A, Spranger T, Reich A, Djahansouzi S, Karten B, Braesen JH, Finckh B, Kohlschutter A, Beisiegel U. Whole plasma oxidation assay as a measure of lipoprotein oxidizability. Biofactors 1997;6:99–109.

92. Konukoglu D, Akcay T, Erdem T. Susceptibility of erythrocyte lipids to oxidation and erythrocyte antioxidant status in myocardial infarction. Clin Biochem 1998;31:667–671.

93. Koramaz I, Pulathan Z, Usta S, Karahan SC, Alver A, Yaris E, Kalyoncu NI, Ozcan F. Cardioprotective effect of cold-blood cardioplegia enriched with N-acetylcysteine during coronary artery bypass grafting. Ann Thorac Surg 2006;81:613–618.

94. Kristal B, Shurtz-Swirski R, Chezar J, Manaster J, Levy R, Shapiro G, Weissman I, Shasha SM, Sela S. Participation of peripheral in the oxidative stress and inflammation in patients with essential hypertension. Am J Hypertension 1998;11:921–928.

95. Lafuente A, Pujol F, Carretero P, Villa JP, Cuchi A. Human glutathione S-transferase m (GST m) deficiency as a marker for the susceptibility to bladder and larynx cancer among smokers. Cancer Lett 1993;68:49–54.

96. Lagrand WK, Visser CA, Hermens WT, Niessen HW, Verheugt FW, Wolbink GJ, Hack CE. C-reactive protein as a cardiovascular risk factor: more than an epiphenomenon? Circulation 1999;100:96–102.

97. Lallas TA, McClain SK, Shahin MS, Buller RE. The glutathione S-transferase M1 genotype in ovarian cancer. Cancer Epidemiol. Biomarkers Prevent. 2000;9: 587–590.

98. Lane J.D, Opara EC, Rose JE, Behm F. Quitting smoking raises whole blood glutathione. Physiol Behav 1996;60:1379–1381.

99. Lang M, Pelkonen O. Metabolism of xenobiotics and chemical carcinogenesis. Chapter 3. In: Ryder W (Ed). Metabolic Polymorphisms and Susceptibility to Cancer. IRAC Scientific Publication No. 148.

100. Lapenna D, de Gioia S, Ciofani G, Mezzetti A, Ucchino S, Calafiore AM, Napolitano AM, Di Ilio C, Cuccurullo F. Glutathione-related antioxidant defenses in human atherosclerotic plaques. Circulation 1998;97:1930–1934.

101. Laplaud PM, Dantoine T, Chapman MJ. Paraoxonase as a risk marker for cardiovascular disease: facts and hypotheses. Clin Chem Lab Med 1998;36:431–441.

102. Lee DH, Silventoinen K, Jacobs Jr DR, Jousilahti P, Tuomileto J. γ-Glutamyltransferase, obesity, and the risk of type 2 diabetes: Observational cohort study among 20,158 middle-aged men and women. J Clin Endocrinol Metab 2004;5410–5414.

103. Lee DH, Blomhoff R, Jacobs Jr DR. Is serum gamma glutamyltransderase a marker of oxidative stress? Free Radical Res 2004;38:535–539.

104. Lemaitre D, Vericel E, Polette A, Lagarde M. Effects of fatty acids on human platelet glutathione peroxidase: possible role of oxidative stress. Biochem Pharmacol 1997;53:479–486.

105. Leopold JA, Loscalzo J. Oxidative enzymopathies and vascular disease. Arterioscler Thromb Vasc Biol 2005;25:1332–1340.

106. Li R, Boerwinkle E, Olshan AF, Chambless LE, Pankow JS, Tyroler HA, Bray M, Pittman GS, Bell DA, Heiss G. Glutathione S-transferase genotype as a susceptibility factor in smoking-related coronary heart disease. Atherosclerosis 2000;49:451–462.

107. Li R, Folsom AR, Sharrett AR, Couper D, Bray M, Tyroler HA. Interaction of the glutathione S-transferase genes and cigarette smoking on risk of lower extremity arterial disease: the Atherosclerosis Risk in Communities (ARIC) study. Atherosclerosis 2001;154:729–738.

108. Lim PS, Wei YH, Yu YL, Kho B. Enhanced oxidative stress in haemodialysis patients receiving intravenous iron therapy. Nephrol Dial Transplant 1999;14:2680–2687.

109. Loeper J, Goy J, Rozensztajn L, Bedu O, Moisson P. Lipid peroxidation and protective enzymes during myocardial infarction. Clinica Chimica Acta 1991;196:119–125.

110. Loeper J, Goy J, Klein JM, Dufour M, Bedu O, Loeper S, Emerit J. The evolution of oxidative stress indicators in the course of myocardial ischemia. Free Radical Res Commun 1991;2:675–680.

111. London SJ, Yuan JM, Chung FL, Gao YT, Coetzee GA, Ross RK, Yu MC. Isothiocyanates, glutathione S-transferase M1 and T1 polymorphisms, and lung-cancer risk: A prospective study of men in Shanghai, China Lancet 2000;356:724–729.

112. Maddipati KR, Marnett LJ. Characterization of the major hydroperoxide-reducing activity of human plasma. Purification and properties of a selenium-dependent glutathione peroxidase. J Biol Chem 1987;262:17398–17403.

113. Markovic S, Dordevic J, Majkic-Singh N, Vasiljevic Z, Petrovic M, Glavinic L, Letic S, Milosevic A. The importance of antioxidant enzyme and total antioxidant status of patients with acute myocardial infarction on thrombolytic therapy. Clin Lab 2000;46:495–499.

114. Maser RL, Magenheimer BS, Calvet JP. Mouse plasma glutathione peroxidase: dDna sequence analysis and renal proximal tubular expression and secretion. J Biol Chem 1994;269:27066–27073.

115. Matetzky S, Freimark D, Ben-Ami S, Goldenberg I, Leor J, Doolman R, Novikov I, Eldar M, Hod H. Association of elevated homocysteine levels with a higher risk of recurrent coronary events and mortality in patients with acute myocardial infarction. Arch Int Med 2003;163:1933–1942.

116. Matteucci E, Giampietro O. Oxidative stress in families of type 1 diabetic patients. Diabetes Care 2000;23:1182–1106.

117. McMurray J, Chopra M, Abdullah I, Smith WE, Dargie HJ. Evidence for oxidative stress in unstable angina. Br Heart J 1992;68:454–457.

118. McWilliams JE, Sanderson BJS, Harris EL, Richert-Boe KE, Henner WD. Glutathione S-transferase M1 (GSTM1) deficiency and lung cancer risk. Cancer Epidemol. Biomarkers Prevent 1995;4:589–584.

119. Mezzetti A, Lapenna D, Calafiore AM, Proietti-Franceschilli G, Porreca E, De Cesare D, Neri M, Di Ilio C, Cuccurullo F. Glutathione-related enzyme activities and lipoperoxide levels in human internal mammary artery and ascending aorta. Relations with serum lipids. Arteriosc Thromb 1992;12:92–98.

120. Michelet F, Gueguen R, Leroy P, Wellman M, Nicolas A, Siest G. Blood and plasma glutathione measured in healthy subjects by HPLC: Relation to sex, aging, biological variables, and life habits. Clin Chem 1995;41:1509–1517.

121. Mills BJ, Weiss MM, Lang CA, Liu MC, Ziegler C. Blood glutathione and cysteine changes in cardiovascular disease. J Lab Clin Med 2000;135:396–401.

122. Minekura H, Kumagai T, Kawamoto Y, Nara F, Uchida K. 4-Hydroxy-2-nonenal is a powerful endogenous inhibitor of endothelial response. Biochem Biophys Res Commun 2001;282:557–561.

123. Miyazawa T, Saeki R, Inaba H. Detection of chemiluminescence in lipid peroxidation of biological systems and its application to HPLC. J Biolumin Chemilumin 1990;4: 475–478.

124. Miyazawa T. Determination of phospholipid hydroperoxides in human blood plasma by a chemiluminescence-HPLC assay. Free Radic Biol Med 1989;7:209–217.

125. Miyazawa T, Fujimoto K, Oikawa S. Determination of lipid hydroperoxides in low density lipoprotein from human plasma using high performance liquid chromatography with chemiluminescence detection. Biomed. Chromatogr 1990;4:131–134.

126. Moat SJ, Bonham JR, Cragg RA, Powers HJ. Elevated plasma homocysteine elicits an increase in antioxidant enzyme activity. Free Rad Res 2000;32:171–179.

127. Moghadasian MH, McManus BM, Frohlich JJ. Homocyst(e)ine and coronary artery disease. Clinical evidence and genetic and metabolic background. Arch Intern Med 1997;157: 2299–2308.

128. Molcanyiova A, Stancakova A, Javorsky M, Tkac I. Beneficial effect of simvastatin treatment on LDL oxidation and antioxidant protection is more pronounced in combined hyperlipidemia than in hypercholesterolemia. Pharmacol Res 2006;54:203–307.

129. Morrison JA, Jacobsen DW, Sprecher DL, Robinson K, Khoury P, Daniels SR. Serum glutathione in adolescent males predicts parental coronary heart disease. Circulation 1999;300:2244–2247.

130. Mullenbach GT, Tabrizi A, Irvine BD, Bell GI, Hallewel RA. Sequence of a cDNA coding for human glutathione peroxidase confirms TGA encodes active site selenocysteine. Nucleic Acids Res 1987;15:5484.

131. Nuttall SL, Martin U, Sinclair AJ, Kendall MJ. Glutathione: in sickness and in health. Lancet 1998;351:645–466.

132. Nourooz-Zadeh J, Tajaddini-Sarmadi J, Ling K-L, Wolff SP. Low-density lipoprotein is the major carrier of lipid hydroperoxides in plasma. Relevance to determination of total plasma lipid hydroperoxide concentrations. Biochem J 1996;313:781–786.

133. Nygard O, Nordrehaug JE, Refsum H, Ueland PM, Farstad M, Vollset SE. Plasma homocysteine levels and mortality in patients with coronary artery disease. N Engl J Med 1997;337:230–236.

134. Oen LH, Utomo H, Suyatna F, Hanafiah A, Asikin N. Plasma lipid peroxides in coronary heart disease. Int J Clin Pharmacol Ther Toxicol 1992;30:77–80.

135. Okkels H, Sigsgaard T, Wolf H, Autrup H. Glutathione S-transferase m as a risk factor in bladder tumours. Pharmacogenetics 1996;6:251–256.

136. Olshan AF, Li R, Pankow JS, Bray M, Tyroler HA, Chambless LE, Boerwinkle E, Pittman GS, Bell DA. Risk of atherosclerosis: interaction of smoking and glutathione S-transferase genes. Epidemiology 2003;14:321–327.

137. Oude Ophuis MB, van Lieshout EM, Roelofs HM, Peters WH, Manni JJ. Glutathione S-transferase M1 and T1 and Cytochrome P4501A1 polymorphisms in relation to the risk for benign and malignant head and neck lesions. Cancer 1998;82:936–943.

138. Ozden S, Dildar K, Kadir YH, Gulizar K. The effects of hormone replacement therapy on lipid peroxidation and antioxidant status. Maturitas 1997;38:165–170.

139. Ozden M, Maral H, Akaydin D, Cetinalp P, Kalender B. Erythrocyte glutathione peroxidase activity, plasma malondialdehyde and erythrocyte glutathione levels in hemodialysis and CAPD patients. Clin Biochem 2002;35:269–273.

140. Palanduz S, Ademoglu E, Gokkusu C, Tamer S. Plasma antioxidants and type 2 diabetes mellitus. Res Commun Mol Pathol Pharmacol 2001;109:309–318.

141. Pandey NR, Kaur G, Chandra M, Sanwal GG, Misra MK. Enzymatic oxidant and antioxidants of human blood platelets in unstable angina and myocardial infarction. Int J Cardiol 2000;76:33–38.

142. Parthasarathy S, Young SG, Witztum JL, Pittman RC, Steinberg D. Probucol inhibits oxidative modification of low density lipoprotein. J Clin Invest 1986;77:641–644.

143. Parthasarathy S, Khoo JC, Miller E, Barnett J, Witztum JL, Steinberg D. Low density lipoprotein rich in oleic acid is protected against oxidative modification: implications for dietary prevention of atherosclerosis. Proc Natl Acad Sci USA 1990;87:3894–3898.

144. Pasaoglu H, Sancak B, Bukan N. Lipid peroxidation and resistance to oxidation in patients with type 2 diabetes mellitus. Tohoku J Exp Med 2004;203:211–218.

145. Pereira EC, Bertolami MC, Faludi AA, Sevanian A, Abdalla DS. Antioxidant effect of simvastatin is not enhanced by its association with alpha-tocopherol in hypercholesterolemic patients. Free Radical Biol Med 2004;37:1440–1448.

146. Perera FP. Molecular epidemiology and prevention of cancer. Environ. Health Perspect. 1995;103(Suppl 8):233–236.

147. Pessah-Rasmussen H, Jerntorp P, Stavenow L, Elmstahl S, Hansen F, Seidegard J, Galvard H, Brattstrom L, Hampelt A. Eighty-year-old men without cardiovascular disease in the community of Malmo. Part II. Smoking characteristics and ultrasound findings with special reference to glutathione transferase and pyridoxal-5-phosphate. J Intern Med 1990;228: 17–22.

148. Pessah-Rasmussen H, Stavenow L, Seidegard J, Solem JO, Israelsson B. Lack of glutathione transferase activity in intermittent claudication. Int Angiol 1990;9:70–74.

149. Porter M, Pearson DJ, Suarez-Mendez VJ, Blann AD. Plasma, platelet and erythrocyte glutathione peroxidases as risk factors in ischaemic heart disease in man. Clin Sci 1992;83: 343–345.

150. Rangaswamy S, Penn MS, Saidel GM, Chisolm GM. Exogenous oxidized low-density lipoprotein injures and alters the barrier function of endothelium in rats in vivo. Circ Res 1997;80:37–41.

151. Ridker PM. Evaluating novel cardiovascular risk factors: can we better predict heart attacks?. Ann Intern Med 1999;130:933–937.

152. Rothman N, Hayes RB. Using biomarkers of genetic susceptibility to enhance the study of cancer etiology. Environ. Health Perspect 1995;103(Suppl 8):291–295.

153. Roxborough HE, Mercer C, McMaster D, Maxwell AP, Young IS. Plasma glutathione peroxidase activity is reduced in haemodialysis patients. Nephron 1999;81:278–283.

154. Rozenberg O, Shih DM, Aviram M. Paraoxonase 1 (PON1) attenuates macrophage oxidative status: studies in PON1 transfected cells and in PON1 transgenic mice. Atherosclerosis 2005;181:9–18.

155. Rubins HB, Robins SJ, Collins D, Fye CL, Anderson JW, Elam MB, Faas FH, Linares E, Schaefer EJ, Schectman G, Wilt TJ, Wittes J. Gemfibrozil for the secondary prevention of coronary heart disease in men with low levels of high-density lipoprotein cholesterol. N Engl J Med 1999;341:410–418.

156. Ruiz C, Alegria A, Barbera R, Farre R, Lagarda MJ. Lipid peroxidation and antioxidant enzyme activities in patients with type 1 diabetes mellitus. Scand J Clin Lab Invest 1999;59: 99–105.

157. Ruiz MC, Medina A, Moreno JM, Gomez I, Ruiz N, Bueno P, Asensio C, Osuna A. Relationship between oxidative stress parameters and atherosclerotic signs in the carotid artery of stable renal transplant patients. Transplant Proceed 2005;37:3796–3798.

158. Ruttmann E, Brant LJ, Concin H, Diem G, Rapp K, Ulmer H. the Vorarlberg Health Monitoring and Promotion Program Study Group. γ-Glutamyltransferase as a risk factor for cardiovascular disease mortality; An epdiemiological investigation in a cohort of 163,944 Austrian adults. Circulation 2005;112:130–2137.

159. Sakamaki R, Nagano S, Yamazaki S, Ozawa N, Tateishi M, Okuda H, Watabe T. Existence of 7 alpha- and 7 beta-hydroperoxycholest-5-en-3 beta-ols in lipoproteins from diabetic patients and normal subjects. J Atheroscler Thromb 1994;1:80–86.

160. Salonen JT, Yla-Herttuala Yamamoto R, Butler S, Korpela H, Salonen R, Nyyssonen K, Palinski W, Witztum JL. Autoantibodies against oxidised LDL and progression of carotid atherosclerosis. Lancet 1992;339:883–887.

161. Seidegard J, Pero RW. The hereditary transmission of high glutathione transferase activity towards tran-stilbene oxide in human mononuclear leukocytes from human blood. Human Genet 198569:66–68.

162. Seidegard J, Pero RW, Miller DG, Beattie EJ. A glutathione transferase in human leukocytes as a marker for the susceptibility to lung cancer. Carcinogenesis 1986;7:751–753.

163. Sela S, Shurtz-Swirski R, Awad J, Shapiro G, Nasser L, Shasha SM, Kristal B. The involvement of peripheral polymorphonuclear leukocytes in the oxidative stress and inflammation among cigarette smokers. Israel Med Assoc J 2002;4:1015–1019.

164. Serdar Z, Aslan K, Dirican M, Sarandol E, Yesilbursa D, Serdar A. Lipid and protein oxidation and antioxidant status in patients with angiographically proven coronary artery disease. Clin Biochem 2006;39:794–803.

165. Sevanian A, Bittolo-Bon G, Cazzolato G, Hodis H, Hwang J, Zamburlini A, Maiorino M, Ursini F. LDL- is a lipid hydroperoxide-enriched circulating lipoprotein. J Lipid Res 1997;38:419–428.

166. Shen L, Sevanian A. OxLDL induces macrophage gamma-GCS-HS protein expression: a role for oxLDL-associated lipid hydroperoxide in GSH synthesis. J Lipid Res 2001;42: 813–823.

167. Shih DM, Gu L, Xia YR, Navab M, Li WF, Hama S, Castellani LW, Furlong CE, Costa LG, Fogelman AM, Lusis AJ. Mice lacking serum paraoxonase are susceptible to organophosphate toxicity and atherosclerosis. Nature 1998;394:284–287.

168. Shurtz-Swirski R, Sela S, Herskovits AT, Shasha SM, Shapiro G, Nasser L, Kristal B. Involvement of peripheral polymorphonuclear leukocytes in oxidative stress and inflammation in type 2 diabetic patients. Diabetes Care 2001;24:104–110.

169. Siemianowicz K, Gminski J, Francuz T, Wojcik A, Posielezna B. Activity of antioxidant enzymes in children from families at high risk of premature coronary heart disease. Scand J Clin Lab Invest 2003;63:151–158.

170. Simic D, Mimic-Oka J, Pljesa M, Milanovic D, Radojevic S, Ivanovic B, Kalimanovska-Ostric D, Matic D, Simic T. Time course of erythrocyte antioxidant activity in patients treated by thrombolysis for acute myocardial infarction. Jpn Heart J 2003;44:823–832.

171. Sneddon AA, Wu HC, Farquharson A, Grant I, Arthur JR, Rotondo D, Choe SN, Wahle KW. Regulation of selenoprotein GPx4 expression and activity in human endothelial cells by fatty acids, cytokines and antioxidants. Atherosclerosis 2003;171:57–65.

172. Solak ZA, Kabaroglu C, Cok G, Parildar Z, Bayindir U, Ozmen D, Bayindir O. Effect of different levels of cigarette smoking on lipid peroxidation, glutathione enzymes and paraoxonase 1 activity in healthy people. Clin Exp Med 2005;5:99–105.

173. Steinberg D, Parthasarathy S, Carew TE, Khoo JC, Witztum JL. Beyond cholesterol: Modifications of low-density lipoprotein that increase its atherogenicity. N Engl J Med 1998;320:915–924.

174. Stickel F, Osterricher CH, Datz C, Ferinci P, Wolfel M, Norgauer W, Kraus MR, Wrba F, Hellerbrand C, Schuppan D. Prediction of progression to cirrhosis by glutathione S-transferase P1 polymorphism in subjects with hereditary hemochromatosis. Arch Int Med 2005;165:1835–1840.

175. Sutken E, Inal M, Ozdemir F. Effects of vitamin E and gemfibrozil on lipid profiles, lipid peroxidation and antioxidant status in the elderly and young hyperlipidemic subjects. Saudi Med J 2006;27:453–459.

176. Takahashi K, Avissar N, Whitin J, Cohen H. Purification and characterization of human plasma glutathione peroxidase: a selenoglycoprotein distinct from the known cellular enzymes. Arch Biochem Biophys 1987;256:677–686.

177. Takahashi K, Akasaka M, Yamamoto Y, Kobayashi C, Mizoguchi J, Koyama J. Primary structure of human plasma glutathione peroxidase deduced from cDNA sequences. J Biochem (Tokyo) 1990;108:145–148.

178. Tamer L, Sucu N, Polat G, Ercan B, Aytacoglu B, Yucebilgic G, Unlu A, Dikmengil M, Atik U. Decreased serum total antioxidant status and erythrocyte-reduced glutathione levels are associated with increased serum malondialdehyde in atherosclerotic patients. Arch Med Res 2002;33:257–260.

179. Tamer L, Ercan B, Camsari A, Yildirim H, Cicek D, Sucu N, Ates NA, Atik U. Glutathione S-transferase gene polymorphism as a susceptibility factor in smoking-related coronary artery disease. Basic Res Cardiol 2004;99:223–229.

180. Telci A, Cakatay U, Kayali R, Erdogan C, Orhan Y, Sivas A, Akcay T. Oxidative protein damage in plasma of type 2 diabetic patients. Hormone Metab Res 2000;32:40–43.

181. Tenkanen L, Manttari M, Kpvanen PT, Virkkunen H, Manninen V. Gemfibrozil in the treatment of dyslipidemia: An 18 year follow-up of the Helsinki Heart Study. Arch Intern Med 2006;166:743–748.

182. Thirman MJ, Albrecht JH, Krueger MA, Erickson RR, Cherwitz DL, Park SS, Gelboin HV, Holtzman JL. Induction of Cytochrome CYPIA1 and Formation of Toxic Metabolites of Benzo[a]pyrene by Rat Aorta: A Possible Role in Atherogenesis. Proc Natl Acad Sci USA 1994;91:5397–5401.

183. Tkac I, Molcanyiova A, Javorsky M, Kozarova M. Fenofibrate treatment reduces circulating conjugated diene level and increases glutathione peroxidase activity. Pharmacol Res 2006;53:261–264.

184. United Kingdom Prospective Diabetes Study United Kingdom Prospective Diabetes Study (UKPDS) 13: relative efficacy of randomly allocated diet, sulfonylurea, insulin or metformin

in patients with newly diagnosed non-insulin dependent diabetes followed for three years. Brit Med J 1995;310:83–88.

185. Ursini F, Maiorino M, Valente M, Ferri L, Gregolin C. Purification from pig liver of a protein which protects liposomes and biomembranes from peroxidative degradation and exhibits glutathione peroxidase activity on phosphatidylcholine hydroperoxides. Biochim Biophys Acta 1982;710:197–211.

186. van Schooten FJ, Hirvonen A, Maas LM, de Mol BA, Kleinjan JCS, Bell DA, Durrer JD, Putative susceptibility markers of coronary artery disease: association between VDR genotype, smoking and aromatic DNA adduct levels in human right artial tissue. FASEB J 1998;12:1409–1417.

187. Valentine RJ, Kaplan HS, Green R, Jacobsen DW, Myers SI, Clagett GP. Lipoprotein (a), homocysteine, and hypercoagulable states in young men with premature peripheral atherosclerosis: a prospective, controlled analysis. J Vasc Surg 1996;23:53–61.

188. Van Remmen H, Qi W, Sabia M, Freeman G, Estlack L, Yang H, Guo ZM, Huano TT, Strong R, Lee S, Epstein CJ, Richardson A. Multiple deficiencies in antioxidant enzymes in mice result in a compound increase in sensitivity to oxidative stress. Free Rad Biol Med 2004;36:1625–1634.

189. Vericel E, Rey C, Calzada C, Haond P, Chapuy PH, Lagarde M. Age-related changes in arachidonic acid peroxidation and glutathione-peroxidase activity in human platelets. Prostaglandins 1992;43:75–85.

190. Vento AE, Nemlander A, Aittomaki J, Salo J, Karhunen J, Ramo OJ. N-acetylcysteine as an additive to crystalloid cardioplegia increased oxidative stress capacity in CABG patients. Scand. Cardiovascular J 2003;37:349–355.

191. Verhoef P, Hennekens CH, Malinow MR, Kok FJ, Willett WC, Stampfer MJ. A prospective study of plasma homocyst(e)ine and risk of ischemic stroke. Stroke 1994;25: 1924–1930.

192. Voetsch B, Jin RC, Bierl C, Benke KS, Kenet G, Simioni P, Ottaviano F, Damasceno BP, Annichino-Bizacchi JM, Handy DE, Loscalzo J. Promoter polymorphisms in the plasma glutathione peroxidase (GPx-3) gene: a novel risk factor for arterial ischemic stroke among young adults and children. Stroke 2007;38:41–49 .

193. Voutilainen S, Morrow JD, Roberts 2nd LJ, Alfthan G, Alho H, Nyyssonen K, Salonen JT. Enhanced in vivo lipid peroxidation at elevated plasma total homocysteine levels. Arterioscler Thromb Vasc Biol 1999;19:1263–1266.

194. Wang XL, Greco M, Sim AS, Duarte N, Wang J, Wilcken DE. Glutathione S-transferase mu1 deficiency, cigarette smoking and coronary artery disease. J Cardiovasc Risk 2002;9: 25–31.

195. Watson AD, Leitinger N, Navab M, Faull KF, Horkko S, Witztum JL, Palinski W, Schwenke D, Salomon RG, Sha W, Subbanagounder G, Fogelman AM, Berliner JA. Structural identification by mass spectrometry of oxidized phospholipids in minimally oxidzed low density lipoprotein that induce monocyte/endothelial interactions and evidence for their presence in vivo. J Biol Chem 1997;272:13597–13607.

196. Wendel A, Cikryt P. The level and half-life of glutathione in human sera. FEBS Lett 1980;120:209–211.

197. Willerson JT. Systemic and local inflammation in patients with unstable atherosclerotic plaques. Prog Cardiovasc Dis 2002;44:469–78.

198. Wilson MH, Grant PJ, Hardie LJ, Wild CP. Glutathione S-transferase M1 null genotype is associated with a decreased risk of myocardial infarction. FASEB J 2000;14:791–796.

199. Wilson MH, Grant PJ, Kain K, Warner DP, Wild CP. Association between the risk of coronary artery disease in South Asians and a deletion polymorphism in glutathione S-transferase M1. Biomarkers 2003;8:43–50.

200. Winter JP, Gong Y, Grant PJ, Wild CP. Glutathione peroxidase 1 genotype is associated with an increased risk of coronary artery disease. Coron Artery Dis 2003;14:149–153.

201. Women's Health Initiative Writing Group. Risks and benefits of estrogen plus progestin in healthy postmenopausal women: Principal results from the Women's Health Initiative randomized controlled trial. JAMA 2002;288:321–333.

202. Yagi K, Komura S, Kojima H, Sun Q, Nagata N, Ohishi N, Nishikimi M. Expression of human phospholipid hydroperoxide glutathione peroxidase gene for protection of host cells from lipid hydroperoxide-mediated injury. Biochem Biophys Res Commun 1996;219: 486–491.

203. Yamamoto Y, Brodsky MH, Baker JC, Ames BN. Detection and characterization of lipid hydroperoxides at picomole levels by high-performance liquid chromatography. Anal Biochem 1987;160:7–13.

204. Yamamoto Y, Takahashi K. Glutathione peroxidase isolated from plasma reduces phospholipid hydroperoxides. Arch Biochem Biophys 1993;305:541–545.

205. Yaqoob M, Patrick AW, McClelland P, Stevenson A, Mason H, White MC, Bell GM. Relationship between markers of endothelial dysfunction, oxidant injury and tubular damage in patients with insulin-dependent diabetes mellitus. Clin Sci 1993;85:557–562.

206. Yasuda M, Narita S. Simultaneous determination of phospholipid hydroperoxides and cholesteryl ester hydroperoxides in human plasma by high-performance liquid chromatography with chemiluminescence detection. J Chromatogr B Biomed Appl 1997;693: 211–217.

207. Yegin A, Yegin H, Aliciguzel Y, Deger N, Semiz E. Erythrocyte selenium-glutathione peroxidase activity is lower in patients with coronary atherosclerosis. Jap Hrt J 1997;38: 793–798.

208. Yilmaz MI, Baykal Y, Kilic M, Sonmez A, Bulucu F, Aydin A, Sayal A, Hakki Kocar IH. Effects of statins on oxidative stress. Biol Trace Element Res 2004;98:119–127.

209. Yla-Herttuala S, Palinski W, Rosenfeld ME, Parthasarathy S, Carew TE, Butler S, Witztum JL, Steinberg D. Evidence of the presence of oxidatively modified low density lipoprotein in atherosclerotic lesions of rabbit and man. J Clin Invest 1989;84:1086–1095.

210. Yoshida H, Sasaki K, Hirowatari Y, Kurosawa H, Sato N, Furutani N, Tada N. Increased serum iron may contribute to enhanced oxidation of low-density lipoprotein in smokers in part through changes in lipoxygenase and catalase. Clinica Chimica Acta 2004;345:161–170.

211. Zamburlini A, Maiorino M, Barbera P, Roveri A, Ursini F. Direct measurement by single photon counting of lipid hydroperoxides in human plasma and lipoproteins. Anal Biochem 1995;232:107–113.

212. Zebrack JS, Anderson JL. The role of inflammation and infection in the pathogenesis and evolution of coronary artery disease. Curr Cardiol Rep 2002;4:278–288.

213. Zaltzberg H, Kanter Y, Aviram M, Levy Y. Increased plasma oxidizability and decreased erythrocyte and plasma antioxidative capacity in patients with NIDDM. Israel Med Assoc J 1999;1:228–231.

214. Zitouni K, Nourooz-Zadeh J, Harry D, Kerry SM, Betteridge DJ, Cappuccio FP, Earle KA. Race-specific differences in antioxidant enzyme activity in patients with type 2 diabetes: a potential association with the risk of developing nephropathy. Diabetes Care 2005;28: 1698–1703

Index

Printed in the United States of America.